T0226420

Endocrine Tumors

Editor

DOUGLAS L. FRAKER

SURGICAL ONCOLOGY
CLINICS OF NORTH AMERICA

www.surgonc.theclinics.com

Consulting Editor
NICHOLAS J. PETRELLI

January 2016 • Volume 25 • Number 1

ELSEVIER

1600 John F. Kennedy Boulevard • Suite 1800 • Philadelphia, Pennsylvania, 19103-2899

http://www.theclinics.com

SURGICAL ONCOLOGY CLINICS OF NORTH AMERICA Volume 25, Number 1
January 2016 ISSN 1055-3207, ISBN-13: 978-0-323-41472-2

Editor: John Vassallo
Developmental Editor: Meredith Clinton

Surgical Oncology Clinics of North America (ISSN 1055-3207) is published quarterly by Elsevier Inc., 360 Park Avenue South, New York, NY 10010-1710. Months of publication are January, April, July, and October. Business and Editorial Offices: 1600 John F. Kennedy Blvd., Ste. 1800, Philadelphia, PA 19103-2899. Customer Service Office: 3251 Riverport Lane, Maryland Heights, MO 63043. Periodicals postage paid at New York, NY and additional mailing offices. Subscription prices are $290.00 per year (US individuals), $471.00 (US institutions) $100.00 (US student/resident), $330.00 (Canadian individuals), $596.00 (Canadian institutions), $205.00 (Canadian student/resident), $410.00 (foreign individuals), $596.00 (foreign institutions), and $205.00 (foreign student/resident). Foreign air speed delivery is included in all *Clinics* subscription prices. All prices are subject to change without notice. **POSTMASTER**: Send address changes to *Surgical Oncology Clinics of North America*, Elsevier Health Science Division, Subscription Customer Service, 3251 Riverport Lane, Maryland Heights, MO 63043. **Customer Service: 1-800-654-2452 (US and Canada). 314-447-8871 (outside US and Canada). Fax: 314-447-8029. E-mail: journalscustomerservice-usa@elsevier.com (for print support); journalsonline support-usa@elsevier.com (for online support).**

Reprints. For copies of 100 or more, of articles in this publication, please contact the Commercial Reprints Department, Elsevier Inc., 360 Park Avenue South, New York, New York 10010-1710. Tel. 212-633-3874; Fax: 212-633-3820; E-mail: reprints@elsevier.com.

Surgical Oncology Clinics of North America is covered in *MEDLINE/PubMed (Index Medicus)* and *EMBASE/ Excerpta Medica, Current Contents/Clinical Medicine,* and *ISI/BIOMED.*

Contributors

CONSULTING EDITOR

NICHOLAS J. PETRELLI, MD, FACS
Bank of America Endowed Medical Director, Helen F. Graham Cancer Center and Research Institute, Christiana Care Health System, Newark, Delaware; Professor of Surgery, Thomas Jefferson University, Philadelphia, Pennsylvania

EDITOR

DOUGLAS L. FRAKER, MD, FACS
Jonathan E. Rhoads Professor of Surgical Science, Vice Chairman, Research Chief, Division of Endocrine Surgery and Surgical Oncology, Department of Surgery, University of Pennsylvania, Philadelphia, Pennsylvania

AUTHORS

COURTNEY J. BALENTINE, MD, MPH
Department of Surgery, University of Wisconsin, Madison, Wisconsin

AZADEH A. CARR, MD
Assistant Professor, Section of Endocrine Surgery, Division of Surgical Oncology, Department of Surgery, Medical College of Wisconsin, Milwaukee, Wisconsin

RAUL CASO, BS
MD/MSc Candidate, New York University School of Medicine, New York, New York

JASHODEEP DATTA, MD
Division of Endocrine and Oncologic Surgery, Department of Surgery, University of Pennsylvania Perelman School of Medicine, Philadelphia, Pennsylvania

DINA ELARAJ, MD
Associate Professor of Surgery, Division of Endocrine Surgery, Department of Surgery, Northwestern University, Chicago, Illinois

HEATHER A. FARLEY, MD
Division of Surgical Oncology, Oregon Health and Science University, Portland, Oregon

GUSTAVO G. FERNANDEZ RANVIER, MD
Assistant Professor of Surgery, Division of Metabolic, Endocrine and Minimally Invasive Surgery, Department of Surgery, Mount Sinai Hospital, Icahn School of Medicine at Mount Sinai, New York, New York

JAMES R. HOWE, MD
Department of General Surgery, University of Iowa Hospitals and Clinics, University of Iowa Carver College of Medicine, Iowa City, Iowa

WILLIAM B. INABNET III, MD, FACS
Eugene W Friedman Professor of Surgery, Chairman, Department of Surgery, Mount Sinai Beth Israel, Icahn School of Medicine at Mount Sinai, New York, New York

RACHEL R. KELZ, MD, MSCE, FACS
Associate Professor of Surgery, Division of Endocrine and Oncologic Surgery, Department of Surgery, Hospital of the University of Pennsylvania, Philadelphia, Pennsylvania

COLLEEN M. KIERNAN, MD, MPH
General Surgery Resident, Division of Surgical Oncology and Endocrine Surgery, Vanderbilt University Medical Center, Nashville, Tennessee

LINDSAY E. KUO, MD, MBA
Clinical Instructor, Department of Surgery, Hospital of the University of Pennsylvania, Philadelphia, Pennsylvania

AMANDA M. LAIRD, MD
Assistant Professor of Surgery, Montefiore Medical Center, Albert Einstein College of Medicine, Bronx, New York

STEVEN K. LIBUTTI, MD
Director, Montefiore Medical Center for Cancer Care; Professor of Surgery and Genetics, Montefiore Medical Center, Albert Einstein College of Medicine, Bronx, New York

JESSICA E. MAXWELL, MD, MBA
Department of General Surgery, University of Iowa Hospitals and Clinics, University of Iowa Carver College of Medicine, Iowa City, Iowa

THOMAS M. O'DORISIO, MD
Department of Internal Medicine, University of Iowa Hospitals and Clinics, University of Iowa Carver College of Medicine, Iowa City, Iowa

KEPAL N. PATEL, MD, FACS
Associate Professor, Director, Division of Endocrine Surgery, Departments of Surgery, Biochemistry and Molecular Pharmacology and Otolaryngology, New York University Langone Medical Center, New York, New York

RODNEY F. POMMIER, MD
Division of Surgical Oncology, Oregon Health and Science University, Portland, Oregon

ROBERT E. ROSES, MD
Division of Endocrine and Oncologic Surgery, Department of Surgery, University of Pennsylvania Perelman School of Medicine, Philadelphia, Pennsylvania

DANIEL SHOUHED, MD
Assistant Professor of Surgery, Division of Metabolic, Endocrine and Minimally Invasive Surgery, Department of Surgery, Mount Sinai Hospital, Icahn School of Medicine at Mount Sinai, New York, New York

REBECCA S. SIPPEL, MD
Department of Surgery, University of Wisconsin, Madison, Wisconsin

CARMEN C. SOLÓRZANO, MD, FACS
Chief Division of General Surgery; Professor of Surgery, Ad Interim Chief, Division of Surgical Oncology and Endocrine Surgery, Vanderbilt University Medical Center, Nashville, Tennessee

MICHAEL T. STANG, MD, FACS
Division of Endocrine Surgery, Department of Surgery, University of Pittsburgh, Pittsburgh, Pennsylvania

CORD STURGEON, MD
Associate Professor of Surgery, Division of Endocrine Surgery, Department of Surgery, Northwestern University, Chicago, Illinois

TRACY S. WANG, MD, MPH, FACS
Associate Professor, Chief, Section of Endocrine Surgery, Division of Surgical Oncology, Department of Surgery, Medical College of Wisconsin, Milwaukee, Wisconsin

JAMES X. WU, MD
Section of Endocrine Surgery, University of California, Los Angeles, David Geffen School of Medicine, Los Angeles, California

ANTHONY YANG, MD
Assistant Professor of Surgery, Division of Endocrine Surgery, Department of Surgery, Northwestern University, Chicago, Illinois

MICHAEL W. YEH, MD
Section of Endocrine Surgery, University of California, Los Angeles, David Geffen School of Medicine, Los Angeles, California

JENNY Y. YOO, MD
Division of Endocrine Surgery, Department of Surgery, University of Pittsburgh, Pittsburgh, Pennsylvania

Contents

> Preoperative diagnosis and operative planning for patients with thyroid
> nodules has improved over the last decade. The Bethesda criteria for cyto-
> pathologic classification of thyroid nodule aspirate has enhanced commu-
> nication between pathologists and clinicians. Multiple genetic tests,
> including molecular markers and the Afirma gene expression classifier,
> have been developed and validated. The tests, along with clinical and radio-
> logic information, are most useful in the setting of indeterminate cytology.
> The development of an updated diagnostic and treatment algorithm incor-
> porating all available tests will help standardize the management of patients
> with nodular thyroid disease and reduce variation and inefficiencies in care.

> Although papillary thyroid cancer (PTC) commonly metastasizes to cervical
> lymph nodes, prophylactic central neck dissection is controversial. The pri-
> mary treatment for lymph node metastases is surgical resection. Patients
> diagnosed with PTC should be assessed preoperatively by cervical ultra-
> sound to evaluate central and lateral neck lymph node compartments.
> Sonographically suspicious lymph nodes in the lateral neck should be bio-
> psied for cytology or thyroglobulin levels. Any compartment (central or
> lateral) that has definitive proof of nodal metastases should be formally
> dissected at the time of thyroidectomy.

> Well-differentiated thyroid cancer is increasing in incidence but the
> disease-specific mortality remains very low. The only effective adjuvant
> treatment is radioactive iodine ablation. Guidelines regarding the use
> and dosage of radioactive iodine depend on pathologic features of the pri-
> mary and metastatic tumor that define risk. Long-term treatment includes
> thyroid-stimulating hormone suppression and surveillance with serum
> thyroglobulin, and radiologic assessment for nodal recurrence.

Outpatient thyroid surgery is controversial because of concerns over life-threatening cervical hematoma. Despite this concern, outpatient thyroidectomy is becoming increasingly common, especially among high-volume endocrine surgeons. Multiple studies have now demonstrated that careful patient selection combined with surgeon experience can result in successful and safe surgery without a full inpatient admission. This article reviews the data on safety and outcomes for outpatient thyroidectomy and discusses several techniques used to minimize risk to patients.

Primary hyperparathyroidism (PHPT) is a common disease, with a prevalence as high as 1 in 400 women and 1 in 1000 men, and most are asymptomatic. Patients with PHPT have hypercalcemia with inappropriately normal levels of parathyroid hormone. Parathyroidectomy is the only curative therapy, and the procedure has become more common and more safe. Among asymptomatic patients, parathyroidectomy halts the progression of disease, improves quality of life, and may decrease risk of fracture and adverse cardiovascular outcomes. Thus, surgery should be considered in all patients with asymptomatic PHPT who have minimal perioperative risk and sufficient life expectancy, regardless of chronologic age.

Intraoperative parathyroid hormone (IOPTH) monitoring is a highly accurate surgical adjunct used to determine the extent of surgery in the setting of primary hyperparathyroidism. It is the successful interpretation of changes in parathyroid hormone (PTH) levels that is essential for using this technique in a way to optimize cure. Thus, it is imperative that the surgeon has an understanding of PTH dynamics and carefully chooses the appropriate IOPTH protocol and interpretation criteria that will best predict operative success, minimize unnecessary bilateral exploration, decrease the likelihood of resecting parathyroid glands that are not hypersecreting, and prevent recurrence.

Primary hyperparathyroidism is a disease that is caused by excess parathyroid hormone (PTH) secretion from 1 or more of the parathyroid glands. Surgery is the only cure. Traditional surgical management consists of a 4-gland cervical exploration. Development of imaging specific to identification of parathyroid glands and application of the rapid PTH assay to operative management have made more minimal exploration possible. There are distinct advantages and disadvantages of minimally invasive parathyroidectomy (MIP) and bilateral neck exploration (BNE). The advantages of MIP seem to outweigh those of BNE, and MIP has replaced BNE as the operation of choice by many surgeons.

> Surgical resection remains the treatment of choice for primary pancreatic neuroendocrine tumors (PNETs), because it is associated with increased survival. Minimally invasive procedures are a safe modality for the surgical treatment of PNETs. In malignant PNETs, laparoscopy is not associated with a compromise in terms of oncologic resection, and provides the benefits of decreased postoperative pain, better cosmetic results, shorter hospital stay, and a shorter postoperative recovery period. Further prospective, multicenter, randomized trials are required for the analysis of these minimally invasive surgical techniques for the treatment of PNETs and their comparison with traditional open pancreatic surgery.

> Neuroendocrine tumors are rare and slow-growing malignancies that commonly metastasize to the liver, resulting in hormonal syndromes and death from liver failure. Surgical consultation and liver debulking are key components in management. Traditional surgical resection guidelines do not apply to these tumors as with other cancers. Surgical resection has shown survival benefit even in the event of an incomplete resection. Ablation may be used as an adjunct to resection or in patients who are not candidates for resection. Asymptomatic patients with high-volume disease do as well with intra-arterial therapy as with surgery.

SURGICAL ONCOLOGY CLINICS OF NORTH AMERICA

Foreword

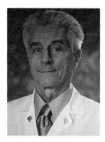

Nicholas J. Petrelli, MD, FACS
Consulting Editor

This issue of the *Surgical Oncology Clinics of North America* is devoted to endocrine tumors. The Guest Editor is Douglas L. Fraker, MD, Chief of the Division of Endocrine and Oncologic Surgery at the Hospital of the University of Pennsylvania, as well as a surgical oncologist and endocrine surgeon who was formerly a senior investigator at the National Cancer Institute. Dr Fraker's research efforts have focused on regional perfusion in treating melanoma and soft tissue sarcomas. His daily clinical practice deals with surgical oncology, including the treatment of melanoma, sarcoma, and liver tumors. He is also an expert in endocrine surgery of the thyroid, parathyroid, adrenal, and pancreas.

Dr Fraker has gathered together an outstanding group of physicians with expertise in endocrine tumors. The article on neuroendocrine liver metastases by Drs Farley and Pommier, from the Division of Surgical Oncology at Oregon Health and Science University, University of Oregon, describes the aggressive surgical approach with this entity. There is also an outstanding article on minimally invasive adrenalectomy by Drs Carr and Wang, from the Section of Endocrine Surgery at the Medical College of Wisconsin, and optimal utilization of intraoperative parathyroid hormone monitoring by Drs Patel and Caso, from the Division of Endocrine Surgery and Department of Otolaryngology at New York University, Langone Medical Center.

I'd like to thank Dr Fraker and his colleagues for an excellent issue of the *Surgical Oncology Clinics of North America*. This is an excellent issue for surgeons in training.

Nicholas J. Petrelli, MD, FACS
Bank of America Endowed Medical Director
Helen F Graham Cancer Center & Research Institute
Christiana Care Health Systems
4701 Ogletown Stanton Road, Suite 1233
Newark, DE 19713, USA

Professor of Surgery
Thomas Jefferson University

E-mail address:
npetrelli@christianacare.org

Surg Oncol Clin N Am 25 (2016) xiii
http://dx.doi.org/10.1016/j.soc.2015.10.002
1055-3207/16/$ – see front matter © 2016 Published by Elsevier Inc.

surgonc.theclinics.com

Preface

Advances in Endocrine Surgery

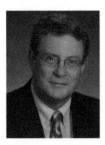

Douglas L. Fraker, MD, FACS
Editor

This issue of *Surgical Oncology Clinics of North America* presents the latest advances in the field of endocrine surgery. Endocrine surgery is the field defined by operative treatment of a variety of benign and malignant neoplasms of the thyroid gland, the parathyroid glands, the adrenal glands, the pancreas, and the gut neuroendocrine tissue. Advances in molecular genetics, hormone assays, and minimally invasive techniques have significantly changed the practice of endocrine surgery over the past decade. Articles in this issue are authored by several national experts across the country who have been instrumental to the development of recent advances in the field of endocrine surgery.

Thyroid cancer is the most common neoplasm treated by endocrine surgeons. Major changes in the molecular genetics available by commercial laboratories in the past three years have very defined likelihood of malignancy in previous lesions with indeterminate cytology. Management of lymph nodes as well as new aspects of postoperative treatment is presented as well. Controversial areas in the treatment of hyperparathyroidism include when to operate, how to use intraoperative parathyroid hormone (PTH) measurements, and what operation to perform, and all of these are described by leaders in the field. There have been several advances in the molecular genetics of pheochromocytomas and paragangliomas that affect both diagnosis and treatment. The operative approach for benign and malignant disease is discussed. Gut and pancreas neuroendocrine tumors reflect a disease that is increasing markedly in incidence in the United States, and the diagnosis, imaging, and surgical treatment are addressed.

This issue of *Surgical Oncology Clinics of North America* covers a wide range of topics that represent the most important advances in the field of endocrine surgery

Surg Oncol Clin N Am 25 (2016) xv–xvi
http://dx.doi.org/10.1016/j.soc.2015.10.001
1055-3207/16/$ – see front matter © 2016 Published by Elsevier Inc.

surgonc.theclinics.com

over the past ten years for surgery of the thyroid, parathyroid, adrenal, and pancreas or gastrointestinal neuroendocrine tumors.

Douglas L. Fraker, MD, FACS
Division of Endocrine Surgery and Surgical Oncology
Department of Surgery
University of Pennsylvania
4 Silverstein
3400 Spruce Street
Philadelphia, PA 19104, USA

E-mail address:
frakerd@uphs.upenn.edu

Management of Thyroid Nodular Disease

Current Cytopathology Classifications and Genetic Testing

Lindsay E. Kuo, MD, MBA[a], Rachel R. Kelz, MD, MSCE[b],*

KEYWORDS

- Thyroid nodules • Molecular markers • Genetic testing • Bethesda classification
- Afirma

KEY POINTS

- The Bethesda system for reporting thyroid cytopathology provides a standardized method of reporting results from fine-needle aspiration of thyroid nodules.
- The Bethesda system for reporting thyroid cytopathology should be applied universally to improve communication between pathologists and clinicians.
- For patients with indeterminate cytology, the Afirma gene expression classifier and tests for genetic mutations may provide helpful diagnostic and prognostic information with which to optimize treatment plans.

INTRODUCTION: NATURE OF THE PROBLEM

Thyroid nodules are common. Reports in the literature suggest a prevalence of 4% to 76% in the general population, depending on the mode of detection and the population studied.[1–3] Autopsy studies have reported similar prevalence rates.[4,5] Increased use of ultrasound technology has led to increased detection of thyroid lesions over the last 30 years.[5–7]

Most thyroid nodules are benign, with only 5% to 10% representing a malignant tumor.[7–11] Evaluation for thyroid malignancy is necessary after the discovery of many thyroid nodules to determine appropriate management recommendations. Nodules greater than 1 to 1.5 cm in size or associated with abnormal lymph node(s) on

The authors have nothing to disclose.
[a] Department of Surgery, Hospital of the University of Pennsylvania, 3400 Spruce Street, 4 Silverstein, Philadelphia, PA 19104, USA; [b] Division of Endocrine and Oncologic Surgery, Department of Surgery, Hospital of the University of Pennsylvania, 3400 Spruce Street, 4 Silverstein, Philadelphia, PA 19104, USA
* Corresponding author.
E-mail address: Rachel.Kelz@uphs.upenn.edu

Surg Oncol Clin N Am 25 (2016) 1–16
http://dx.doi.org/10.1016/j.soc.2015.08.001
1055-3207/16/$ – see front matter © 2016 Elsevier Inc. All rights reserved.

ultrasonography should receive an ultrasound-guided fine-needle aspiration (FNA) to obtain a sample for cytologic evaluation of malignancy.[3,12]

The clinical utility of FNA to guide management decisions occurs when results clearly indicate benign or malignant disease. However, FNA is not a perfect diagnostic tool. Variation in the interpretation of cytopathologic samples can occur between pathologists and across institutions,[13] leading to controversy over management. Moreover, approximately 10% to 25% of FNA evaluations report "indeterminate" results whereby neither benign nor malignant disease can be declared.[3,14] Consequently, thyroid lobectomy is needed to obtain tissue for an accurate diagnosis. However, more than half of these patients are found to have benign disease on formal pathologic evaluation, making their surgery seem unnecessary.[15] For those with malignancy found on surgical pathology, a second operation is usually recommended to improve surveillance for recurrence and to permit additional treatment when necessary. The need for a second operation can be troubling for patients and challenging for surgeons.[16]

Improved characterization of thyroid nodules is necessary to guide appropriate patients to surgery and reduce unnecessary surgeries. A universal cytopathologic classification system and several diagnostic tests have been developed in the last decade to facilitate the decision-making process.

CYTOPATHOLOGIC CLASSIFICATION
Bethesda Classification System

Background
Before 2007, multiple classification systems existed describing the results of FNA of thyroid nodules. Discordance between these classification systems led to inconsistent reporting of FNA results, creating confusion among clinicians and limiting the effectiveness of the test.[17,18] At the National Cancer Institute conference in the fall of 2007, a leading group of pathologists and clinicians proposed a 6-tiered classification scheme,[19] known as The Bethesda System for Reporting Cytopathology ("the Bethesda system"). The goal of the system was to provide a consistent means of reporting clinically relevant information so that physicians could best advise patients[17] (**Table 1**).

The classification system
A description of each category follows, along with the clinical recommendations put forth by the Bethesda group. Similar information is available in **Table 1** for ease of review. The chart is designed to be printed and posted in the surgical office setting, and can be especially helpful in an academic setting to raise awareness of the standard of care and encourage appropriate treatment decisions.

Class I: nondiagnostic or unsatisfactory FNA samples may have blood obscuring the specimen, a thick smear, smears that are improperly dried, or an insufficient quantity of cells.[17] The malignancy risk in nondiagnostic or unsatisfactory samples is 1% to 4%. Repeated aspiration of the nodule with ultrasound guidance should lead to a diagnostic result in 50% to 88% of cases; for nodules that remain nondiagnostic or unsatisfactory after repeat aspiration, excisional biopsy leads to a malignant result in 10%.[17] *Recommendation:* Repeat FNA under ultrasound guidance is suggested.

Class II: benign Thyroid FNAs are benign in 60% to 70% of cases. The false-negative rate of a benign result is 0% to 3%. Patients with a benign FNA should be followed clinically for 6 to 18 months, and repeat ultrasound, FNA, or both performed if clinical changes are noted.[17] *Recommendation:* Ultrasonographic surveillance every 6 to 18 months to assess stability. Change warrants repeat FNA.[12]

Table 1
Bethesda system for reporting cytopathology

Category		Includes	Risk of Malignancy (%)	Recommended Action
I	Nondiagnostic/unsatisfactory	Result of limited cellularity, lack of follicular cells, or poor fixation and preservation of sample	1–4	Repeat FNA with ultrasound guidance
II	Benign	Nodular goiter; hyperplastic or adenomatous nodule; chronic lymphocytic thyroiditis	0–3	Clinical follow-up
III	Follicular lesion of undetermined significance/atypia of undetermined significance	Cases that cannot be classified as either benign or a follicular neoplasm	5–15	Repeat FNA, correlate with clinical and radiologic findings. Consider molecular marker testing
IV	Follicular neoplasm/suspicious for follicular neoplasm	Includes nonpapillary follicular lesions and Hurthle cell lesions or neoplasms	15–30	Consider clinical and radiologic findings to determine between diagnostic lobectomy or near-total thyroidectomy[1]
V	Suspicious for malignancy	Suspicious for papillary carcinoma, medullary carcinoma, lymphoma, metastatic disease. May be due to presence of necrosis in specimen	60–75	Surgical lobectomy ± intraoperative frozen section to determine extent of surgery or near-total thyroidectomy for definitive diagnosis and treatment[a]
VI	Malignant	Evidence of papillary carcinoma and its variants, medullary carcinoma, lymphoma, anaplastic carcinoma, metastases	97–99	Near-total thyroidectomy for definitive management[b]

[a] Lateral neck ultrasonography should be performed preoperatively to examine for suspicious nodes and appropriate treatment determined pending results.
[b] Ultrasonography of entire thyroid gland and the cervical lymph node compartments should be performed preoperatively to examine for suspicious nodes and possible malignancy in contralateral lobe. Appropriate treatment is determined pending results.
Adapted from Refs.[3,12,17,19]

Class III: atypia of undetermined significance/follicular lesion of undetermined significance This category encompasses lesions that are not readily categorized as benign, malignant, or suspicious. This result occurs in 3% to 6% of FNAs, and should prompt performance of a repeat FNA. Repeated FNA will result in categorization in 80% of aspirates, but 20% will remain classified as atypia of undetermined significance (AUS)/follicular lesion of undetermined significance (FLUS). Because all patients with AUS/FLUS do not receive surgical resection, determination of the rate of potential malignancy is difficult. However, in AUS/FLUS specimens with concerning features on ultrasonography or physical examination, 20% to 25% are found to harbor malignancy.[17] The risk of malignancy for all AUS/FLUS specimens is likely lower. *Recommendation:* Repeat FNA under ultrasound guidance with consideration of molecular marker testing.[12]

Class IV: follicular neoplasm/suspicious for follicular neoplasm This category includes lesions that are concerning for follicular carcinoma, which cannot be diagnosed on FNA. Approximately 15% to 30% of these FNAs will be malignant on pathologic evaluation after surgical resection, diagnosed as either follicular carcinomas or follicular variants of papillary thyroid carcinomas. FNAs with a predominance of Hurthle cells may be reported as suspicious for Hurthle cell neoplasm, and 15% to 45% of these are malignant.[17] Surgical resection is needed to make a definitive diagnosis following categorization of a sample as follicular neoplasm (FN)/suspicious for follicular neoplasm (SFN). *Recommendation:* Diagnostic lobectomy or total thyroidectomy, depending on the clinical scenario, is appropriate.[17,19]

Class V: suspicious for malignancy Aspirates with some characteristics of malignancy but not definitively malignant are grouped into this category. Surgical resection is needed to diagnose malignancy, which is found in 60% to 75% of cases. The most common diagnosis is papillary carcinoma, follicular variant.[17] *Recommendation:* Surgical resection is indicated. Lobectomy with intraoperative frozen section or total thyroidectomy is appropriate.[3,20]

Class VI: malignant This classification describes samples that are definitively malignant, which occurs in 3% to 7% of FNAs, most of which are papillary thyroid carcinomas.[17] *Recommendation:* Surgical resection is indicated.

Accuracy and efficacy of the Bethesda system
One stated goal of the Bethesda system was to reduce confusion between pathologists and clinicians, and provide a standardized approach to patient care. Meta-analysis of the literature on the accuracy of the Bethesda system found correlations between each diagnostic category and the risk of malignant disease,[21] indicating that the diagnostic scheme is valid. In one study of patients with indeterminate lesions, implementation of the Bethesda criteria resulted in lower rates of malignancy in thyroidectomy specimens, suggesting that the Bethesda system has improved diagnostic accuracy.[22] However, in that study the calculated rate of malignancy in specimens classified as benign was higher, at 3.7%. This figure exceeded the rate suggested as appropriate by the Bethesda group, but did fall within the American Thyroid Association guideline recommendations.[21]

The effect of the Bethesda criteria on reducing unnecessary surgery is unclear: the number of patients receiving surgery after FNA varied greatly between institutions reviewed in the meta-analysis.[21] However, a 2011 single-institution review found a lower rate of surgical resection after implementation of the Bethesda criteria. The decline in surgical resection was attributed to a decline in the rate of surgical resection among patients with benign findings.[18]

A novel category introduced by the Bethesda system was AUS/FLUS. Despite the goal of reporting this result in only 3% to 6% of cases,[17] a meta-analysis found this category used in 9.6% of cases and with an associated 15.9% malignancy rate.[21] Sullivan and colleagues[23] found heterogeneous reporting rates of AUS/FLUS between institutions, with some institutions reporting this categorization in 29% of aspirates. This variation may be due to the inability to precisely define morphologic criteria for atypia.[21] Methods for limiting the overuse of this classification are under consideration. One suggestion is to implement the ratio of AUS/FLUS to malignant tumor as a performance metric, with a goal range of 1 to 3.[24]

Although the Bethesda group recommended performing repeat FNA after an AUS/FLUS classification, management following reporting of AUS/FLUS is also variable: some patients receive repeat FNA, whereas others proceed to surgical resection.[18,21,25] A 2010 review of thyroidectomy rates for indeterminate lesions at a single institution before and after implementation of the Bethesda criteria demonstrated no change in rates of thyroidectomy performance.[22] This variation in practice may be due to initial hesitancy to follow a less aggressive (nonsurgical) approach despite the Bethesda system recommendations, or may result from differing published guidelines by national societies. For example, the 2009 management guidelines published by the American Thyroid Association recommend pursuing molecular markers (see later discussion) for aspirates classified as indeterminate.[12] Of note, Heller and colleagues[25] performed a cost-effective analysis on repeat FNA for AUS/FLUS lesions, and found repeat FNA to be less costly and more effective than diagnostic lobectomy.

Overall, the Bethesda classification has improved communication between providers and across institutions that adopted its use. Moving forward, establishment of additional criteria to help resolve indeterminate results is under way to further encourage the selective use of surgery as a diagnostic modality when not required for treatment purposes.

MOLECULAR TESTS
Afirma

The Afirma test, produced by Veracyte (San Francisco, CA, USA) is a gene expression classifier (GEC) for use on cytologically indeterminate (AUS/FLUS and FN/SFN) nodules. The Afirma test is primarily used to rule in a benign diagnosis for thyroid nodules, and is only approved for nodules at least 1 cm in size. Clinical characteristics including maximal tumor size should also be considered before Afirma testing.

Test procedures
During an FNA of a thyroid nodule, in addition to obtaining aspirates for cytopathologic examination, 2 needle passes are dedicated to obtaining specimens for Afirma analysis. These specimens are immediately stored in a nucleic acid preservative. Most physicians send FNA specimens to Thyroid Cytopathology Partners (TCP) (Austin, TX, USA), a Veracyte partner. TCP then performs cytopathologic review of the FNA sample, and only if this cytopathologic analysis results in an indeterminate diagnosis is the Afirma test run. Several academic medical centers are designated an "Enabled Center," which allows the center to send samples for Afirma GEC testing based on in-house cytopathology results, instead of sending samples to TCP.[26]

If cytopathologic evaluation of the FNA specimen yields an indeterminate result (AUS/FLUS or FN/SFN) based on the Bethesda criteria, the Afirma test is performed on the preserved sample. If cytopathologic evaluation reveals any other diagnosis, the preserved sample is discarded.

During the Afirma GEC test RNA is extracted, amplified, and hybridized to a custom microarray to examine for gene patterns. The sample is compared with a proprietary panel of 167 mRNA gene expression patterns, which are derived from 142 genes. Results of the test lead to either a "benign" or "suspicious" test result. If the result is "suspicious," a "malignancy classifier" test can then be performed to examine for specific genetic mutations. Insufficient RNA in the sample leads to a "no result" conclusion in approximately 10% of cases.[27]

Validity of the Afirma test

In 2012, Alexander and colleagues[28] examined 265 indeterminate FNA samples, and found sensitivity of 92%, specificity of 52%, a positive predictive value (PPV) of 38%, and a negative predictive value (NPV) of 93%. For fine-needle aspirates classified as AUS/FLUS the NPV was 95%, whereas for aspirates classified as FN/SFN the NPV was 94%. As a result, the risk of malignancy in a nodule with a benign result on the Afirma test is estimated at 5% to 6%, which is considered equivalent to the risk of malignancy in a lesion diagnosed as "benign" on the Bethesda cytopathologic classification.[28] However, for aspirates designated suspicious for malignancy (SM) on cytopathologic testing, the calculated NPV of the Afirma test was lower, at 85%, indicating that these nodules continue to require surgical resection for diagnosis. Performance of the Afirma test is therefore not indicated for SM nodules.

A second multi-institution study was performed by Alexander and colleagues[29] in which cytopathologic investigation was performed at institutional Enabled Centers instead of at TCP. This study examined 346 indeterminate nodules, and reported results similar to those of the original study. Furthermore, this study had a 51% rate of benign Afirma, and reported a 76% reduction in surgical performance among patients who would have received surgery without the Afirma test. Li and colleagues[30] performed a cost-effectiveness analysis of the Afirma test, assuming 74% fewer thyroidectomies based on Afirma results, and calculated an incremental cost saving of $1453 per patient and an increase of 0.07 quality-adjusted life years (QALYs) over 5 years when compared with clinical practice based on cytopathologic findings alone.

However, these promising results have not been borne out in all studies conducted on the Afirma GEC. In a third study, in which cytopathologic analysis was performed at a single institution, McIver and colleagues[26] examined 72 indeterminate nodules and reported a much lower benign result rate of only 27%. Consequently, the calculated NPV of the Afirma test in this study was only 75%; the PPV was also significantly lower, at 15.6%. Based on these results, 4 Afirma tests would be needed to prevent 1 unnecessary surgery, instead of 2, as suggested by the 51% benign result noted by McIver and colleagues.[26] Lastly, Harrell and Bimston[31] studied 58 indeterminate nodules, all of which underwent evaluation at TCP, and found a benign diagnosis rate of 34%, an NPV of 80% to 90%, and a PPV of 38% to 57%.

The varying results of these studies may be due to the differing pretest probabilities of malignancy used in each study: as the pretest probability of malignancy increases, the PPV increases while the NPV decreases[26]; this can also be seen graphically in **Fig. 1**. Further studies are needed to clarify the diagnostic utility of the Afirma test, and the downstream effects on thyroidectomy rates and costs of care. Regardless, it is important to remember the 5% to 6% risk of malignancy in patients with a benign Afirma result. Careful observation of these patients is warranted. Furthermore, because the PPV of the test is only 38% at best, a "suspicious" result does not mean that the patient has cancer. Individual risk assessments for each patient should be performed, incorporating all available information, to lead to a recommended course of action.

GENETIC MUTATIONS

Some 60% to 70% of thyroid cancers harbor DNA mutations, but not all mutations are associated with malignancy. FNA samples and thyroid tissue can be tested for genetic mutations. Although genetic mutation tests are highly specific for the presence of thyroid malignancy, they are not sensitive: in other words, the tests possess high PPV but low NPV. However, genetic marker testing can improve the accuracy of the cytopathologic diagnosis, particularly for nodules classified as indeterminate.

BRAFV600E

Mutations in the *BRAF* gene are the most common genetic mutations in thyroid cancer.[32,33] The *BRAF* gene is located on chromosome 7, and mutations cause activation of the RAS/RAF/mitogen-activated protein kinase/extracellular-signal-regulated kinase-signal transduction pathway, leading to increased mitotic activity.[34] There are more than 40 mutations associated with the *BRAF* gene, the most common of which is *BRAF*V600E. Mutations in *BRAF* are highly specific for detection of papillary thyroid carcinoma (PTC).[34,35] *BRAF*V600E mutations are found in up to 87% of PTCs, including the classic subtype, but are also found in 15% to 20% of follicular variants of PTC (FVPTC) and 50% to 100% of tall cell variants.[36,37] *BRAF*V600E mutations are also found in anaplastic thyroid carcinoma and other poorly differentiated thyroid carcinomas.[38] The *BRAF*K601E mutation, less common than the V600E mutation, has also been described and is typically found in FVPTC[39] (**Table 2**).

In cytologically indeterminate nodules on FNA, a positive *BRAF*V600E mutation is associated with malignancy in 100% of cases.[33,40] However, absence of the mutation does not rule out carcinoma, particularly nonpapillary thyroid carcinoma.[34]

Some studies have shown that the *BRAF*V600E mutation is associated with an increased prevalence of extrathyroidal extension, thyroid capsular invasion, lymph node metastasis, and a poorer response to radioactive iodine treatment.[36] Other studies have demonstrated that the *BRAF*V600E mutation is a prognostic factor for recurrent and persistent disease, and is associated with an increased rate of mortality in PTC patients.[36,41,42] However, recent literature has not agreed with these findings,[43,44] and determination of the clinical significance of the *BRAF*V600E mutation is of ongoing interest.

Because of the potential aggressiveness of PTC with *BRAF*V600E mutations, preoperative discovery of the *BRAF*V600E mutation could lead to more aggressive initial surgical management. However, a retrospective study of the *BRAF*V600E mutation in cytologically indeterminate nodules found that identification of the *BRAF* mutation did not alter the surgical management of these patients.[45] Moreover, in a cost-utility analysis of *BRAF* testing, Lee and colleagues[46] found that preoperative *BRAF* testing followed by total thyroidectomy and central neck dissection resulted in overall outcomes similar to those of routine care without *BRAF* testing, and was associated with increased costs. Both treatments resulted in an additional 23.60 QALYs per patient, but treatment without *BRAF* testing was associated with $801.51 lower costs. Higher costs associated with *BRAF* testing stemmed from the cost of the test itself, increased operative and hospital costs related to a more complex procedure, and increased postoperative complication rates.[46] However, both costs and QALYs are affected by the low recurrence rate of *BRAF*-positive carcinoma used in study calculations. In a population with more aggressive disease and higher recurrence rates, BRAF testing will be a useful, cost-effective adjunct to triage.

In summary, the prognostic relationship between *BRAF*V600E mutation positivity and more aggressive thyroid cancer is unclear. However, *BRAF* mutations are highly specific for PTC, and when found may help guide treatment decisions.

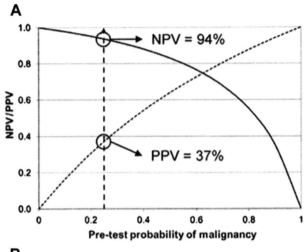

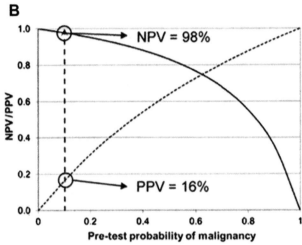

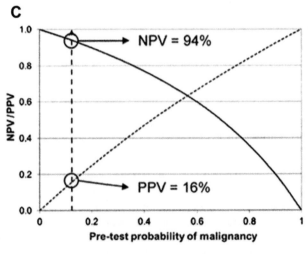

Table 2
Prevalence of gene mutations in thyroid cancer, by type

Mutation	Type of Carcinoma	Prevalence (%)	Positive Predictive Value (%)
BRAF V600E	Classic papillary thyroid carcinoma (PTC)	45	100
	Follicular variant of PTC	15–20[36]	
	Tall cell variant of PTC	50–100[36]	
	Anaplastic thyroid carcinoma	25	
RAS (H-ras, K-ras, N-ras)	Follicular adenoma	20–25	74–87
	Follicular thyroid carcinoma (FTC)	25–45[32]	
	Follicular variant of PTC	10–45[39]	
	Poorly differentiated thyroid carcinoma	20–40	
	Anaplastic thyroid carcinoma	20–50[39]	
RET/PTC	PTC	20–30[38]	100
PAX8/PPAR	FTC	29–56[56–59]	100
	Follicular variant of PTC	5[39]	
	Follicular adenoma	7[39]	
Mutation panel	All	70–75	88

Adapted from Xing M. Molecular pathogenesis and mechanisms of thyroid cancer. Nat Rev Cancer 2013;13(3):187; with permission from Macmillan Publishers Ltd.

RAS

RAS mutations are the second most common mutation in thyroid cancers. The *ras* family of proto-oncogenes includes the H-*ras*, K-*ras*, and N-*ras* genes. The *ras* genes code for membrane proteins that transduce mitogenic signals from growth hormone receptors to intracellular activity; mutation leads to constant "on" activity by these proteins, resulting in oncogenesis.[47] Although most human malignancies contain only 1 *ras* mutation, all 3 mutations have been reported in thyroid carcinoma.[47]

RAS mutations are seen in 40% to 50% of follicular thyroid carcinomas (FTC), 10% to 20% of PTC, and 20% to 40% of poorly differentiated and anaplastic carcinomas.[48,49] A *ras* mutation in an FNA sample is associated with an 87.5% risk of malignancy, including an approximately 25% risk of FTC and a 62.5% risk of PTC.[32,40] *RAS*-positive tumors are most often diagnosed to be FVPTC on surgical resection.[48]

◄────────────────────────────────

Fig. 1. Relationship between the pretest probability of malignancy and the NPV and PPV of the Afirma GEC. (*A*) The NPV and PPV for Afirma GEC for FN/SFN, as a function of the pretest probability of malignancy, based on sensitivity and specificity reported by Alexander and colleagues.[28] The Afirma GEC has a reported sensitivity of 90% and specificity of 48% in FN/HCN, which results in a PPV of 38% and NPV of 94%. (*B*) At the same sensitivity and specificity, but with a lower pretest probability of malignancy, estimated at 10% in the study illustrated here, the PPV decreases to 16%, whereas NPV is expected to increase to 98%. (*C*) Data from the study imply a specificity of 39% and sensitivity of 83% if there are no additional false-negatives among the Afirma GEC–benign nodules.[26] This changes the shape of the curves relating PPV and NPV to pretest the probability of malignancy changes, as shown. Sensitivity of 38%, specificity of 83%, and a 12% pretest probability of malignancy yield the observed PPV of 16% and NPV of 94%. (*From* McIver B, Castro MR, Morris JC, et al. An independent study of a gene expression classifier (Afirma) in the evaluation of cytologically indeterminate thyroid nodules. J Clin Endocrinol Metab 2014;99(11):4075; with permission.)

RAS mutations are also seen in 68.0% of *ret*-negative sporadic medullary thyroid cancer (MTC), but are rarely seen in *ret*-positive MTC.[50] RAS mutations may also offer prognostic information; the presence of the *ras* mutation in thyroid carcinomas has been shown to be associated with increased rates of disease-related death.[51]

The *ras* mutation may also be present in benign lesions, such as follicular adenomas or hyperplastic nodules.[32,33,48] As the potential for a follicular adenoma to develop into an FTC is unclear, discovery of a follicular adenoma with a mutation in *ras* should prompt a thorough discussion with the patient about the risk of malignancy and surgical management.[40]

The high prevalence of *ras* mutations in FTC has the potential to change surgical management, as these carcinomas are difficult to diagnose on FNA cytopathology and typically require lobectomy for diagnosis, followed by completion thyroidectomy. However, because *ras* mutations are not specific for malignancy, the PPV of *ras* for malignancy is just 74% to 87%.[49] Consequently, total thyroidectomy as an initial surgical procedure is not indicated following identification of a *ras* mutation.

RET/PTC

Somatic rearrangements in the *RET* tyrosine kinase gene are associated with papillary thyroid cancer, both classic and follicular variants. These rearrangements are collectively known as *RET/PTC*, and are different from germline mutations in *RET* associated with multiple endocrine neoplasia-2 syndromes. Rearrangements in the *RET* gene result in constitutional activation of the tyrosine kinase, which is involved with intracellular signal transduction.[52] The 2 most common *RET/PTC* mutations are *RET/PTC1* and *RET/PTC3*; there are more than 10 types of translocations overall.[37]

The prevalence of *RET/PTC* in papillary thyroid carcinomas varies widely in the literature, from 8% to 92.3%.[37,49] This variation is due in part to differing sensitivities in the methods of detection,[52,53] in addition to geographic location, patient age, and exposure to ionizing radiation. On average, *RET/PTC* is found in 20% of sporadic PTCs.[38] Clonal *RET/PTC* rearrangements are described by Zhu and colleagues[52] as prevalent in most tumor cells and the only genetic mutation present, signifying malignant transformation from a single cell. Such mutations are found in 10% to 20% of PTCs. Clonal *RET/PTC* rearrangements are highly specific for PTC.[49]

Nonclonal *RET/PTC* rearrangements, defined as occurring in a minority of tumor cells and therefore not an indicator of a neoplasm from a single cell, may be seen in malignant thyroid lesions.[49,52] However, nonclonal *RET/PTC* rearrangements are also seen in 10% to 45% of patients with benign thyroid disease.[49] The clinical implications of these findings are unclear.[53] Discovery of a *RET/PTC* transformation in a patient with benign disease should prompt careful follow-up, as the clinical significance of this finding has yet to be determined. However, because nonclonal *RET/PTC* rearrangements are not specific for PTC, identification of nonclonal mutations provides no diagnostic information.

Despite the high specificity of clonal *RET/PTC* mutations for thyroid carcinoma, the utility of the test is uncertain. In one investigation of cytologically indeterminate nodules, the prevalence of *RET/PTC* rearrangements was only 0.83%.[40] Furthermore, the low prevalence of the *RET/PTC* rearrangements in PTC prevents the test from being an independent useful marker of malignancy. No cost-effectiveness analyses of the test have been carried out. Because of the high specificity of the rearrangement for PTC and the unclear significance of the positive result in a benign tumor, testing for the rearrangement can be useful when combined with other mutation tests.

PAX8/PPARγ

The PAX8/PPARγ fusion protein is caused by a somatic tumor genetic rearrangement resulting in the chromosomal translocation t(2;3) (q13;p25).[54] The exact mechanism of the PAX8/PPARγ fusion protein that leads to tumorigenesis is unknown.[55]

PAX8/PPARγ is found in 29% to 56% of FTCs,[56–59] and may be related to radiation exposure.[56] It is also found in 37.5% of FVPTCs.[57] In FVPTC patients the translocation is associated with multifocality and vascular invasion, suggesting that the rearrangement leads to higher malignant potential.[57]

The PAX8/PPARγ translocation is also found in 4% to 33.3% of follicular thyroid adenomas.[56–59] The unclear prevalence of the PAX8/PPARγ translocation in both malignant and benign disease affects the specificity of the test to rule in malignancy. However, in a small number of cytologically indeterminate samples studied the translocation possesses 100% specificity,[32,40] suggesting it has the potential to be a useful diagnostic tool.

Other Mutations

Many other genetic alterations associated with thyroid cancer have been discovered, including deletions of PTEN, mutations of PTEN, p53, β-catenin, anaplastic lymphoma kinase (ALK), isocitrate dehydrogenase 1 (IDH1), and NADH dehydrogenase 1α subcomplex 13 (NDUFA13).[37] Amplification of the PIK3CA, PIK3CB, 3-phosphoinositide–dependent protein kinase 1 (PDPK1), AKT1, and AKT2 genes may also occur in thyroid tumorigenesis.[37] Many of these genetic aberrations, in addition to those described in detail herein, affect one of a few specific signaling pathways, and may have cumulative effects the conversion of benign thyroid tissue to malignant tissue, or the change from well-differentiated to poorly differentiated thyroid carcinoma.[37] The exact effects of these genetic alterations, their interactions with each other, and the prevalence of the alternations in thyroid cancer are areas for future investigation.

Mutation Panels

No one mutation has 100% sensitivity for thyroid cancer; therefore, a negative result on a genetic test does not rule out malignancy. The diagnostic utility of testing for genetic markers of thyroid cancer can be improved by testing for several mutations and rearrangements at once.

Three studies have examined testing for panels of 5 or more genetic markers.

In 2009, Nikiforov and colleagues[32] investigated the combination of the BRAFV600E, BRAFK601E, and ras mutations and the RET/PTC and PAX8/PPARγ rearrangements, and found specificity of 100% for malignancy in indeterminate nodules. Overall accuracy of the panel in diagnosing malignancy was improved in comparison with FNA alone (97% vs 93%).[32] When examining the same combination of genetic alterations, Cantara and colleagues[33] determined that the PPV of cytology plus molecular analysis for malignancy in indeterminate or suspicious nodules was 89.7%, up from 85.2% for cytology alone. The combination of these 5 genetic tests correctly identified 78.2% of all thyroid malignancies, compared with 58.9% found on cytology alone.[33] Ohori and colleagues[60] examined the diagnostic utility of the same panel in FNA samples categorized as Bethesda III (AUS/FLUS). The PPV and specificity of the gene panel were 100%. Moreover, genetic analysis discovered more malignant nodules than did repeat FNA. Although each of these studies used different methods to detect genetic abnormalities, they collectively demonstrate that genetic analysis provides increased diagnostic information over cytology alone.

However, the sensitivity of these 4 studies ranges from 38% to 85.7%,[61] indicating that mutation panels should not be used as a screening test.

Most recently, Yip and colleagues[62] examined the effect of the aforementioned mutation panel on the choice of initial surgical procedure. One patient cohort did not receive a mutation panel, and underwent an initial lobectomy or total thyroidectomy based on existing American Thyroid Association guidelines. A second patient cohort received a mutation panel, positive results of which mandated initial total thyroidectomy, whereas negative results indicated treatment following current guidelines. Performance of the mutation panel led to a higher rate of malignancy on total thyroidectomy and a lower rate of malignancy after lobectomy. Patients with indeterminate cytology who did not receive a mutation panel were significantly more likely to require a 2-stage thyroidectomy than those who did receive the panel.[62] There were no differences in the rates of total thyroidectomy performed for ultimately benign disease between patients who received the mutation panel and patients who did not. This study demonstrated the utility of regular mutation panel performance in guiding treatment decisions.

In a different study, Yip and colleagues[63] analyzed the cost-effectiveness of a panel including BRAFV6003, BRAFK601E, and 3 ras mutations, and the RET/PTC and PAX8/PPARγ rearrangements, in aspirates classified as Bethesda II or III. Use of the panel decreased the rate of diagnostic lobectomy by 20% (from 11.6% with standard care to 9.7% with molecular testing), and increased the rate of total thyroidectomy from 16.1% to 18.2%. The cumulative cost of performing the molecular panel followed by total thyroidectomy for a positive result ($16,414) was less than performing an initial lobectomy plus completion thyroidectomy when indicated ($19,638).[63] However, the investigators noted that the cost savings only existed because the panel cost $650; if the panel cost $870 or more, performance of the panel would not result in overall cost savings. Furthermore, the study did not account for deferral of surgical intervention in appropriate FLUS/AUS patients and potential associated costs.

In the most recently published management guidelines, the American Thyroid Association recommended consideration of molecular marker testing in patients with indeterminate FNA cytology.[12] The results of Yip and colleagues[62,63] strongly suggest that regular mutation panel testing may help guide initial surgical management.

Barriers to Regular Testing

Testing indeterminate FNA samples for genetic mutations or rearrangements can provide additional diagnostic and prognostic information, potentially altering surgical management and leading to reduced costs. However, these tests are not yet widely performed.

Performing routine genetic studies on FNA samples will require the development of a process that allows easy DNA, mRNA, or micro-RNA extraction from the samples.[61] At present, genetic mutations are tested with polymerase chain reaction (PCR)-based methods, whereas gene rearrangements are detected through reverse-transcriptase PCR methods or fluorescence in situ hybridization. Collection of sufficient material to complete all testing, and processing the material correctly to allow for testing, are 2 obstacles to routine genetic testing.[39]

Lastly, additional molecular markers are needed to fill the gap in the diagnostic sensitivity of the current genetic testing methods, as up to 30% of thyroid cancers have no known genetic mutation or rearrangement.[61] So although a positive result on a mutation panel is nearly 100% predictive of malignancy, a negative result provides no additional diagnostic or prognostic information. Development of an algorithm to help rule out malignancy is necessary.[39]

SUMMARY

Several important developments have been made in the last decade to assist in the preoperative diagnosis and operative planning for patients with thyroid nodules. Use of the Bethesda criteria for cytopathologic classification of thyroid nodule aspirates has improved communication between pathologists and clinicians, and has helped to simplify decision making based on the operative findings.

Multiple genetic tests, including testing for molecular markers and the Afirma GEC, have been developed and validated. However, none of these tests is both 100% sensitive and 100% specific for thyroid malignancies. Genetic tests and molecular markers can be useful adjuncts to standard clinical and radiologic information in the evaluation of thyroid nodules, especially in the setting of indeterminate cytology. The development of an updated diagnostic and treatment algorithm incorporating the full armamentarium of available tests for use in the management of thyroid nodules will help to standardize the management of patients with nodular thyroid disease, and reduce variation and inefficiencies in care.

REFERENCES

1. Vander JB, Gaston EA, Dawber TR. The significance of nontoxic thyroid nodules: final report of a 15-year study of the incidence of thyroid malignancy. Ann Intern Med 1965;69:537–40.
2. Ezzat S, Sarti DA, Cain DR, et al. Thyroid incidentalomas. Prevalence by palpation and ultrasonography. Arch Intern Med 1994;154(16):1838–40.
3. Gharib H, Papini E, Paschke R, et al. American Association of Clinical Endocrinologists, Associazione Medici Endocrinologi, and European Thyroid Association medical guidelines for clinical practice for the diagnosis and management of thyroid nodules. Endocr Pract 2010;16(Suppl 1):1–43.
4. Mortenson JD, Woolner LB, Bennett WA. Gross and microscopic findings in clinically normal thyroid glands. J Clin Endocrinol Metab 1955;15:1270–80.
5. Davies L, Welch HG. Increasing Incidence of thyroid cancer in the United States, 1973-2002. JAMA 2006;295:2164–7.
6. Mitchell J, Parangi S. The thyroid incidentaloma: an increasingly frequent consequence of radiologic imaging. Semin Ultrasound CT MRI 2005;26:37–46.
7. Roman SA. Endocrine tumors: evaluation of the thyroid nodule. Curr Opin Oncol 2003;15:66–70.
8. Hegedus L. The thyroid nodule. N Engl J Med 2004;351:1764–71.
9. Ajmal S, Rapoport S, Ramirez Batlle H, et al. The natural history of the benign thyroid nodule: what is the appropriate follow-up strategy? J Am Coll Surg 2015;220: 987–92.
10. Mandel SJ. A 64-year-old woman with a thyroid nodule. JAMA 2004;292(21): 2632–42.
11. Papini E, Guglielmi R, Bianchini A, et al. Risk of malignancy in nonpalpable thyroid nodules: predictive value of ultrasound and color-Doppler features. J Clin Endocrinol Metab 2002;87(5):1941–6.
12. American Thyroid Association (ATA) Guidelines Taskforce on Thyroid Nodules and Differentiated Thyroid Cancer, Cooper DS, Doherty GM, et al. Revised American Thyroid Association management guidelines for patients with thyroid nodules and differentiated thyroid cancer. Thyroid 2009;19(11):1167–214.
13. Wang CC, Friedman L, Kennedy GC. A large multicenter correlation study of thyroid nodule cytopathology and histopathology. Thyroid 2011;21(3): 243–51.

14. Duick DS. Overview of molecular biomarkers for enhancing the management of cytologically indeterminate thyroid nodules and thyroid cancer. Endocr Pract 2012;19(4):611–5.
15. Yassa L, Cibas ES, Benson CB. Long-term assessment of a multidisciplinary approach to thyroid nodule diagnostic evaluation. Cancer 2007;111(6):508–16.
16. Lefevre JH, Tresallet C, Leenhardt L, et al. Reoperative surgery for thyroid disease. Langenbecks Arch Surg 2007;392(6):685–91.
17. Cibas ES, Ali SZ. The Bethesda system for reporting thyroid cytopathology. Am J Clin Pathol 2009;132:658–65.
18. Crowe A, Linder A, Hameed O, et al. The impact of implementation of the Bethesda system for reporting thyroid cytopathology on the quality of reporting, "risk" of malignancy, surgical rate, and rate of frozen sections requested for thyroid lesions. Cancer Cytopathol 2011;119:315–21.
19. Baloch ZW, LiVolsi VA, Asa SL, et al. Diagnostic terminology and morphologic criteria for cytologic diagnosis of thyroid lesions: a synopsis of the National Cancer Institute thyroid fine-needle aspiration state of the science conference. Diagn Cytopathol 2008;36(6):425–37.
20. Haymart MR, Greenblatt DY, Elson DF, et al. The role of intraoperative frozen section if suspicious for papillary thyroid cancer. Thyroid 2008;18(4):419–23.
21. Bongiovanni M, Spitale A, Faquin WC, et al. The Bethesda system for reporting thyroid cytopathology: a meta-analysis. Acta Cytol 2012;56:333–9.
22. Rabaglia JL, Kabbani W, Wallace L, et al. Effect of the Bethesda system for reporting thyroid cytopathology on thyroidectomy rates and malignancy risk in cytologically indeterminate lesions. Surgery 2010;148:1267–73.
23. Sullivan PS, Hirschowitz SL, Fung PC, et al. The impact of atypia/follicular lesion of undetermined significance and repeated fine-needle aspiration: 5 years before and after implementation of the Bethesda system. Cancer Cytopathol 2014;122:866–72.
24. Krane JF, Vanderlaan PA, Faquin WC, et al. The atypia of undetermined significance/follicular lesion of undetermined significance:malignant ratio: a proposed performance measure for reporting in the Bethesda system for thyroid cytopathology. Cancer Cytopathol 2012;120:111–6.
25. Heller M, Zanocco K, Zydowicz S, et al. Cost-effectiveness of analysis of repeat fine-needle aspiration for thyroid biopsies read as atypia of undetermined significance. Surgery 2012;152:423–30.
26. McIver B, Castro MR, Morris JC, et al. An independent study of a gene expression classifier (Afirma) in the evaluation of cytologically indeterminate thyroid nodules. J Clin Endocrinol Metab 2014;99(11):4069–77.
27. Duick DS, Klopper JP, Diggans JC, et al. The impact of benign gene expression classifier test results on the endocrinologist-patient decision to operate on patients with thyroid nodules with indeterminate fine-needle aspiration cytopathology. Thyroid 2012;22(10):996–1001.
28. Alexander EK, Kennedy GC, Baloch ZW, et al. Preoperative diagnosis of benign thyroid nodules with indeterminate cytology. N Engl J Med 2012;367:705–15.
29. Alexander EK, Schorr M, Klopper J, et al. Multicenter clinical experience with the Afirma Gene expression classifier. J Clin Endocrinol Metab 2014;99:119–25.
30. Li H, Robinson KA, Anton B, et al. Cost-effectiveness of a novel molecular test for cytologically indeterminate thyroid nodules. J Clin Endocrinol Metab 2011;96:E1719–26.

31. Harrell RM, Bimston DN. Surgical utility of Afirma: effects of high cancer prevalence and oncocytic cell types in patients with indeterminate thyroid cytology. Endocr Pract 2014;20(4):364–9.
32. Nikiforov YE, Steward DL, Robinson-Smith TM, et al. Molecular testing for mutations in improving the fine-needle aspiration diagnosis of thyroid nodules. J Clin Endocrinol Metab 2009;94:2092–8.
33. Cantara S, Capezzone M, Marchisotta S, et al. Impact of proto-oncogene mutation detection in cytological specimens from thyroid nodules improves the diagnostic accuracy of cytology. J Clin Endocrinol Metab 2010;96:1365–9.
34. Cohen Y, Rosenbaum E, Clark DP, et al. Mutational analysis of BRAF in fine needle aspiration biopsies of the thyroid: a potential application for the preoperative assessment of thyroid nodules. Clin Cancer Res 2004;10:2761–5.
35. Trovisco V, Vieira de Castro I, Soares P, et al. BRAF mutations are associated with some histological types of papillary thyroid carcinoma. J Pathol 2004;202:247–51.
36. Tufano RP, Teixeira GV, Bishop J, et al. BRAF mutation in papillary thyroid cancer and its value in tailoring initial treatment. A systemic review and meta-analysis. Medicine 2012;91:274–86.
37. Xing M. Molecular pathogenesis and mechanisms of thyroid cancer. Nat Rev Cancer 2013;13:184–99.
38. Nikiforov YE. Thyroid carcinoma: molecular pathways and therapeutic targets. Mod Pathol 2008;21:S37–43.
39. Hassell LA, Gillies EM, Dunn ST. Cytologic and molecular diagnosis of thyroid cancers. Is it time for routine reflex testing? Cancer Cytopathol 2012;120:7–17.
40. Nikiforov YE, Ohori NP, Hodak SP, et al. Impact of mutational testing on the diagnosis and management of patients with cytologically indeterminate thyroid nodules: a prospective analysis of 1056 FNA samples. J Clin Endocrinol Metab 2011;96:3390–7.
41. Kebebew E, Weng J, Bauer J, et al. The prevalence and prognostic value of BRAF mutation in thyroid cancer. Ann Surg 2007;246:466–71.
42. Xing M, Alzahrani AS, Carson KA, et al. Association between BRAF V600E mutation and mortality in patients with papillary thyroid cancer. JAMA 2013;309(14):1493–501.
43. Niederer-Wust SM, Jochum W, Förbs D, et al. Impact of clinical risk scores and BRAF V600E mutation status on outcome in papillary thyroid cancer. Surgery 2015;157:119–25.
44. Gouviea C, Can NT, Bostrom A, et al. Lack of association of BRAF mutation with negative prognostic indicators in papillary thyroid carcinoma. The University of California, San Francisco, experience. JAMA Otolaryngol Head Neck Surg 2013;139(11):1164–70.
45. Kleiman DA, Sporn MJ, Beninato T, et al. Preoperative BRAF(V600E) mutation screening is unlikely to alter initial surgical treatment of patients with indeterminate thyroid nodules. Cancer 2013;119:1495–502.
46. Lee WS, Palmer BJ, Garcia A, et al. BRAF mutation in papillary thyroid cancer: a cost-utility analysis of preoperative testing. Surgery 2014;156:1569–78.
47. Escapa CT, Johnson SJ, Kendall-Taylor P, et al. Prevalence of RAS mutations in thyroid neoplasia. Clin Endocrinol 1999;50:529–35.
48. Gupta N, Dasyam AK, Carty SE, et al. RAS mutations in thyroid FNA specimens are highly predictive of low-risk follicular-pattern cancers. J Clin Endocrinol Metab 2013;98:E914–22.
49. Nikiforov YE, Nikiforova MN. Molecular genetics and diagnosis of thyroid cancer. Nat Rev Endocrinol 2011;7:569–80.

50. Moura MM, Cavaco BM, Pinto AE, et al. High prevalence of RAS mutations in RET-negative sporadic medullary thyroid carcinomas. J Clin Endocrinol Metab 2011;96:E863–8.
51. Garcia-Rostan G, Zhao H, Camp RL, et al. RAS mutations are associated with aggressive tumor phenotypes and poor prognosis in thyroid cancer. J Clin Oncol 2003;21:3226–35.
52. Zhu Z, Ciampi R, Nikiforova MN, et al. Prevalence of RET/PTC rearrangements in thyroid papillary carcinomas: effects of the detection methods and genetic heterogeneity. J Clin Endocrinol Metab 2006;91(9):3603–10.
53. Guerra A, Sapio MR, Marotta V, et al. Prevalence of RET/PTC rearrangement in benign and malignant thyroid nodules and its clinical application. Endocrinol Jpn 2011;58(1):31–8.
54. Kroll TG, Sarraf P, Pecciarini L, et al. PAX8-PPARG1 fusion oncogene in human thyroid carcinoma. Science 2000;289:1357–60.
55. Eberhardt NL, Grebe SK, McIver B, et al. The role of the PAX8/PPARG fusion oncogene in the pathogenesis of follicular thyroid cancer. Mol Cell Endocrinol 2010;321:50–6.
56. Dwight T, Thoppe SR, Foukakis T, et al. Involvement of the PAX8/Peroxisome proliferator-activated receptor gamma rearrangement in follicular thyroid tumors. J Clin Endocrinol Metab 2003;88:4440–5.
57. Castro P, Rebocho AP, Soares RJ, et al. PAX8-PPARG rearrangement is frequently detected in the follicular variant of papillary thyroid carcinoma. J Clin Endocrinol Metab 2006;91:213–20.
58. Nikiforova MN, Lynch RA, Biddinger PW, et al. RAS point mutations and PAX8-PPARG rearrangement in thyroid tumors: evidence for distinct molecular pathways in thyroid follicular carcinoma. J Clin Endocrinol Metab 2003;88:2318–26.
59. Marques AR, Espadinha C, Catarino AL, et al. Expression of PAX8-PPARG1 rearrangements in both follicular thyroid carcinomas and adenomas. J Clin Endocrinol Metab 2002;87:3947–52.
60. Ohori NP, Nikiforova MN, Schoedel KE, et al. Contribution of molecular testing to thyroid fine-needle aspiration cytology of "follicular lesion of undetermined significant/atypia of undetermined significance". Cancer Cytopathol 2010;118:17–23.
61. Ferraz C, Eszlinger M, Paschke R. Current state and future perspective of molecular diagnosis of fine-needle aspiration biopsy of thyroid nodules. J Clin Endocrinol Metab 2011;96:2016–26.
62. Yip L, Wharry LI, Armstrong MJ, et al. A clinical algorithm for fine-needle aspiration molecular testing effectively guides the appropriate extent of initial thyroidectomy. Ann Surg 2014;260:163–8.
63. Yip L, Farris C, Kabaker AS, et al. Cost impact of molecular testing for indeterminate thyroid nodule fine-needle aspiration biopsies. J Clin Endocrinol Metab 2012;97(6):1905–12.

Surgical Management of Lymph Node Compartments in Papillary Thyroid Cancer

Cord Sturgeon, MD*, Anthony Yang, MD, Dina Elaraj, MD

KEYWORDS

- Papillary thyroid cancer • Lymph node dissection • Recurrent thyroid cancer
- Lymph node metastases • Central neck lymph node dissection

KEY POINTS

- When central or lateral compartment cervical lymph node metastases are clinically evident at the time of the index thyroid operation for PTC, formal surgical clearance of the affected nodal basin is the optimal management.
- Prophylactic central neck dissection for PTC is practiced by some high-volume surgeons with low complication rates, but is considered controversial because there appears to be a higher risk of complications with an uncertain clinical benefit.
- When a clinically significant recurrence is detected in a previously undissected central or lateral cervical compartment, a comprehensive surgical clearance of the lateral compartment is the preferred treatment.
- When a nodal recurrence is found in a previously dissected central or lateral neck field, the reoperation may focus on the areas where recurrence is demonstrated.

INTRODUCTION

In endocrine surgery, controversy abounds. It is difficult, in fact, to find a topic in surgical endocrinology for which there is little or no controversy. The management of cervical nodal metastases from papillary thyroid cancer (PTC) is no exception. Fortunately, there is widespread agreement regarding the management of clinically evident nodal metastases. It seems clear, based on the risks of persistent or recurrent disease, that the optimal management is formal surgical clearance of the affected nodal basin or basins when cervical nodal metastases are clinically evident at the

The authors have nothing to disclose.
Division of Endocrine Surgery, Department of Surgery, Northwestern University, 676 North Saint Clair Street, Suite 650, Chicago, IL 60611, USA
* Corresponding author.
E-mail address: csturgeo@nm.org

time of the index thyroid operation. On the other hand, because of the high frequency and uncertain clinical significance of occult nodal metastases from PTC, considerable controversy surrounds the management of the clinically negative central compartment, and the performance of so-called prophylactic central neck dissection (CND). Likewise, there is uncertainty regarding the thresholds for recommending remedial CND, given the attendant risks of the procedure and uncertain benefits. Within this contribution to the *Surgical Oncology Clinics of North America*, the data relevant to the surgical management of the lymph nodes of the central and lateral compartments of the neck in PTC are reviewed and discussed.

NOMENCLATURE: PROPHYLACTIC VERSUS THERAPEUTIC

As defined in the American Thyroid Association (ATA) consensus statement on the terminology and classification of CND for thyroid cancer,[1] a therapeutic neck dissection is one that is performed for clinically apparent nodal metastases, whether they are recognized before or during an operation, and regardless of the methodology used to detect the nodal metastases (eg, imaging, physical examination, frozen section). A prophylactic neck dissection is one that is performed on a nodal basin for which there is no clinical or imaging study evidence of nodal metastases. Prophylactic neck dissection is also synonymous with elective neck dissection.

EPIDEMIOLOGY OF CENTRAL NECK METASTASES

Metastases from PTC are frequently found in the central compartment lymph nodes. Nodal metastases from PTC are found in the central compartment in 12% to 81% of cases, depending on the completeness of the nodal dissection by the surgeon and the level of scrutiny to identify lymph nodes by the pathologist.[2] In surgical series of patients with PTC treated with prophylactic CND, occult positive central compartment nodes are found in at least one-third, and up to two-thirds of cases.[2,3] Given the high frequency of nodal metastases in the central compartment, some experts routinely clear the central compartment in a prophylactic fashion.

CONTROVERSY REGARDING PROPHYLACTIC CENTRAL NECK DISSECTION

Routine prophylactic CND for patients with clinically node-negative PTC is controversial. The controversy is centered on the fact that there is risk associated with the performance of a prophylactic CND, and that it is unclear if there is any survival or quality-of-life benefit. Furthermore, the finding of occult nodal disease will upstage patients older than 45 and may influence the usage of radioiodine.

Given the high rate of occult nodal metastases, some experts recommend that a thyroidectomy for PTC be accompanied by at least an ipsilateral central compartment nodal dissection. Proponents of prophylactic CND argue that because of the high rate of occult central nodal metastasis, prophylactic CND should decrease the need for reoperative neck surgery by reducing locoregional recurrence and simplify follow-up by lowering postoperative serum thyroglobulin.[4–6] In a study of 134 patients with PTC wherein all patients underwent a CND, the authors found that 29% of patients undergoing primary surgery for PTC had ipsilateral central neck metastases and also 29% had ipsilateral lateral neck metastases.[3] These authors recommended routine central and ipsilateral lateral nodal compartment dissection for patients undergoing primary surgery for PTC with a T1b or larger primary tumor. Other experts cite the higher complication rate when thyroidectomy is combined with CND, with no apparent improvement in survival, as rationale against prophylactic CND.[4] They maintain that prophylactic CND exposes patients to the additional risks of recurrent laryngeal nerve (RLN) injury and hypoparathyroidism without proven benefit.

Several recent retrospective analyses have compared outcomes of PTC patients who underwent total thyroidectomy with and without CND.[5,7–9] In one study, 20 prophylactic CNDs were required to prevent one central compartment reoperation.[5] A meta-analysis performed on studies that evaluated recurrence and complications associated with prophylactic CND found that the number needed to treat to prevent one recurrence was 31.[10] Two meta-analyses have demonstrated an increased rate of transient hypocalcemia following prophylactic CND without showing a difference in permanent hypoparathyroidism or RLN injury.[7,9] In most studies, prophylactic CND is associated with a higher rate of temporary hypocalcemia and parathyroid gland removal.[11] In most formal cost-effectiveness analysis studies, prophylactic CND has not been found to be cost-effective for PTC.[12,13]

The presence of nodal metastases may have a significant impact on the stage of disease based on the current American Joint Commission on Cancer (AJCC) TNM staging for thyroid cancer.[14] Patients 45 years of age or older are upstaged to stage III for any central neck nodal metastases regardless of the size and number of metastases found. Prophylactic neck dissection is therefore likely to upstage many patients to stage III for subclinical disease. Because the AJCC staging system for differentiated thyroid cancer was not derived or validated during an era of widespread CND, it is not clear if patients upstaged for subclinical metastases found during prophylactic dissection will have the same prognosis as patients with clinically evident central neck metastases.

It is also not certain how the practice of prophylactic nodal dissection might affect the likelihood to receive therapeutic doses of radioactive iodine (RAI). Some studies indicate that patients are more likely to receive RAI after total thyroidectomy with CND.[11] One hypothesis is that a greater frequency of detection of nodal metastases, and the associated upstaging of disease, leads to a greater utilization of RAI. Other studies show that prophylactic CND is associated with a lower probability of receiving RAI.[15] This finding, in turn, may be due to the fact that a more complete surgical clearance of the central compartment may lead to lower preablation thyroglobulin levels, and consequently, to a lower utilization of RAI. In a study by Lang and colleagues,[16] 51% of the patients who underwent prophylactic CND had undetectable preablative thyroglobulin.

A recent single-institution randomized controlled trial of total thyroidectomy with or without prophylactic CND in patients with PTC without evidence of preoperative or intraoperative lymph node metastases has been reported by Viola and colleagues[15] from Pisa, Italy. Their study of 181 patients with a median follow-up of 5 years found that clinically node-negative patients treated with prophylactic CND had a reduced necessity for repeat RAI treatments compared with those patients who did not undergo CND. However, the prophylactic CND patients also had a significantly higher prevalence of permanent postoperative hypoparathyroidism (19.4 vs 8.0%).

PREOPERATIVE ASSESSMENT OF THE CERVICAL NODAL COMPARTMENTS

The assessment of lymph node status before an operation for PTC is necessary because the presence and location of metastatic lymph nodes may not be clinically apparent, and the identification of nodal metastases will frequently alter the planned procedure. All patients should undergo a comprehensive history and physical examination focused on determining the extent of disease. Unfortunately, physical examination is notoriously unreliable for the exclusion of cervical nodal metastases.

Imaging studies, however, can detect abnormal lymph nodes in patients who have no palpable lymphadenopathy and may also yield information that alters the extent of the operation, even when overt nodal metastases are present.

Imaging Studies

Routine preoperative sonographic imaging of the cervical nodal basins changes the extent of surgery in as many as 41% of patients.[17,18] In a retrospective cohort study of 486 patients who underwent neck ultrasound before initial operation for PTC, ultrasound detected abnormal lymph nodes in 16% of patients who had nonpalpable lymph nodes on physical examination and changed the extent of surgery in 15 of 37 (41%) patients who had palpable lymph nodes on physical examination.[18] Similarly, in a retrospective study of 151 patients who underwent neck ultrasound before initial operation for differentiated thyroid cancer, ultrasound detected abnormal lymph nodes in 52 (34%) patients who had nonpalpable lymph nodes on physical examination.[17] Most patients with PTC who have lymph node metastases will have them in the inferior aspect of the neck. In a retrospective study of 578 lymph nodes that underwent fine needle aspiration (FNA) biopsy in 588 patients with differentiated thyroid cancer, 67% of malignant lymph nodes were found in the inferior third of the neck, whereas 46% of lymph nodes biopsied in the superior third of the neck were benign.[19]

Multiple imaging modalities have been studied for the preoperative staging of patients with PTC. Computed tomography (CT) is the preferred imaging modality for the preoperative staging of patients with head and neck squamous cell cancers, but is not used routinely for the staging of PTC. Nonetheless, CT can characterize the size, shape, appearance, and contrast enhancement pattern of lymph nodes and may be helpful in the prognostication of cervical lymph nodes in patients with PTC. CT features of malignant lymph nodes include size greater than 1.5 cm in levels I or II, greater than 0.8 in the retropharyngeal space, and greater than 1.0 cm in other locations; spherical shape; cystic change; presence of calcifications; and abnormal contrast enhancement.[20–22] In the setting of a known head and neck squamous cell cancer, CT has approximately 80% sensitivity and specificity for the detection of lymph node metastases.[20] There is no established size criterion for metastatic lymph nodes in PTC, however, and the sensitivity of CT may be lower in patients with PTC due to the higher rates of micrometastatic disease, which may not cause a change in the appearance of these lymph nodes on CT. In large retrospective studies evaluating the accuracy of CT in detecting metastatic lymphadenopathy in patients with PTC, CT has a sensitivity of 50% to 67% and specificity of 76% to 91% for detecting metastatic lymph nodes in the central compartment of the neck. Likewise, CT has a sensitivity of 59% to 82% and a specificity of 71% to 100% for detecting metastatic lymph nodes in the lateral compartment in PTC.[21,23,24]

The ATA guidelines on the management of thyroid cancer recommend against the routine use of preoperative imaging studies, such as CT, MRI, or PET, for the initial staging of PTC.[6] In some cases, however, these imaging modalities may play an important role in the preoperative evaluation of the patient. CT has been the most widely studied cross-sectional imaging modality, and its main advantages are that it is not operator dependent and that it generates high-resolution images with the ability to perform multiplanar image reconstructions. Its main limitation is that the iodine load associated with the intravenous contrast given during the scan may reduce RAI uptake for several weeks after administration.[25,26] CT can be particularly helpful in the evaluation and surgical planning for patients with advanced PTC, or those with large, fixed, or substernal cancers. In such cases, CT may accurately demonstrate extension of disease into the mediastinum, invasion into adjacent structures such as the aerodigestive tract, or reveal lymph node metastases in areas that are poorly assessed by ultrasound (retropharyngeal/retrotracheal space, low-level VI/superior mediastinum).[21,23,27] MRI has not been found to be particularly help-ful in the identification of cervical nodal metastases from thyroid cancer due to poor sensitivity and only moderate interobserver agreement.[28] PET scanning is useful for imaging patients with poorly differentiated thyroid cancers, but adds little to the im-aging of well-differentiated thyroid cancers.

The ATA and National Comprehensive Cancer Network (NCCN) guidelines recom-mend comprehensive neck ultrasound for the preoperative staging of PTC.[6,27] High-resolution neck ultrasound has been reported to have sensitivity of 52% to 93% and specificity of 79% to 100% for the detection of abnormal lymph nodes in pa-tients with PTC, in both index and reoperative settings.[17,18,29] Sensitivities vary widely between studies, while specificities are consistently high. Sensitivity is higher for the detection of abnormal lymph nodes in the lateral compartment of the neck compared with the central compartment of the neck, as the assessment of the central neck may be affected by surrounding structures, such as the tracheal air shadow, clavicle, and sternum.[17,29,30] Cervical sonography has several advantages over other imaging mo-dalities. Compared with CT, ultrasound is less costly, does not expose the patient to radiation, can be performed repeatedly in children and pregnant women, is painless and noninvasive, does not require intravenous access, does not generally precipitate claustrophobic reactions, and does not have a maximum weight limit. Limitations of ultrasound include that it is operator dependent and that it may be limited in evaluating lymph nodes in patients with high body mass index or in certain locations, such as the retropharyngeal, paratracheal, or retrotracheal spaces, level VI, and the superior mediastinum.[21,23]

Ultrasound can help characterize a lymph node as benign or malignant based on size, shape, and appearance. Sonographic features of benign lymph nodes include flattened elongated shape, smooth border, and hyperechoic hilum.[19] Sonographic features of malignant lymph nodes include enlarged size, rounded shape, loss of hilar architecture, cystic change, hyperechoic punctate microcalcifications, and hypervas-cularity.[19,31,32] No single sonographic feature, however, has adequate sensitivity and specificity for the detection of metastatic disease. In a prospective study of 103 sus-picious lymph nodes detected on ultrasound in 18 patients who underwent operation for recurrence of differentiated thyroid cancer, Leboulleux and colleagues[32] found that the criterion of long axis greater than 1 cm had only 68% sensitivity and 75% speci-ficity for the detection of a lymph node metastasis. It should be noted that benign reac-tive lymphadenopathy is frequently encountered in the submental, submandibular, subdigastric, and high jugular regions; consequently, under normal conditions, lymph nodes in these areas may be considerably larger than lymph nodes in the remainder of the lateral neck. In Leboulleux's study as well as another similar prospective study of 350 lymph nodes evaluated in 112 patients with PTC by Rosario and colleagues,[31] loss of fatty hilum had 88% to 100% sensitivity and 29% to 90% specificity, and cystic appearance and hyperechoic punctate calcifications each had 100% specificity but only 11% to 20% and 46% to 50% sensitivity, respectively, for the detection of lymph node metastases.[32]

Image-Guided Needle Biopsy

A definitive diagnosis of malignancy in a cervical lymph node is best obtained by ultrasound-guided FNA biopsy. Cytology from FNA has high sensitivity (73%–86%) and specificity (100%) for the detection of metastatic PTC, but can be limited by non-diagnostic or inadequate samples.[33,34] Measurement of thyroglobulin in the FNA biopsy aspirate fluid has been developed as an adjunct to the cytologic evaluation of suspicious-appearing cervical lymph nodes. This technique is semiquantitative in that it involves rinsing the needle used for the aspirate into 1 mL of saline and assaying the thyroglobulin level in that fluid by immunoradiometric or chemiluminescent assay.[33] Some reports describe rinsing the needle in thyroglobulin-free serum; however, a study by Frasoldati and colleagues[33] demonstrated that using normal saline as the washout fluid yielded equivalent results. The addition of the aspirate thyroglobulin level to the cytologic assessment can improve the diagnostic sensitivity of FNA to 86% to 100%, and can be diagnostic even when the number of cells is insufficient for standard cytologic analysis.[33,34] Several authors have proposed threshold values which, when exceeded, indicate metastatic thyroid cancer; however, universal agreement has not been achieved. Because it has been recognized that the aspirate thyroglobulin level is correlated to the serum TSH and serum thyroglobulin levels, it may be prudent to obtain all 3 samples in the same setting.[35,36] In one report, an aspirate thyroglobulin greater than 36 ng/mL in a patient with a thyroid gland and greater than 1.7 ng/mL in a patient without a thyroid gland was defined as being indicative of metastasis.[37] However, many studies suggest that much lower thresholds might be more sensitive. In one study, the threshold of 1.0 ng/mL was optimal for making the diagnosis of metastatic PTC with a sensitivity of 93.2% and a specificity of 95.9%.[35] Another investigator used the same thresholds of 1 ng/mL for patients with serum thyroglobulin less than 1 ng/mL and found that the sensitivity and specificity were 93% and 100%, respectively. The same study demonstrated that an aspirate to serum thyroglobulin ratio threshold of 0.5 for patients with a serum thyroglobulin greater than 1 ng/mL had a sensitivity of 98% and specificity of 98% for the detection of metastatic PTC.[36] In another study, an aspirate thyroglobulin threshold value of 0.2 ng/mL had a sensitivity of 100% and specificity of 87.5%.[38]

Although approximately 25% of patients with thyroid cancer have circulating antibodies that interfere with the assays used to detect thyroglobulin, these antithyroglobulin antibodies have not been found to interfere with the detection of thyroglobulin in FNA aspirate specimens.[37] Clearly, thyroglobulin only has utility as a tumor marker in patients with differentiated thyroid cancers of follicular cell origin. Consequently, an important limitation of this technique is in the evaluation of lymph node metastases from medullary thyroid cancer, or poorly differentiated or undifferentiated thyroid cancer. Thyroglobulin assay also has no role in the prognostication of thyroid nodules.

Implications for Surgical Planning

Systematic compartment-oriented dissection is indicated when cervical nodal metastases are identified. Formal clearance of the nodal basin has been shown to improve both recurrence rates and survival.[39] Selective lymph node removal ("berry picking") is not recommended, because this leaves behind lymph nodes that are at risk for developing recurrent disease, which would then be more difficult to remove in a reoperative field.

INTRAOPERATIVE ASSESSMENT OF LYMPH NODE STATUS

The role of prophylactic CND during thyroidectomy for PTC remains controversial. Some surgeons perform prophylactic CND routinely; some surgeons perform prophylactic CND only if there is metastatic disease in the lateral compartment, and some surgeons rely on intraoperative assessment of the lymph nodes in the central compartment and perform CND selectively. In this section, the methods of intraoperative assessment of the central and lateral compartments are described.

Intraoperative Inspection, Palpation, and Frozen Section

Many strategies exist for the intraoperative assessment of central compartment lymph nodes, including inspection and palpation and intraoperative frozen section. The accuracy of intraoperative inspection and palpation to assess the status of the central compartment lymph nodes was examined in a prospective study of 47 patients with PTC who underwent thyroidectomy with routine prophylactic CND. This study demonstrated poor sensitivity (49%–59%) and specificity (67%–83%) of inspection and palpation in identifying metastatic central neck lymph nodes regardless of level of surgeon experience (senior surgeon, fellow, or resident).[40] Some surgeons use the results of intraoperative frozen section of a central neck lymph node to decide on the necessity or extent of formal CND. The most common lymph nodes evaluated in this manner are the prelaryngeal, precricoid, or pretracheal nodes.

The Delphian lymph node is the eponymous term for a precricoid lymph node with potential for harboring metastatic PTC. The precricoid lymph nodes have been studied as predictors of advanced disease in thyroid cancer. Although the significance of a positive node is controversial, large, retrospective studies examining this issue have found that 20% to 25% of patients with PTC who had precricoid lymph nodes examined had a positive Delphian lymph node. Furthermore, a positive Delphian lymph node was associated with larger primary tumor size, multicentric PTC, extrathyroidal extension, lymphovascular invasion, and more nodal disease.[41–43] A positive Delphian node has also been found to predict additional central neck lymph node metastases with a sensitivity and specificity of 41% to 100% and 37% to 95%, respectively, and predicts lateral neck lymph node metastases with a sensitivity and specificity of 50% to 85% and 76% to 88%, respectively.[41–43] Because of the relationship between the Delphian lymph node and the status of the remainder of the central compartment, some surgeons will perform a CND whenever a Delphian node is identified. Caution must be exercised in interpreting these data, however, because not all studies examining this issue performed CND routinely, and therefore, the true negative predictive value of a benign precricoid lymph node is not known.

Intraoperative Assessment of the Lateral Compartments

Although the performance of routine prophylactic CND is controversial, there is little controversy regarding prophylactic lateral compartment lymph node dissection for PTC. Prophylactic dissection of the lateral compartments is not indicated for PTC. The sensitivity and specificity of high-resolution ultrasound for the evaluation of the lateral compartment of the neck are sufficient to rule out clinically significant nodal disease in the lateral compartment, and therefore, it is not necessary to explore the lateral compartment of the neck intraoperatively if the preoperative ultrasound is normal. Lateral compartment lymph node dissection is recommended only for therapeutic purposes, such as clinically apparent or biopsy-proven lymph node metastases.[6,27]

As an adjunct, some surgeons advocate intraoperative ultrasound after the completion of the lateral neck dissection to assess for residual disease. A prospective study of intraoperative ultrasound after lateral neck dissection in 25 patients with thyroid cancer (23 PTC, 2 medullary thyroid cancer) demonstrated that intraoperative ultrasound identified residual abnormal lymph nodes in 16% of patients.[44] Moreover, a retrospective study of 101 patients with PTC showed a statistically significant difference in the rate of residual/recurrent tumor in patients who underwent surgery with or without ultrasound guidance (2 vs 12%, $P<.05$).[45]

COMPARTMENTAL ANATOMY
Definition of the Central Neck Compartment

The first broadly accepted contemporary report to attempt to standardize CND terminology was by Robbins and colleagues[46] in 1991. In 2009, the ATA convened a multidisciplinary panel of experts and developed a consensus statement on the terminology and classification of CND for thyroid cancer.[1] The definitions from this consensus guideline are the most widely accepted standards and will thus be referenced in the following anatomic and procedural descriptions.

The nomenclature used to describe the neck nodal basins was originally developed by the Memorial Sloan-Kettering Head and Neck Surgery Service and modified and updated by the American Academy of Otolaryngology–Head and Neck Surgery.[47] The neck is divided into 7 node-bearing levels, and each is referred to by Roman numeral. Six sublevels have been described and are designated by the letters A or B. The central neck compartment (also known as the anterior compartment) is designated level VI. It is bounded by the hyoid bone superiorly, the suprasternal notch inferiorly, the common carotid artery (or lateral border of the sternohyoid muscle) laterally, the deep layer of the deep cervical fascia posteriorly, and the superficial layer of the deep cervical fascia anteriorly (**Fig. 1, Table 1**). Included in level VI are the precricoid

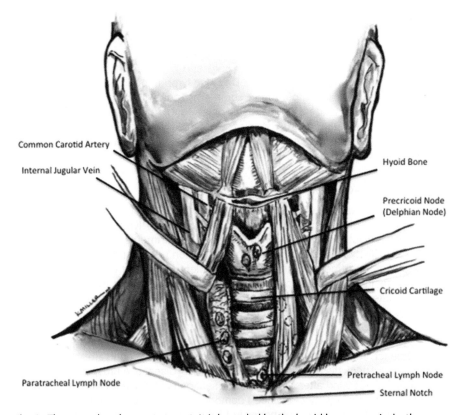

Fig. 1. The central neck compartment. It is bounded by the hyoid bone superiorly, the suprasternal notch inferiorly, the common carotid artery laterally, the deep layer of the deep cervical fascia posteriorly, and the superficial layer of the deep cervical fascia anteriorly. Lymph nodes in the precricoid and paratracheal areas are illustrated.

Table 1
Anatomic neck levels

Level	Anatomic Designation	Boundaries	Sublevel Designation/ Notable Contents
I	Submental (IA)	Triangular boundary from the anterior belly of the digastric muscles and hyoid bone	IA
	Submandibular (IB)	Anterior belly of digastric muscle to stylohyoid muscle to the body of the mandible. Includes: submandibular gland	IB Marginal mandibular nerve
II	Upper jugular	Upper third of the IJV and CN XI (superior) to the level of the hyoid bone (inferior), the stylohyoid muscle (anterior/ medial), and the posterior border of the SCM (posterior/lateral)	IIA: LN-bearing tissue anterior (medial) to CN XI IIB: LN-bearing tissue posterior (lateral) to CN XI Marginal mandibular nerve, IJV, CN XI, phrenic nerve, vagus nerve, cervical sympathetic trunk
III	Middle jugular	Middle third of IJV from inferior border of hyoid bone (superior) to inferior border of cricoid cartilage (inferior), lateral border of SHM (anterior/medial), and posterior border of SCM (posterior/lateral)	IJV, CN XI, phrenic nerve, vagus nerve, cervical sympathetic trunk, brachial plexus
IV	Lower jugular	Lower third of IJV from inferior border of cricoid cartilage (superior) to clavicle (inferior), lateral border of SHM (anterior/medial), and posterior border of SCM (posterior/lateral)	Virchow' node, IJV, CN XI, phrenic nerve, vagus nerve, cervical sympathetic trunk, brachial plexus, thoracic duct/right neck cervical lymphatic duct
V	Posterior triangle/ supraclavicular	Convergence of SCM and trapezius (superior) to clavicle (inferior), posterior border of SCM (anterior/ medial), anterior border of trapezius (posterior/lateral).	VA[a]: (superior) lymph nodes along CN XI VB[a]: (inferior) transverse cervical and supraclavicular lymph nodes
VI	Anterior (central) compartment	Hyoid bone (superior) to suprasternal notch (inferior) to common carotid arteries (lateral)	Delphian (precricoid) node, pretracheal, and paratracheal lymph nodes along the RLNs

Abbreviation: SHM, sternohyoid muscle.

[a] VA and VB are separated by a horizontal plane marking the inferior border of the anterior arch of the cricoid cartilage.

Adapted from Robbins KT, Clayman G, Levine PA, et al. Neck dissection classification update: revisions proposed by the American Head and Neck Society and the American Academy of Otolaryngology-Head and Neck Surgery. Arch Otolaryngol Head Neck Surg 2002;128(7):751–8; and Ferris R, Goldenberg D, Haymart MR, et al. American thyroid association consensus review of the anatomy, terminology and rationale for lateral neck dissection in differentiated thyroid cancer. Thyroid 2012;22(5):501–8.

lymph nodes, pretracheal lymph nodes, and the paratracheal lymph nodes both anterior and posterior to the RLNs; these 3 lymph node packets are the most commonly involved central compartment lymph nodes in PTC. The ATA consensus statement on CND includes level VII in the definition of the central neck compartment, which is bounded superiorly by the suprasternal notch, and inferiorly by the innominate artery, and contains lymph nodes and thymic tissue.[1]

Definition of the Lateral Neck Compartments

In 2012, the ATA published a consensus statement regarding the anatomy, terminology, and rationale for lateral neck dissection in differentiated thyroid cancer.[48] The important anatomic structures located within each level are enumerated in **Table 1** and are discussed in the section on technique of lateral neck dissection.

Roman numerals I through V are used to define the lateral neck lymph node levels and sublevels (**Fig. 2**; see **Table 1**). Level I includes the submandibular and submental lymph nodes. Level I is divided into sublevels IA and IB. Level IA (submental) nodes are located in the midline between the anterior bellies of the digastric muscles and the hyoid bone. Level IB (submandibular) nodes are located in a triangular field bounded

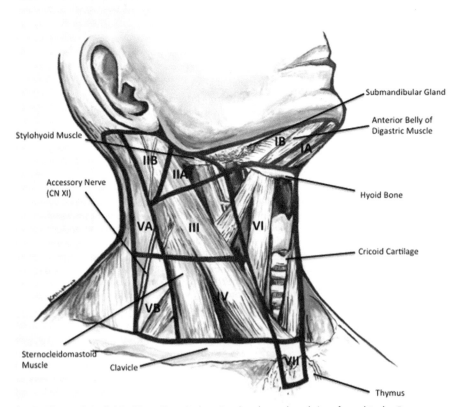

Fig. 2. The neck is divided into 7 node-bearing levels, and each is referred to by Roman numeral. Six sublevels have been described and are designated by the letters A or B. Levels I–V define the lateral neck. The central compartment is designated as level VI, and the region between the suprasternal notch and innominate is level VII.

superiorly by the body of the mandible, posteriorly by the stylohyoid muscle, and anteriorly by the anterior belly of the digastric muscle. Level IB contains the submandibular gland and associated lymph node–bearing tissue.

In aggregate, levels II, III, and IV describe the lymph node–bearing tissue in the quadrangle bounded superiorly by the skull base, inferiorly by the subclavian vein, anteromedially by the lateral border of the sternohyoid muscle, and laterally by the posterior border of the sternocleidomastoid muscle (SCM). Level II (upper jugular) lymph nodes are located along the superior third of the internal jugular vein (IJV) from the skull base superiorly to the hyoid bone inferiorly. Level II contains the jugulodigastric lymph nodes and the proximal portion of cranial nerve (CN) XI. The oblique course of this nerve divides this compartment into level IIA (anterior and inferior to CN XI) and level IIB (posterior and superior to CN XI). Level III (middle jugular) lymph nodes lie along the IJV extending from the lower body of the hyoid bone superiorly to the lower margin of the cricoid cartilage inferiorly. Level IV (lower jugular) lymph nodes are located in the region bordered by the lower margin of the cricoid cartilage superiorly to the level of the subclavian vein inferiorly.

Level V (posterior triangle) lymph nodes are found in a triangular-shaped compartment bounded by the posterior border of the SCM anteriorly, the anterior border of the trapezius muscle posteriorly, the subclavian vein inferiorly, and the apex of where the SCM and trapezius muscles meet superiorly. Level V is also divided into sublevel VA (superior) and VB (inferior) by a horizontal plane at the inferior border of the cricoid cartilage.

TECHNIQUE OF CENTRAL NECK DISSECTION
Timing and Indications for Central Neck Dissection

The efficacy of therapeutic CND is well established and is considered standard practice for patients with resectable lymph node metastases that are known at the time of the operation. The role of prophylactic CND is more controversial because there is a higher risk of complications and there are conflicting data on the impact of prophylactic CND on recurrence and survival.

It is well-established that a formal compartment-oriented dissection including the prelaryngeal, pretracheal, and paratracheal lymph nodes should be performed when nodal metastases from thyroid cancer are clinically evident at the index operation. The practice of "berry picking" only clinically apparent lymph node metastases is an oncologically inadequate operation and may be associated with higher recurrence rates and morbidity related to reoperation after recurrence.[1] The practice of "berry picking" central compartment lymph nodes is not synonymous with a selective, compartment-oriented dissection and is eschewed by most endocrine surgeons.

CND is most often performed at the time of the index thyroid operation. CND can be performed en bloc with the thyroidectomy specimen[49] or the nodal packet may be resected as a separate specimen. At the authors' institution, they begin with resection of the precricoid (Delphian) lymph node packet as part of the exposure of the thyroid gland. Frozen section analysis is used in cases where the clinical information gained might alter the surgical approach. A standard extracapsular total or near-total thyroidectomy then proceeds in standard fashion without division of the isthmus.

Surgical Technique of Central Neck Dissection

Dissection of the central compartment begins with a careful inspection and palpation of the dissection field in order to determine the location and viability of the parathyroid glands, the anatomic relationship between the RLN and the inferior thyroid artery, and if there is clinical evidence of metastatic lymphadenopathy.

Before the compartmental dissection, any parathyroid gland that has been devascularized should be autotransplanted. Because inspection of the parathyroid gland is notoriously inaccurate in determining viability, many experts recommend piercing or cutting the capsule of the gland to determine if there is continued perfusion, as evidenced by the presence of brisk bleeding. The authors advocate liberal use of autotransplantation of any parathyroid gland in which ischemia is suspected, because this may prevent or significantly mitigate the risk of permanent postoperative hypoparathyroidism. Following the CND, parathyroid glands remaining in situ are again examined for evidence of ischemia and autotransplanted if necessary. The inferior glands are at highest risk for devascularization and are routinely autotransplanted by some experts.

The RLN must always be identified and traced from its insertion through its entire course as it passes caudally through the central neck compartment. Full visualization of the RLN is maintained throughout the dissection. Atraumatic technique with only gentle manipulation and minimal traction of the nearby tissues should be used during dissection along the RLN. When bulky lymphadenopathy exists, the position of the RLN may be displaced by the adenopathy; this is particularly true on the right side, where adenopathy may be located deep to the RLN.

The paratracheal lymph node packet is removed as one specimen. The dissection is usually performed in a cephalad to caudad manner, removing all the node-bearing fibrofatty tissue from the level of the hyoid bone superiorly down to the innominate artery inferiorly. The width of the dissection field extends from the carotid artery laterally to the anterior midpoint of the trachea medially. The pretracheal lymph nodes inferior to the thyroid gland should always be included within the dissection specimen. Thymectomy is not necessary during CND.[50] The dissection specimen should be clearly labeled and oriented to site and side. The operative note should clearly describe the levels included in the dissection and their borders, the disposition of the parathyroid glands, and if any anatomic variants were identified.

Some investigators have reported that very little node-bearing tissue is ever found above the level of the insertion of the RLN and have questioned the necessity of extending the paratracheal dissection field above the level RLN insertion. In one study of 31 paratracheal neck dissections for thyroid cancer in 27 patients, no lymph nodes, lymphatic tissue, or metastatic disease was identified in any upper paratracheal specimens retrieved above the level of the cricoid cartilage.[51] All benign and metastatic lymph nodes were located in the lower paratracheal specimens. Accordingly, it may be reasonable to use the level of the cricoid cartilage as the superior border of the CND in the absence of clinically apparent or biopsy-proven metastatic disease in the region between the cricoid and the hyoid bone. Furthermore, limiting the superior extent of the CND to the level of the cricoid might decrease the likelihood of devascularizing the superior parathyroid glands while not compromising the oncologic outcome of the operation.

Complications of Central Neck Dissection

Complications of CND are mainly related to injury to the RLN and external branch of the superior laryngeal nerve, and devascularization of the parathyroid glands. As described above, permanent postoperative hypoparathyroidism rates from CND can be as high as nearly 20%.[15] In experienced hands, the incidence of permanent RLN injury should be low, on the order of 1% to 6%.[52] Meticulous hemostatic dissection technique and operative experience are significant contributors to minimizing these complications.

TECHNIQUE OF LATERAL NECK DISSECTION
Timing and Indications for Lateral Neck Dissection

Dissection of the lateral cervical compartments is performed only for therapeutic purposes when there is evidence of nodal metastatic disease from PTC.[48] Unlike the central compartment, metastatic disease in the lateral compartment is usually demonstrable with standard sonographic imaging. Because it is possible to accurately survey the lateral neck for clinically significant nodal disease, prophylactic lateral neck dissection is not used for differentiated thyroid cancer. This more cautious approach to lateral neck dissection is due to the fact that the lateral neck is undisturbed during a thyroid operation, and there are significant risks to opening and dissecting the lateral compartment, including greater cosmetic deformity, chronic neck pain or numbness, chyle leak or fistula, and cranial nerve injury.

The controversial topic in lateral neck dissection for differentiated thyroid cancer is the extent of the dissection. The classic radical neck dissection described by Crile, which included sacrifice of the SCM, IJV, and CN XI, is rarely required for PTC and, instead, modified or selective neck dissections are performed wherein one or more of these structures are preserved (see **Table 1**). Because level I is rarely involved by metastatic thyroid cancer, this level is not usually included in the dissection. There is controversy regarding the inclusion or exclusion of levels IIB and VA. Dissection in levels II and V places CN XI at risk of injury. The ATA consensus statement on the rationale for lateral neck dissection leaves dissection of IIB and VA to the discretion of the surgeon and states that IIB dissection is not required unless there are suspicious lymph nodes in that region. Similarly, dissection of level VA should be reserved for cases where sonographic evaluation reveals metastatic disease in that sublevel. The ATA consensus statement recommends that selective lateral neck dissection for differentiated thyroid cancer metastases include levels IIA, III, IV, and VB. "Berry picking" is not recommended in the lateral neck, or any cervical compartment for metastatic thyroid cancer.[48]

General Principles of Incision and Exposure

Multiple incisions have been described for exposure of the lateral compartment. A long, low Kocher incision with a vertical extension along the posterior border of the SCM up to the mastoid process offers excellent exposure to all levels of the lateral neck. The lateral compartments can also be approached through just a long Kocher incision, which allows access to all but the highest level II lymph nodes. Another alternative approach is a parallel counterincision placed more cephalad and lateral to the Kocher incision.

Regardless of the incision used, subplatysmal flaps are raised with care taken to stay superficial to the external jugular vein. This site is the first point at which the great auricular nerve can be injured. The great auricular nerve arises from the second and third cervical nerve rami, curves around the posterior border of the SCM, and then ascends toward the ear on the anterior surface of the SCM, parallel to the external jugular vein. Injury to the great auricular nerve is one of the most common complications of lateral node dissection (LND), causing pain or numbness of the ear, which is often significantly bothersome to the patient. The marginal mandibular branch of the facial nerve (CN VII) can be injured during the dissection as well. The marginal mandibular branch runs along the inferior border of the mandible anterior to the facial artery and vein. Attention should be paid to retraction of the skin flaps in this area because compression of the marginal mandibular branch of the facial nerve can lead to palsy of the ipsilateral circumoral musculature and may be caused by retraction of the superior skin flap alone.

The SCM can almost always be preserved during a selective or modified radical neck dissection. The SCM is mobilized by sharply dissecting the muscle free of the underlying deep cervical fascia. If necessary, the SCM can be nearly circumferentially dissected, and encircled with a Penrose drain to aid with retraction and exposure. Branches of the transverse cervical cutaneous nerves are divided while mobilizing the SCM, which causes hypesthesia of the skin of the neck.

To complete the exposure of the lateral compartments, the omohyoid muscle is mobilized and may be divided, and the second layer of deep cervical fascia is incised in order to expose the lymph node–bearing fatty tissue packet.

The dissection of the lymph node packet can be performed by starting in level IV and continuing in a superomedial direction, or by starting in level II and then continuing in an inferolateral direction. For simplicity, the technique of caudad to cephalad dissection beginning in level IV is described.

Level IV Dissection

Level IV is the region bordered by a line at the level of the cricoid cartilage superiorly, the subclavian vein inferiorly, the sternohyoid muscle anteromedially, and the posterior edge of the SCM posterolaterally. The cervical lymphatics coursing between the level IV nodes and the thoracic duct should be identified at the junction of the IJV and the subclavian vein and ligated individually with a painstaking delicate technique. In the authors' experience, clips are not usually adequate to secure these lymphatics. The thoracic duct itself does not usually need to be ligated. The thoracic duct usually drains into the posterior left subclavian vein just proximal to its confluence with the left IJV. The right thoracic duct has a similar course in the neck, but is much smaller than the left. A Valsalva maneuver, or compression of the surrounding tissue, can distend the duct and lymphatic tributaries and aid with identification. If there is suspicion that the thoracic duct has been injured, it should be ligated to prevent a chylous leak or fistula, which can be difficult to manage and may lead to life-threatening complications, such as fluid and electrolyte disturbances, hypoalbuminemia, coagulopathy, immunoglobulin deficiency, wound infection, malnutrition, and chylothorax. When dissecting level IV, it should be kept in mind that lymph nodes lie in the soft tissue posterior to the IJV and retraction and possibly circumferential dissection of the IJV may be required in order to obtain an adequate dissection in this region. The deep border of the dissection of this lymph node packet should be superficial to the third layer of deep cervical fascia and will lessen the risk of injury to the phrenic nerve, which courses along the anterior surface of the anterior scalene muscle, and the brachial plexus, which emanates between the anterior and medial scalene muscles. Once the cervical lymphatics are ligated, the soft tissue packet should be sharply dissected off of the scalenes. The vagus nerve is quite large and should be easily identified and preserved along the medial margin of the dissection. Likewise, the phrenic nerve should be easily identified and preserved along the posterior margin of the dissection. The transverse cervical artery and vein are also preserved along the posterior border of the dissection field. The subclavian vein should be clearly visible at the inferior border of the dissection field, and care should be taken to avoid injury to the subclavian vessels or pleura in this region.

Level V Dissection

Level V is also known as the posterior triangle and is bounded by the posterior border of the SCM anteriorly, the trapezius muscle posteriorly, the subclavian vein inferiorly, and the apex of where the SCM and trapezius muscles meet superiorly. Level V is divided into sublevels VA (superior) and VB (inferior) by a horizontal plane extending laterally from the cricoid cartilage. Level VA contains the lymph nodes along the distal portion of the spinal accessory nerve (CN XI). Level VB contains the transverse cervical vessels and associated lymph nodes as well as the supraclavicular lymph nodes.

If only level VB is to be dissected, then the lymph node–bearing fatty tissue along the transverse cervical vessels and in the supraclavicular region should be removed en bloc with the specimen. Care should be taken to identify CN XI and avoid injury to it even if the level VA lymph node packet is not included in the dissection.

If level VA is included, the anterior border of the trapezius muscle (the posterior-lateral border of level V) is identified and incised approximately 1 cm anterior to the border of the muscle. This incision will allow for easier and safer identification of CN XI as it inserts into the trapezius muscle. CN XI will be found coursing over the levator scapulae muscle and will be approximately parallel to the trapezius muscle itself. Much of the lymph node–bearing tissue in level VB (and level II) will be around CN XI, and thus, it must be clearly identified and carefully manipulated. As CN XI is dissected in a superomedial direction toward the upper posterior border of the SCM, a plexus of cervical nerve branches will be encountered at the posterior border of the SCM. The great auricular nerve can be found here just inferior to CN XI as it courses underneath the SCM. Often referred to as Erb point,[53] this plexus is a useful landmark to identify CN XI in a more superior and medial location.

Level III Dissection

Level III extends from the superior border of level IV to the hyoid bone. The medial and lateral borders are the same as level IV. Dissection of the node-bearing fibrofatty tissue packet should continue sharply over the scalene muscles and along the IJV through level III, with continued care taken to directly visualize and avoid injury to the phrenic and vagus nerves. Cervical sensory nerve fibers should be preserved if preservation will not compromise the oncologic outcome of the operation. The common trunk of the supraclavicular nerve can be identified beneath the SCM and should be preserved to avoid lateral neck, shoulder, and anterior chest numbness postoperatively. Staying superficial to the third layer of deep cervical fascia will lessen the likelihood of injury to all of the nerve structures except for the vagus nerve. The cervical sensory plexus can be used as a landmark that the superior portion of the dissection has almost been completed.

Level II Dissection

Level II extends from the superior border of level III to the skull base superiorly. The anteromedial border is the stylohyoid muscle and the lateral border is the posterior edge of the SCM. CN XI divides level II into level IIA and level IIB. If only level IIA is to be dissected, then identification of CN XI will represent the posterosuperior limit of the dissection, and the dissection specimen is sharply dissected from the IJV and CN XI and truncated at the apex of these 2 structures. If level IIB is to be included, the dissection should continue to the level of the posterior belly of the digastric muscle.

Once the dissection has been completed, the dissection specimen should be clearly labeled and oriented. The operative procedure note should clearly describe the levels included in the dissection and the borders. Drain placement is at the discretion of the surgeon.

Complications of Lateral Neck Dissection

The common and major complications of lateral neck dissection have been described above in relation to the steps of the procedure. In summary, the most common complications are sensory deficits related to injury to the great auricular nerve or cervical sensory nerve fibers. Major, avoidable complications include chylous leak or chylothorax related to unrecognized injuries of the thoracic duct or other major lymphatic branches, shoulder weakness resulting from injury to CN XI, lip droop related to marginal mandibular nerve injury, and symptoms related to injuries to the other relevant nerves (phrenic, vagus, hypoglossal). Rough handling of major vascular structures such as the carotid artery and IJV can lead to vascular injuries, bleeding, embolic stroke (including air embolism), and carotid dissection. Clear visualization of the nervous, lymphatic, and vascular structures, delicate dissection technique, and meticulous hemostasis will minimize complications.

IMPACT OF NODAL CLEARANCE ON RECURRENCE AND SURVIVAL
Impact of Nodal Basin Clearance on Recurrence and Survival

Regional lymph node metastases at the time of presentation are relatively common in PTC.[17,54] There has been a long-standing controversy over the clinical significance of lymph node metastases in PTC in low-risk patients. However, the controversy over the significance of lymph node metastases in high-risk patients is less questioned. Multiple studies have shown that lymph node metastases are an independent predictor of poor outcome. Although the overall survival differences may be slight (82% for node-negative disease vs 79% for node-positive disease at 14 years), they are statistically significant,[1,55] and there is also an increased risk of recurrence in patients with lymph node metastases in PTC. Although there are fewer patients presenting with lateral neck metastases, there is evidence that lateral neck metastases are associated with a poorer outcome, namely increased risk of recurrence and possibly decreased survival.[17,56,57]

Clearance of the affected nodal basins of metastatic disease may offer other benefits beyond a small improvement in survival. First of all is the reduction in recurrence after CND or LND. Although there is a paucity of randomized controlled or other matched control studies in the literature, multiple studies have shown recurrence rates on the order of 10% after total thyroidectomy with CND in patients with or without known preoperative central neck lymph node metastases.[58,59] Multiple studies indicate that CND or LND can successfully control persistent or recurrent disease as reflected by meaningful decreases in serum thyroglobulin levels, with some studies finding that a substantial number of patients can have undetectable preablative thyroglobulin levels after surgery.[16,60] Recurrence after CND (and in patients who have not undergone CND) tends to occur in the lateral neck lymph node basins, particularly levels III and IV, rather than in the central neck compartment.[58,59] Prognostic factors for local recurrence include increasing number of metastatic lymph nodes and extracapsular lymph node extension on pathologic analysis.[1]

Prophylactic CND remains controversial because multiple studies indicate that the incidence of both temporary[61–63] and permanent[15,58] hypoparathyroidism is increased with CND. Furthermore, CND is associated with a higher incidence of RLN injury, most of which is temporary.[58,61,63] Multiple studies have shown that complication rates are lower in operations for thyroid cancer, including CND and LND, when the procedure is performed by a high-volume thyroid surgeon.[6] Therefore, the ATA consensus statements recommend that the surgeon's skill level be considered when making the decision whether a patient who requires CND or LND should remain in that surgeon's hands or be referred to a high-volume thyroid surgery center.[1,6,64]

RECURRENT NODAL METASTASES
A Comparison of Surveillance Strategies Recommended by the American Thyroid Association and National Comprehensive Cancer Network

Most patients who have been treated for PTC undergo long-term surveillance. The primary goals of long-term follow-up are the early and accurate detection of recurrent disease and the longitudinal monitoring of thyroxine replacement and TSH.[6] The ATA recommends that following total thyroidectomy, serum thyroglobulin and anti-thyroglobulin antibodies should be measured every 6 to 12 months in the same laboratory using the same assay. Rising thyroglobulin values over time are considered suspicious for recurrence. Periodic neck ultrasound is also recommended. In low-risk patients with no detectable tumor, the ATA recommends that a TSH-stimulated thyroglobulin be measured 12 months after radioiodine ablation to verify that there is no recurrent or persistent disease. For those patients who have no detectable stimulated thyroglobulin, the ATA recommends yearly clinical examination and unstimulated thyroglobulin.[6]

The NCCN guidelines recommend physical examination, TSH, thyroglobulin, and antithyroglobulin antibodies at 6 and 12 months and then annually thereafter if the patient is considered disease-free. Similar to the ATA recommendations, neck ultrasound is also recommended on a periodic basis by the NCCN.[27] The NCCN recommends that stimulated thyroglobulin be measured in patients who underwent radioiodine ablation and in those who have undetectable unstimulated thyroglobulin and no antithyroglobulin antibodies. Furthermore, TSH-stimulated radioiodine scanning should be considered for patients with detectable stimulated or unstimulated thyroglobulin, sonographic evidence of persistent or recurrent disease, rising antithyroglobulin antibody titer, or with radioiodine avid metastases, or in patients considered high risk. In patients with high-risk radioiodine avid tumors, especially those with detectable thyroglobulin, distant metastases, or extension into the soft tissues, the NCCN recommends radioiodine imaging every 1 to 2 years.

Ultrasound and Serum Thyroglobulin Measurement Are Highly Accurate at Detecting Recurrence

Sonographic cervical imaging has been found to be more accurate than radioiodine scanning for the detection of recurrent or persistent disease. In addition, the measurement of stimulated thyroglobulin has been found to be complementary to cervical sonography, increasing the accuracy of the surveillance strategy. In a series of 340 consecutive patients with differentiated thyroid cancer who underwent near-total thyroidectomy and radioiodine ablation, the combination of stimulated thyroglobulin and cervical sonography had the greatest accuracy at detecting persistent disease (sensitivity 96.3% and negative predictive value of 99.5%).[65] In a series of 80 consecutive patients with PTC microcarcinoma who underwent near-total thyroidectomy but did not undergo radioiodine ablation, cervical ultrasound was found to be more accurate than radioiodine scanning for the detection of persistent disease.[66] Although radioiodine scanning showed no pathologic uptake in any patient, cervical sonography identified nodal metastases in patients with or without detectable thyroglobulin. The authors concluded that in this low-risk population, ultrasound should be the primary screening modality, stimulated thyroglobulin was indicative of remnant normal thyroid tissue, and radioiodine scanning was not valuable for the detection of persistent disease. These findings support the recommendations from the ATA and NCCN that surveillance be conducted primarily via cervical sonography and measurement of serum thyroglobulin, and that radioiodine scanning be reserved for higher-risk patients with radioiodine avid disease.

Surveillance Frequently Reveals Recurrent or Persistent Disease

The ATA defines absence of disease using 3 criteria: no clinically detectable tumor recurrence, no evidence of recurrence on imaging, and undetectable stimulated and unstimulated thyroglobulin (when interfering antibodies are absent).[6] Unfortunately, because of the stringency of these criteria and the high sensitivity of current imaging modalities and methods for detection of thyroglobulin, many patients will not satisfy these criteria, especially if they have not undergone radioiodine ablation of the thyroid remnant.

The recurrence rate is relatively high in PTC and is related to the sensitivity of the tests used to conduct surveillance, the biology of PTC, and the initial treatment. Biologic variables that impact recurrence include the number of positive nodes, tumor burden, and the presence of extranodal extension.[2,67–70] Patients who are pathologically N0 are at lowest risk of recurrence. Patients with microscopic N1a disease are at an intermediate risk.[71] Patients with clinically positive or macroscopic N1 disease are at high risk. Patients with extranodal extension are at the highest risk. A recent meta-analysis stratified patients into risk groups based on the number of positive nodes. They found that the risk of recurrence was 4% with fewer than 5 positive nodes, 19% with more than 5 positive nodes, and 24% with clinically apparent nodes with extranodal extension.[2]

For patients with stable, low levels of detectable thyroglobulin whose disease cannot be detected on imaging, it is considered acceptable to continue active surveillance. For patients with recurrent or persistent disease that can be imaged, surgical resection is the preferred treatment.

Recommendations for Surveillance of the Lateral Neck

Metastases to the lateral compartment are common and are therefore one of the focal points of surveillance for patients with PTC. Ultrasound is the imaging modality of choice for the detection of lateral neck nodal metastases when performing surveillance. Sonographic surveillance of the lateral neck should be performed periodically depending on the likelihood of recurrent or persistent disease. The entire neck should be imaged (levels I through VII) by a sonographer experienced in surveillance of PTC. Special attention should be paid to the nodal basins ipsilateral to the primary tumor, because they are the most likely a location for recurrent or persistent disease.

Establishing the Diagnosis of Recurrent or Persistent Disease

The ATA published a consensus statement on the anatomy, terminology, and indications for lateral neck dissection in PTC.[64] They concluded that the initial modality should be ultrasound and that FNA of suspicious lymph nodes is the best way to establish the diagnosis of nodal metastases. In addition, the ATA Statement on Preoperative Imaging for Thyroid Cancer Surgery recommends that suspicious masses or lymph nodes be biopsied before a reoperation for persistent or recurrent disease.[72] Ultrasound has been shown to accurately detect the presence of central and lateral nodal metastases and has been found to alter the extent of surgery in up to 40% of index and reoperative cases.[18] Therefore, in the course of surveillance for PTC, sonographically suspicious lymph nodes should be interrogated with FNA biopsy. The aspirate may be assayed for thyroglobulin in order to increase the sensitivity and specificity for metastatic disease.

Is Positive Imaging Alone Ever Sufficient?

The 2009 ATA guidelines state that lateral neck dissection should not be performed prophylactically, but should be performed as a "therapeutic intervention for known disease."[6] This statement raises the question of whether imaging alone would be sufficient to confirm the presence of metastatic disease. In some cases, the location of the lymph node may not be amenable to needle biopsy or patients may refuse needle biopsy. The ATA Subcommittee on Lateral Neck Dissection indicated in their recent review that lateral neck lymph nodes not amenable to FNA biopsy may be followed for growth by serial imaging. If the inaccessible node grows during follow-up, an open biopsy should be performed with conversion to formal lateral neck dissection if the frozen section is positive. The ATA Statement on Preoperative Imaging for Thyroid Cancer Surgery states that preoperative FNA may not be required under the following 2 conditions: "(a) abnormal lymph nodes are inaccessible or anatomically risky to biopsy, usually due to their location with respect to major vessels, and (b) unequivocally abnormal lymph nodes are found on imaging and surgery would be recommended regardless of FNA results."[72]

The Treatment of Recurrent or Persistent Nodal Disease

The management of low-volume recurrent or persistent nodal metastases is controversial. The 2 most reasonable treatment options are surgical resection and active surveillance.[73] The preferred treatment for locoregional recurrence, according to the NCCN, is surgical resection. Radioiodine therapy and external beam radiotherapy are alternative treatment options for tumors that either do or do not concentrate radioiodine, respectively. The NCCN recommends that clinically significant nodal metastases in a previously undissected nodal basin be treated with a formal compartmental clearance of the nodal basin involved. For recurrence in the central neck in a patient with no prior CND, a complete dissection of that ipsilateral central compartment is indicated. Likewise, recurrence discovered in a previously undissected lateral compartment should be treated with a formal modified radical neck dissection, including levels II, III, IV, and VB. Conversely, recurrence in a previously dissected central or lateral compartment should be adequately treated with a focused dissection of the region containing the nodal metastasis.[27]

The 2009 ATA guidelines for DTC state that the "preferred hierarchy of treatment for metastatic disease" is surgical resection for potentially curable patients with locoregional disease, radioiodine therapy for patients with iodine-avid disease, external beam radiation therapy, active surveillance in patients with stable or slowly progressive asymptomatic disease, and experimental trials.[6] They also indicate that more nontraditional management may also benefit selected patients, such as ethanol ablation, radiofrequency ablation, or chemoembolization. Furthermore, active surveillance is presented as a reasonable option for patients with stable asymptomatic disease that does not involve the central nervous system. Similar to NCCN, the ATA guidelines support a comprehensive dissection of previously unexplored cervical compartments harboring metastatic disease, and a more limited or focused dissection of previously operated compartments. Clinically significant nodal metastases are defined as those greater than 0.8 cm in size. The treatment of cervical nodal metastases in patients with untreatable distant metastases may be considered for palliation or avoidance of aerodigestive tract invasion.

SUMMARY

When central or lateral compartment cervical lymph node metastases are clinically evident at the time of the index thyroid operation for PTC, formal surgical clearance of the affected nodal basin is the optimal management. Prophylactic CND for PTC is practiced by some high-volume surgeons with low complication rates, but is considered controversial because there appears to be higher risk of complications with an uncertain clinical benefit. Long-term surveillance strategies are performed for most PTC patients after their initial treatment, and due to the high sensitivity of both the imaging modalities used and thyroglobulin measurement, approximately 20% of patients will be found to have persistent or recurrent disease. It is unclear what exactly constitutes a clinically significant recurrence, but the most commonly used definition is a lymph node greater than 0.8 cm. Surgical resection and active surveillance strategies may both be used depending on the clinical context. When a clinically significant recurrence is detected in a previously undissected central or lateral cervical compartment, a comprehensive surgical clearance of the lateral compartment is the preferred treatment. When a nodal recurrence is found in a previously dissected central or lateral neck field, the reoperation should focus on the areas where recurrence is demonstrated.

ACKNOWLEDGMENTS

The authors thank Kyle Miller, MD for the original illustrations that accompany the text.

REFERENCES

1. Carty SE, Cooper DS, Doherty GM, et al. Consensus statement on the terminology and classification of central neck dissection for thyroid cancer. Thyroid 2009;19(11):1153–8.
2. Randolph GW, Duh QY, Heller KS, et al. The prognostic significance of nodal metastases from papillary thyroid carcinoma can be stratified based on the size and number of metastatic lymph nodes, as well as the presence of extranodal extension. Thyroid 2012;22(11):1144–52.
3. Machens A, Hinze R, Thomusch O, et al. Pattern of nodal metastasis for primary and reoperative thyroid cancer. World J Surg 2002;26(1):22–8.
4. Carling T, Carty SE, Ciarleglio MM, et al. American Thyroid Association design and feasibility of a prospective randomized controlled trial of prophylactic central lymph node dissection for papillary thyroid carcinoma. Thyroid 2012;22(3): 237–44.
5. Popadich A, Levin O, Lee JC, et al. A multicenter cohort study of total thyroidectomy and routine central lymph node dissection for cN0 papillary thyroid cancer. Surgery 2011;150(6):1048–57.
6. Cooper DS, Doherty GM, Haugen BR, et al. Revised American Thyroid Association management guidelines for patients with thyroid nodules and differentiated thyroid cancer. Thyroid 2009;19(11):1167–214.
7. Chisholm EJ, Kulinskaya E, Tolley NS. Systematic review and meta-analysis of the adverse effects of thyroidectomy combined with central neck dissection as compared with thyroidectomy alone. Laryngoscope 2009;119(6):1135–9.
8. Hughes DT, White ML, Miller BS, et al. Influence of prophylactic central lymph node dissection on postoperative thyroglobulin levels and radioiodine treatment in papillary thyroid cancer. Surgery 2010;148(6):1100–6 [discussion: 1006–7].
9. Zetoune T, Keutgen X, Buitrago D, et al. Prophylactic central neck dissection and local recurrence in papillary thyroid cancer: a meta-analysis. Ann Surg Oncol 2010;17(12):3287–93.
10. Wang TS, Cheung K, Farrokhyar F, et al. A meta-analysis of the effect of prophylactic central compartment neck dissection on locoregional recurrence rates in patients with papillary thyroid cancer. Ann Surg Oncol 2013;20(11):3477–83.

11. Moo TA, McGill J, Allendorf J, et al. Impact of prophylactic central neck lymph node dissection on early recurrence in papillary thyroid carcinoma. World J Surg 2010;34(6):1187–91.
12. Zanocco K, Elaraj D, Sturgeon C. Routine prophylactic central neck dissection for low-risk papillary thyroid cancer: a cost-effectiveness analysis. Surgery 2013; 154(6):1148–55 [discussion: 1154–5].
13. Garcia A, Palmer BJ, Parks NA, et al. Routine prophylactic central neck dissection for low-risk papillary thyroid cancer is not cost-effective. Clin Endocrinol (Oxf) 2014;81(5):754–61.
14. Edge SB, American Joint Committee on Cancer. AJCC cancer staging manual. 7th edition. New York: Springer; 2010.
15. Viola D, Materazzi G, Valerio L, et al. Prophylactic central compartment lymph node dissection in papillary thyroid carcinoma: clinical implications derived from the first prospective randomized controlled single institution study. J Clin Endocrinol Metab 2015;100(4):1316–24.
16. Lang BH, Wong KP, Wan KY, et al. Impact of routine unilateral central neck dissection on preablative and postablative stimulated thyroglobulin levels after total thyroidectomy in papillary thyroid carcinoma. Ann Surg Oncol 2012;19(1): 60–7.
17. Kouvaraki MA, Shapiro SE, Fornage BD, et al. Role of preoperative ultrasonography in the surgical management of patients with thyroid cancer. Surgery 2003; 134(6):946–54 [discussion: 954–5].
18. Stulak JM, Grant CS, Farley DR, et al. Value of preoperative ultrasonography in the surgical management of initial and reoperative papillary thyroid cancer. Arch Surg 2006;141(5):489–94 [discussion: 494–6].
19. Kuna SK, Bracic I, Tesic V, et al. Ultrasonographic differentiation of benign from malignant neck lymphadenopathy in thyroid cancer. J Ultrasound Med 2006; 25(12):1531–7 [quiz: 1538–40].
20. Eisenmenger LB, Wiggins RH 3rd. Imaging of head and neck lymph nodes. Radiol Clin North Am 2015;53(1):115–32.
21. Soler ZM, Hamilton BE, Schuff KG, et al. Utility of computed tomography in the detection of subclinical nodal disease in papillary thyroid carcinoma. Arch Otolaryngol Head Neck Surg 2008;134(9):973–8.
22. Som PM, Brandwein M, Lidov M, et al. The varied presentations of papillary thyroid carcinoma cervical nodal disease: CT and MR findings. AJNR Am J Neuroradiol 1994;15(6):1123–8.
23. Kim E, Park JS, Son KR, et al. Preoperative diagnosis of cervical metastatic lymph nodes in papillary thyroid carcinoma: comparison of ultrasound, computed tomography, and combined ultrasound with computed tomography. Thyroid 2008;18(4):411–8.
24. Choi JS, Kim J, Kwak JY, et al. Preoperative staging of papillary thyroid carcinoma: comparison of ultrasound imaging and CT. AJR Am J Roentgenol 2009;193(3): 871–8.
25. Nygaard B, Nygaard T, Jensen LI, et al. Iohexol: effects on uptake of radioactive iodine in the thyroid and on thyroid function. Acad Radiol 1998;5(6):409–14.
26. Laurie AJ, Lyon SG, Lasser EC. Contrast material iodides: potential effects on radioactive iodine thyroid uptake. J Nucl Med 1992;33(2):237–8.
27. Tuttle R, Haddad R, Ball D, et al. National Comprehensive Cancer Network Clinical Practice Guidelines in Oncology: Thyroid Carcinoma v.2.2014. 2014. Available at: http://www.nccn.org/professionals/physician_gls/pdf/thyroid.pdf. Accessed April 25, 2015.

28. Chen Q, Raghavan P, Mukherjee S, et al. Accuracy of MRI for the diagnosis of metastatic cervical lymphadenopathy in patients with thyroid cancer. Radiol Med 2015. [Epub ahead of print].
29. Roh JL, Park JY, Kim JM, et al. Use of preoperative ultrasonography as guidance for neck dissection in patients with papillary thyroid carcinoma. J Surg Oncol 2009;99(1):28–31.
30. Choi JS, Chung WY, Kwak JY, et al. Staging of papillary thyroid carcinoma with ultrasonography: performance in a large series. Ann Surg Oncol 2011;18(13): 3572–8.
31. Rosario PW, de Faria S, Bicalho L, et al. Ultrasonographic differentiation between metastatic and benign lymph nodes in patients with papillary thyroid carcinoma. J Ultrasound Med 2005;24(10):1385–9.
32. Leboulleux S, Girard E, Rose M, et al. Ultrasound criteria of malignancy for cervical lymph nodes in patients followed up for differentiated thyroid cancer. J Clin Endocrinol Metab 2007;92(9):3590–4.
33. Frasoldati A, Toschi E, Zini M, et al. Role of thyroglobulin measurement in fine-needle aspiration biopsies of cervical lymph nodes in patients with differentiated thyroid cancer. Thyroid 1999;9(2):105–11.
34. Pacini F, Fugazzola L, Lippi F, et al. Detection of thyroglobulin in fine needle aspirates of nonthyroidal neck masses: a clue to the diagnosis of metastatic differentiated thyroid cancer. J Clin Endocrinol Metab 1992;74(6):1401–4.
35. Moon JH, Kim YI, Lim JA, et al. Thyroglobulin in washout fluid from lymph node fine-needle aspiration biopsy in papillary thyroid cancer: large-scale validation of the cutoff value to determine malignancy and evaluation of discrepant results. J Clin Endocrinol Metab 2013;98(3):1061–8.
36. Jeon MJ, Kim WG, Jang EK, et al. Thyroglobulin level in fine-needle aspirates for preoperative diagnosis of cervical lymph node metastasis in patients with papillary thyroid carcinoma: two different cutoff values according to serum thyroglobulin level. Thyroid 2015;25(4):410–6.
37. Boi F, Baghino G, Atzeni F, et al. The diagnostic value for differentiated thyroid carcinoma metastases of thyroglobulin (Tg) measurement in washout fluid from fine-needle aspiration biopsy of neck lymph nodes is maintained in the presence of circulating anti-Tg antibodies. J Clin Endocrinol Metab 2006; 91(4):1364–9.
38. Holmes BJ, Sokoll LJ, Li QK. Measurement of fine-needle aspiration thyroglobulin levels increases the detection of metastatic papillary thyroid carcinoma in cystic neck lesions. Cancer Cytopathol 2014;122(7):521–6.
39. Scheumann GF, Gimm O, Wegener G, et al. Prognostic significance and surgical management of locoregional lymph node metastases in papillary thyroid cancer. World J Surg 1994;18(4):559–67 [discussion: 567–8].
40. Scherl S, Mehra S, Clain J, et al. The effect of surgeon experience on the detection of metastatic lymph nodes in the central compartment and the pathologic features of clinically unapparent metastatic lymph nodes: what are we missing when we don't perform a prophylactic dissection of central compartment lymph nodes in papillary thyroid cancer? Thyroid 2014;24(8):1282–8.
41. Isaacs JD, Lundgren CI, Sidhu SB, et al. The Delphian lymph node in thyroid cancer. Ann Surg 2008;247(3):477–82.
42. Iyer NG, Kumar A, Nixon IJ, et al. Incidence and significance of Delphian node metastasis in papillary thyroid cancer. Ann Surg 2011;253(5):988–91.
43. Oh EM, Chung YS, Lee YD. Clinical significance of Delphian lymph node metastasis in papillary thyroid carcinoma. World J Surg 2013;37(11):2594–9.

44. Agcaoglu O, Aliyev S, Taskin HE, et al. The utility of intraoperative ultrasound in modified radical neck dissection: a pilot study. Surg Innov 2014;21(2):166–9.
45. Ertas B, Kaya H, Kurtulmus N, et al. Intraoperative ultrasonography is useful in surgical management of neck metastases in differentiated thyroid cancers. Endocrine 2015;48(1):248–53.
46. Robbins KT, Medina JE, Wolfe GT, et al. Standardizing neck dissection terminology. Official report of the Academy's Committee for Head and Neck Surgery and Oncology. Arch Otolaryngol Head Neck Surg 1991;117(6):601–5.
47. Robbins KT, Clayman G, Levine PA, et al. Neck dissection classification update: revisions proposed by the American Head and Neck Society and the American Academy of Otolaryngology-Head and Neck Surgery. Arch Otolaryngol Head Neck Surg 2002;128(7):751–8.
48. Ferris R, Goldenberg D, Haymart MR, et al. American Thyroid Association consensus review of the anatomy, terminology and rationale for lateral neck dissection in differentiated thyroid cancer. American Thyroid Association Surgical Affairs Committee. Thyroid 2012;22(5):501–8.
49. Hamming JF, Roukema JA. Management of regional lymph nodes in papillary, follicular, and medullary thyroid cancer. In: Clark OH, Duh Q, Kebebew E, editors. Textbook of endocrine surgery. 2nd edition. Philadelphia: Elsevier Saunders; 2005. p. 195–206.
50. El Khatib Z, Lamblin J, Aubert S, et al. Is thymectomy worthwhile in central lymph node dissection for differentiated thyroid cancer? World J Surg 2010;34(6):1181–6.
51. Holostenco V, Khafif A. The upper limits of central neck dissection. JAMA Otolaryngol Head Neck Surg 2014;140(8):731–5.
52. Carling T, Long WD 3rd, Udelsman R. Controversy surrounding the role for routine central lymph node dissection for differentiated thyroid cancer. Curr Opin Oncol 2010;22(1):30–4.
53. Landers JT, Maino K. Clarifying Erb's point as an anatomic landmark in the posterior cervical triangle. Dermatol Surg 2012;38(6):954–7.
54. Grebe SK, Hay ID. Thyroid cancer nodal metastases: biologic significance and therapeutic considerations. Surg Oncol Clin N Am 1996;5(1):43–63.
55. Podnos YD, Smith D, Wagman LD, et al. The implication of lymph node metastasis on survival in patients with well-differentiated thyroid cancer. Am Surg 2005;71(9):731–4.
56. Gemsenjager E, Perren A, Seifert B, et al. Lymph node surgery in papillary thyroid carcinoma. J Am Coll Surg 2003;197(2):182–90.
57. Ito Y, Tomoda C, Uruno T, et al. Preoperative ultrasonographic examination for lymph node metastasis: usefulness when designing lymph node dissection for papillary microcarcinoma of the thyroid. World J Surg 2004;28(5):498–501.
58. Ahn D, Sohn JH, Park JY. Surgical complications and recurrence after central neck dissection in cN0 papillary thyroid carcinoma. Auris Nasus Larynx 2014;41(1):63–8.
59. Forest VI, Clark JR, Ebrahimi A, et al. Central compartment dissection in thyroid papillary carcinoma. Ann Surg 2011;253(1):123–30.
60. Hughes DT, Laird AM, Miller BS, et al. Reoperative lymph node dissection for recurrent papillary thyroid cancer and effect on serum thyroglobulin. Ann Surg Oncol 2012;19(9):2951–7.
61. Cavicchi O, Piccin O, Caliceti U, et al. Transient hypoparathyroidism following thyroidectomy: a prospective study and multivariate analysis of 604 consecutive patients. Otolaryngol Head Neck Surg 2007;137(4):654–8.

62. Lee YS, Kim SW, Kim SW, et al. Extent of routine central lymph node dissection with small papillary thyroid carcinoma. World J Surg 2007;31(10):1954–9.

63. Roh JL, Park JY, Park CI. Total thyroidectomy plus neck dissection in differentiated papillary thyroid carcinoma patients: pattern of nodal metastasis, morbidity, recurrence, and postoperative levels of serum parathyroid hormone. Ann Surg 2007;245(4):604–10.

64. Stack BC Jr, Ferris RL, Goldenberg D, et al. American Thyroid Association consensus review and statement regarding the anatomy, terminology, and rationale for lateral neck dissection in differentiated thyroid cancer. Thyroid 2012; 22(5):501–8.

65. Pacini F, Molinaro E, Castagna MG, et al. Recombinant human thyrotropin-stimulated serum thyroglobulin combined with neck ultrasonography has the highest sensitivity in monitoring differentiated thyroid carcinoma. J Clin Endocrinol Metab 2003;88(8):3668–73.

66. Torlontano M, Crocetti U, Augello G, et al. Comparative evaluation of recombinant human thyrotropin-stimulated thyroglobulin levels, 131I whole-body scintigraphy, and neck ultrasonography in the follow-up of patients with papillary thyroid microcarcinoma who have not undergone radioiodine therapy. J Clin Endocrinol Metab 2006;91(1):60–3.

67. Wang LY, Palmer FL, Nixon IJ, et al. Lateral neck lymph node characteristics prognostic of outcome in patients with clinically evident n1b papillary thyroid cancer. Ann Surg Oncol 2015. [Epub ahead of print].

68. Wang LY, Palmer FL, Nixon IJ, et al. Central lymph node characteristics predictive of outcome in patients with differentiated thyroid cancer. Thyroid 2014;24(12): 1790–5.

69. Wu MH, Shen WT, Gosnell J, et al. Prognostic significance of extranodal extension of regional lymph node metastasis in papillary thyroid cancer. Head Neck 2015;37(9):1336–43.

70. Shah PK, Shah KK, Karakousis GC, et al. Regional recurrence after lymphadenectomy for clinically evident lymph node metastases from papillary thyroid cancer: a cohort study. Ann Surg Oncol 2012;19(5):1453–9.

71. Bardet S, Ciappuccini R, Quak E, et al. Prognostic value of microscopic lymph node involvement in patients with papillary thyroid cancer. J Clin Endocrinol Metab 2015;100(1):132–40.

72. Yeh MW, Bauer AJ, Bernet VA, et al. American Thyroid Association statement on preoperative imaging for thyroid cancer surgery. Thyroid 2015;25(1):3–14.

73. Tufano RP, Clayman G, Heller KS, et al. Management of recurrent/persistent nodal disease in patients with differentiated thyroid cancer: a critical review of the risks and benefits of surgical intervention versus active surveillance. Thyroid 2015; 25(1):15–27.

Current Guidelines for Postoperative Treatment and Follow-Up of Well-Differentiated Thyroid Cancer

Jenny Y. Yoo, MD, Michael T. Stang, MD*

KEYWORDS

- Thyroid cancer • Radioactive iodine • I^{131} • TSH suppression

KEY POINTS

- The pathology and demographics of well-differential thyroid cancer patients define specific risk groups.
- Adjuvant radioactive iodine is recommended for moderate- to high-risk patients after surgical resection.
- Administration of thyroxine to suppress TSH levels is a cornerstone of long-term therapy.
- Long-term follow-up is guided by serum thyroglobulin measurements and cervical ultrasound to detect recurrent disease.

Well-differentiated thyroid carcinoma (WDTC) is predominately a surgical disease with respect to the primary tumor, locoregional advanced disease, and the treatment of cervical neck recurrences. However, the multidisciplinary approach to postoperative management of thyroid cancer is central in minimizing the risk of recurrence and surveying patients long-term in a cost-effective manner to detect clinically significant disease recurrence that warrants further treatment. Because long-term survival from WDTC is good with 10-year survival of 93% for papillary thyroid cancer (PTC) inclusive of all stages it is vital to appropriately treat the patients that are at higher risk of complications from their disease burden without overtreating those patients with a low risk of thyroid cancer–related adverse outcome.[1]

For the purpose of this article, the discussion is inclusive of the postoperative treatment of adult differentiated carcinoma processes derived from follicular epithelial cells and comprises PTC, follicular (FCC), and oncocytic follicular (Hürthle or oxyphillic cell [HCC]) subtypes.

The authors have nothing to disclose.
Division of Endocrine Surgery, Department of Surgery, University of Pittsburgh, 3471 Fifth Avenue, Kaufman Building, Suite 101, Pittsburgh, PA 15213, USA
* Corresponding author.
E-mail address: stangmt@upmc.edu

Surg Oncol Clin N Am 25 (2016) 41–59
http://dx.doi.org/10.1016/j.soc.2015.08.002
1055-3207/16/$ – see front matter © 2016 Elsevier Inc. All rights reserved.

In the past two decades, there has been a dramatic and sustained rise in incidence and detection of these well-differentiated thyroid tumors. Most of the rise in incidence is caused by the detection of PTC and likely the consequence of increased sensitivity of imaging modalities and pathologic identification of subclinical microscopic tumors. With the relative rapid increase in the diagnosis of WDTC, clinicians caring for this epidemic of thyroid cancer need guidance in providing algorithmic care from rational guidelines formed out of extensive literature review and consensus expert opinion. In our own clinical treatment of patients with thyroid cancer, postoperative care and surveillance is directed predominately by guidelines laid out by the American Thyroid Association (ATA) as initially published in 2006 and revised in 2009, with the anticipated third iteration due in 2015, and guidelines established through the National Comprehensive Cancer Network® (NCCN®), with the current version published in 2015.[2–4] Use of such guidelines is not to discredit the recommendations made through other vigorous reviews and the expert opinion of very relevant professional organizations involved in promoting improved WDTC care.[5–8]

ASSIGNMENT OF RISK

Most patients with WDTC who have undergone a total thyroidectomy with or without appropriate lymphadenectomy have relatively excellent prognosis for long-term survival and very low disease-specific mortality.[9,10] However, there is an inherent risk of growth of occult persistent disease and this is often reflected as a locoregional cervical neck or mediastinal recurrence.[9,10] This is especially true for PTC, which accounts for most cases of WDTC. As reasoned, the ultimate goal in the postoperative management of patients with WDTC is to maximize disease-free recurrence with appropriate and measured treatments that serve benefit to those patients with a real risk of adverse outcome from recurrent disease while not overtreating most patients that have minimal risk of recurrence following surgical removal of the primary tumor alone.

Specific factors have been identified that permit a more individualized estimation of recurrence rate and survival and help guide long-term oncologic adjuvant treatment and surveillance strategies. Of these, the patient's age at the time of presentation and tumor stage are two of the most important prognostic factors.[11–14] As one would expect, age is an independent variable in the long-term risk of mortality, with older patients more likely to succumb to disease burden. The inflection point of increased risk of death begins in the fourth decade and escalates for those greater than 60 years of age.[9] Risk of tumor recurrence, however, is more bimodal as it pertains to age at diagnosis. The risk of recurrence is highest for those with age less than 20 and greater than 60.[9,12–14] Male sex also portends more aggressive disease when compared with that of female cohorts.[10]

As with any other cancer, tumor biology has a profound influence on the expected long-term outcome. For WDTC, this is best represented by the pathologic features of the primary tumor including tumor size, tumor histology, extrathyroidal extension (ETE), vascular invasion, and the extent of metastatic lymph node involvement. Clearly, small tumors (<1 cm) conventionally referred to as microcarcinomas would be expected to have favorable outcomes and are addressed separately. Larger tumors (>1.5 cm) are associated with a higher risk of recurrence and disease-specific mortality.[9] Indeed, there is an incremental increase in the risk of distant metastasis with increasing tumor size.[15]

Certain histologic variants of WDTC portend a more concerning risk of recurrence and/or disease-specific mortality. Among these are variants of PTC including tall-cell, insular, columnar, and diffuse sclerosing variants.[10,16–20] Conversely, follicular variant PTC carries a very favorable risk profile and is especially true with evidence of clear demarcation or complete encapsulation.[21,22] Conventional follicular and onco-cytic follicular carcinomas are largely considered to have more aggressive tumor biology especially with larger tumors and advanced age.[23–25] However, tumors with evidence of minimal invasion as defined by microscopic capsular disruption are considered to have a favorable biology and low risk of recurrence.[26,27]

Ten percent of WDTC exhibit evidence on anatomic pathology of tumor extension through the outer thyroid capsule into the immediate perithyroidal soft tissue.[9] Such extension is variable and designated as either minimal ETE (American Joint Committee on Cancer [AJCC] T3) or macroscopic and extensive (AJCC T4a). The risk of recurrence significantly correlates to the degree of ETE. For minimal ETE, risk of recurrence is 3% to 9%, whereas recurrence rates for T4a disease is 23% to 40%.[28–33] Further, intrathyroidal extension observed as vascular invasion has been shown to correlate with tumor recurrence (16%–30%), high rate of distant metastasis (12%–35%), and long-term adverse outcomes.[34–38]

Lymph node metastasis in the context of WDTC is common and observed in most patients (62%–81%) when detailed lymph node dissection is performed.[39–42] However, it is clear from large retrospective series and observational studies that not all lymph node metastasis carry the same clinical significance because the real risk of recurrence ranges from 2% to 38%.[41,43–46] To an extent, this holds true even in patients managed without lymph node dissection or adjuvant treatment with radioactive iodine (RAI).[40,46] To more clearly synthesize the abundant and varied data for lymph node metastasis and risk of recurrence or adverse outcome, an ATA taskforce clarified the characteristics of lymph node metastasis to be considered at low risk or higher risk.[47] Micrometastasis (<0.2 cm in largest diameter) in five or fewer nodes are classified as lower-risk disease with an estimated risk of recurrence of 5% without further treatment.[47] More than five metastatic lymph nodes, clinically apparent N1 disease (detected with either preoperative imaging or intraoperatively), or any metastatic focus greater than 3 cm are classified as higher risk of recurrence with risk of recurrence greater than 20%.[47] Identification of extranodal extension is also an important indication of biology and the risk of recurrence is 2% for patients with less than or equal to three lymph nodes exhibiting extranodal extension rising to 38% for those with greater than three lymph nodes demonstrating extranodal extension.[46]

The extent of data available regarding the various risk factors for recurrence and disease-specific morbidity for a given presentation of WDTC has resulted in several different staging systems all establishing a relative prognostic score. The AJCC TNM staging system is considered the most useful for prediction of the risk of death from thyroid cancer.[3,43] However, the AJCC TNM staging system does tend to fall short in its overall clinical relevance in predicting recurrence of WDTC.[13,48] Other common prognostic scoring methodologies used within the literature in analyzing large prospective and retrospective clinical cohorts include AGES (*Age*, tumor *Grade*, *Extent*, and *Size*), AMES (*Age*, *Metastasis*, *Extent*, and *Size*), MACIS (*Metastasis*, *Age*, *Completeness* of resection, *Invasion*, and *Size*), EORTC (European Organization for Research and Treatment of Cancer), and NTCTCS (National Thyroid Cancer Treatment Cooperative Study) among other more institutional-specific scores (Ohio State University and Memorial Sloan Kettering Cancer Center).[9,13,49–53] Such scoring systems alternatively weigh the typical prognostic variables to better define the outcome end point they were designed to measure. Overall, none of the scoring systems have shown over time to provide primacy in the ability to predict outcome whether it is recurrence or disease-specific mortality.[13,27,54,55] A simplified three-tier risk staging system was proposed as part of the 2009 ATA guidelines (**Table 1**) to more specifically address the risk of clinical recurrence and has proved to be well validated in its approach.[56–59] This more relevant risk stratagem provides the basis for the key components in the postoperative care of WDTC patients as it pertains to adjuvant treatment with RAI and thyroid-stimulating hormone (TSH) suppression, in addition to establishing the tempo and intensity of long-term surveillance.

An important consideration in long-term postoperative care of WDTC patients is to be cognizant that the initial staging as specified by the AJCC TNM stage does not change over time; however, because most patients live decades following diagnosis, the biology of the disease may evolve with time. Most WDTC persistent disease remains indolent in nature and escalation of treatment is infrequently needed. For some patients with thyroid cancer, nonetheless, the response to therapy is incomplete and/or the clinical course transforms and with that the ongoing risk of recurrence, disease progression, and risk of disease-specific death may change over time. Thus, the multidisciplinary team tasked with long-term treatment of each patient should provide an ongoing reassessment of the risk of recurrence as their clinical data emerges with the response to therapy and clinical course.[3,36,38]

THE INCIDENTAL PAPILLARY THYROID MICROCARCINOMA

The detection of small PTC lesions (<1 cm), termed microcarcinomas (PTMC), has been steadily increasing over the last four decades and accounts for a large portion of the steady rise observed in overall number of PTC over that same timeframe.[60] These are typically found incidental to the original indication for thyroid surgery and are very-low-risk lesions with essentially zero risk of disease-specific mortality and less than 1% risk of distant metastasis.[61,62] The risk of locoregional recurrence is 2.4% despite studies reporting 60% of PTMC are associated with lymph node metastasis.[42,63] Patients with PTMC have an excellent overall prognosis and most pertinent studies demonstrate no significant improvement in recurrence rate or increased

Table 1
A simplified three-tier risk staging system

Low Risk	Intermediate Risk	High Risk
Absence of local or distant metastasis	Evidence of microscopic extrathyroidal extension into perithyroidal tissue	Macroscopic tumor invasion of perithyroidal structures
Complete macroscopic tumor resection	Presence of cervical lymph node metastasis	Incomplete resection of the primary tumor
No tumor invasion of locoregional tissues or structures	Evidence of aggressive histology[a] or vascular invasion	Distant metastasis
Absence of vascular invasion or predominate aggressive histology[a]	Evidence of I[131] uptake outside the thyroid bed on posttreatment whole-body RAI scan	Serum Tg levels out of proportion to I[131] uptake observed on posttreatment whole-body RAI scan
No I[131] uptake outside the thyroid bed on posttreatment whole-body RAI scan		

[a] Insular, columnar, tall-cell, solid, and diffuse sclerosing variants.
Adapted from Cooper DS, Doherty GM, Haugen BR, et al. American Thyroid Association (ATA) Guidelines Taskforce on Thyroid Nodules and Differentiated Thyroid Cancer Revised American Thyroid Association management guidelines for patients with thyroid nodules and differentiated thyroid cancer. Thyroid 2009;19(11):1180; with permission.

survival after total thyroidectomy versus thyroid lobectomy with or without RAI treatment in the context of PTMC.[64,65] Accordingly, the ATA and NCCN Clinical Practice Guidelines in Oncology (NCCN Guidelines®) do not advocate the use of RAI ablation or completion thyroidectomy for these tumors because of the low risk of recurrence and metastatic potential.[3,4] If PTMC is discovered following diagnostic lobectomy whether unifocal or multifocal, periodic surveillance of the contralateral lobe with high-resolution ultrasound (US) is adequate for postsurgical management.[4]

COMPLETION THYROIDECTOMY

Not all patients have the amenity of a preoperative diagnosis of WDTC and anywhere from 5% to 75% of patients with nondiagnostic, atypia of undetermined significance, follicular lesion, or suspicious for malignancy cytology (Bethesda System for Reporting Thyroid Cytopathology I, III, IV, and V) on fine-needle aspiration (FNA) biopsy have a clinically significant malignancy diagnosed on anatomic pathology following the initial surgical resection.[66] Many of these patients receive a diagnostic lobectomy because of the uncertainty of the indeterminate cytology reporting categories. For these patients, the first step in postoperative care involves the decision to proceed with completion thyroidectomy. This often requires a multidisciplinary approach and clear communication between the endocrine surgeon, endocrinologist, and nuclear medicine specialist involved in posttreatment plans.

Total thyroidectomy for patients with primary tumors greater than or equal to 1 cm yields lower recurrence rates and higher survival rates.[67] As such, the treatment of choice is total thyroidectomy if the tumor is biopsy proved preoperatively. Current guidelines prescribe that if a total thyroidectomy was warranted with a preoperative diagnosis of WDTC, then completion thyroidectomy should be offered.[3] This is especially true for those patients that are to be recommended RAI treatment or those where active surveillance is more of a concern.[3,4] Conversely, patients with low-risk purely intrathyroidal PTC (favorable histology, such as follicular variant <4 cm) and without evidence of ETE or only minimally invasive FCC less than 2 cm may be considered to have definitive therapy with thyroid lobectomy alone.[4,21,44,68]

Treatment or attempt at ablation of the remaining contralateral lobe of the thyroid with RAI is not recommended under circumstances where it can be removed surgically.[3,69] Circumstances that can present a challenge with respect to completion thyroidectomy are cases where the recurrent laryngeal nerve is injured at the initial resection and the patient is left with a vocal fold motion deficit. This also highlights the vital importance of laryngoscopy in the postoperative setting to document any deficit and proceed with treatment if needed.

RADIOACTIVE IODINE TREATMENT

In the context of surgical oncology and adjuvant oncology treatment, there are few treatments that are more "targeted" than that of RAI. A hallmark of follicular-derived thyroid epithelial cells is their ability to import via the sodium-iodine symporter and retain iodine in the process of organification. Such activity provides for a reasonable cellular retention time and potentiates radiopharmacologic imaging and treatment. Postoperative treatment with radioactive I^{131} is primarily applied for three reasons. First, RAI ablates or eliminates any remaining normal thyroid tissue and facilitates the specificity of thyroglobulin (Tg) as a tumor marker in long-term surveillance. This is of more significance in the low-risk and some intermediate-risk group patients that otherwise may never have disease recurrence but could observe an increase in Tg over time because of growth of any normal thyroid remnant tissue from incomplete thyroidectomy. Second, RAI serves as an adjuvant treatment of intermediate-risk patients to destroy remaining occult small foci of WDTC and potentiating a decrease in long-term risk of recurrent disease. Finally, RAI may be administered in a true therapeutic fashion for those high-risk patients with macroscopic residual disease or distant metastatic disease.

The 2009 ATA guidelines and current version of NCCN Guidelines for the treatment of WDTC patients with RAI are reasonably congruent (**Table 2**).[3,4] In general, both sets of guidelines define a set of patients at low risk of recurrence for whom there is little documented benefit in administering either an ablative or adjuvant dose of RAI. Certainly for those patients at high risk of recurrence there is relative uniformity in recommending an empiric therapeutic dose of RAI. For all other WDTC patients in between as either low risk with tumors 1 to 4 cm or intermediate risk with only a low-volume of nodal metastasis, the use becomes more selective and inherently subjective. Furthermore, for those patients in the intermediate-risk group or those with low risk of recurrence but tumors greater than 4 cm the multidisciplinary team must determine the appropriate empiric dose range to treat, whether that is more consistent with an ablative dose (30–100 mCi) or an adjuvant dose (100–200 mCi).

With respect to the less common WDTC histology of FCC and HCC, widely invasive tumors or those exhibiting vascular invasion should prompt RAI treatment in all cases. For tumors greater than 2 cm or those with only a few foci of vascular invasion, consideration of RAI treatment should follow best clinical judgment.[4] Tumors with evidence of minimal invasion as defined by microscopic capsular disruption do not typically warrant RAI treatment.[3,4,26,27]

The actual RAI doses for each of stated intent of simple remnant ablation, adjuvant treatment, and therapeutic dosing vary to a degree across the ATA and NCCN Guidelines.[3,4] However, some generalizations can be made with respect to empiric dosing. An ablative dose is typically 30 to 100 mCi (ATA) with the NCCN favoring more restrained use with 30 mCi for most ablative intents and in some cases of low to intermediate risk of recurrence (see **Table 2**, NCCN Selective Use). Adjuvant and therapeutic treatment dosing tends to overlap and typically ranges from 100 to 200 mCi for those in the intermediate- and high-risk groups, favoring 200 mCi for those at highest risk (ATA).[3] The NCCN Guidelines more specifically recommend doses of 100 to 175 mCi for known lymph node metastasis, 150 to 200 mCi for incompletely resected tumor remaining in the thyroid bed, and 200 mCi for those patients with evidence of distant metastasis.[4] Because of the risk of pulmonary fibrosis, patients with diffuse pulmonary metastasis are recommended not to exceed a dose of 150 mCi.[4] The role of other dosing strategies, such as lesional dosimetry or upper limit blood- and body-based dosimetry, in the initial postoperative treatment is less well defined and is most appropriate to consider for patients with significant distant metastatic disease, diffuse pulmonary metastasis, or medical comorbidities, such as renal failure, that potentiate the possibility of significant toxicity with the upper limits fixed empiric dosing.[3,70,71]

Preparation for RAI imaging and treatment includes induction of an iodine deficient state and elevation of the TSH level to maximize the response of remaining normal thyroid tissue and any persistent tumor burden. It is vital for the multidisciplinary care team to inquire about potential exposures to high levels of iodine, such as intravenous contrast or amiodarone. Spot urine iodine can be measured to guide in the timing of RAI because most patients with urinary iodine concentrations greater than 135 µg/L following high-dose iodine return to baseline within 60 days.[72] Patients are instructed to maintain a low-iodine diet (≤50 µg/day) for at least 1 to 2 weeks before receiving RAI.[3,4,73] Useful resources for patients regarding complying with a low-iodine diet are

Table 2
Recommendations for the use of RAI

	Not Recommended	Selective Use	Recommended	Recommended
		Ablative (30–100 mCi) or adjuvant dosing (100–200 mCi)	Ablative (30–100 mCi) or adjuvant dosing (100–200 mCi)	Therapeutic dosing 100–200 mCi
ATA[c]	Most low risk	Low risk with tumor 1–4 cm[a] Intermediate risk: age <45 nodal metastasis only[a] Intermediate risk: age >45 nodal metastasis only (AJCC T1-2 N1a)[a] Intermediate risk: any age with minimal ETE only (AJCC T3 with tumor <4 cm)[a]	Low risk with tumor >4 cm[a] Most intermediate risk[a]	High risk
[NCCN][d]	PTC: unifocal or multifocal classic variant PTC with all primary tumors <1 cm without ETE, absence of anti-Tg antibodies and unstimulated Tg <1 ng/mL FCC/HCC: primary tumor <2 cm without ETE or vascular invasion, absence of nodal or distant metastasis and absence of anti-Tg antibodies	PTC: tumor 1–4 cm or high-risk histology or lymphovascular invasion or lymph node metastasis or macroscopic multifocal (>1 cm) or positive anti-Tg antibodies or unstimulated Tg 1–5 ng/mL[b] FCC/HCC: primary tumor 2–4 cm or minor vascular invasion or lymph node metastasis or positive anti-Tg antibodies or positive or unstimulated Tg 1–5 ng/mL[b]	PTC: primary tumor >4 cm or gross extrathyroidal extension or unstimulated Tg >5 ng/mL[b] FCC/HCC: primary tumor >4 cm or gross extrathyroidal extension or extensive vascular invasion or unstimulated Tg >5 ng/mL[b]	PTC, FCC, and HCC: known or suspected distant metastasis or incomplete resection or primary tumor

[a] Suspected or known residual disease based on clinical judgment or demonstrated on pretherapy WBS should prompt treatment with 100 to 200 mCi. In the absence of known or suspected residual disease based on clinical judgment or pretherapy WBS, dosing of 30 to 100 mCi should be used.

[b] If pretherapy WBS shows no thyroid bed uptake and Tg <1 ng/mL then follow without ablation. With thyroid bed uptake only proceed with remnant ablation dose of 30 mCi. For patients with proved metastatic disease proceed with empiric dosing 100–200 mCi.

[c] Cooper DS, Doherty GM, Haugen BR, et al. American Thyroid Association (ATA) Guidelines Taskforce on Thyroid Nodules and Differentiated Thyroid Cancer Revised American Thyroid Association management guidelines for patients with thyroid nodules and differentiated thyroid cancer. Thyroid. 2009;19(11):1167–214. PMID: 19860577.

[d] Referenced with permission from the NCCN Clinical Practice Guidelines in Oncology (NCCN Guidelines®) for Thyroid Carcinoma V.2.2015 © National Comprehensive Cancer Network, Inc 2015. All rights reserved. Accessed September 14, 2015. To view the most recent and complete version of the guideline, go online to NCCN.org. NATIONAL COMPREHENSIVE CANCER NETWORK®, NCCN®, NCCN GUIDELINES®, and all other NCCN Content are trademarks owned by the National Comprehensive Cancer Network, Inc.

found through the ATA (http://www.thyroid.org/faq-low-iodine-diet/) and the Thyroid Cancer Survivors Association (http://thyca.org/rai.htm#diet).

Recombinant Human Thyrotropin Versus LT4 Withdrawal in an Iodine Deficient State

Traditionally, RAI had been administered in the setting of levothyroxine (LT4) withdrawal to elevate the TSH level to a goal of greater than 30 mU/L, which is the level shown necessary to adequately concentrate iodine with remnant thyroid and persistent tumor.[3,4] Comparable results are achieved by simply administering recombinant human thyrotropin (rhTSH) before RAI without the need to discontinue LT4. In several randomized controlled trials, low- to intermediate-risk patients demonstrated equivalent ablation with rhTSH versus LT4 withdrawal.[74–78] The role of rhTSH in high-risk patients is less clear and it is still recommended to use LT4 withdrawal in this patient cohort in the absence of medical comorbidities that preclude a prolonged hypothyroid state.[3]

Pretreatment whole body scan (WBS) with either 1.5 to 3 mCi I^{123} or low activity 1 to 3 mCi I^{131} is controversial in whether it confers long-term benefit because it rarely changes the RAI dosing treatment algorithm.[79–82] The concern, typically, is whether iodine administered for the pretreatment WBS "stuns" the targeted tissue and inhibits activity of the impending ablative dose.[83,84] As such, the use of pretreatment scans is selective and recommended if the information gathered is anticipated to change management (ie, low-risk patients undergoing remnant ablation with unexpected uptake outside the thyroid bed may prompt higher empiric dosing of I^{131} or the finding of diffuse pulmonary metastasis limiting RAI dosing in limiting pulmonary toxicity).[3,4] Optimal I^{131} treatment is subsequently administered within 72 hours to maximize treatment.[3,85] Following administration of I^{131}, posttherapy WBS done within 2 to 10 days is strongly recommended to detect clinically unapparent disease, which can be present in 10% to 25% of cases, and guide ongoing assessment of risk of recurrence and subsequent surveillance.[3,4,86,87]

Treatment with I^{131} is well tolerated; however, the multidisciplinary care team needs to be aware of and clinically evaluate all patients administered I^{131} for the potential short- and long-term complications that can arise. The more common side effects of RAI are related to iodine avidity of epithelial cells with the salivary glands and lacrimal ducts. Temporary or permanent dysfunction of these tissues can lead to salivary gland dysfunction, xerostomia, dental carries, dysgeusia, sialadenitis or parotiditis, and lacrimal duct obstruction. The likely best management of such symptoms in the early posttreatment period is adequate hydration.

THYROID-STIMULATING HORMONE SUPPRESSION

The 2009 ATA and current NCCN Guidelines for adults with WDTC recommend TSH suppression as an important adjunct in the long-term treatment of patients at intermediate and high risk of recurrence.[3,4] The upcoming 2015 ATA guidelines will likely continue this recommendation with modification based on the degree of response to therapeutic interventions.[88] The theoretic benefit and goal of therapy is in inducing hyperthyroxemia with oral LT4 suppressing hypothalamic thyrotropin-releasing hormone and subsequent pituitary TSH production. This relative suppression of TSH relegates its potential to stimulate the growth of nascent disease. The rationale for this treatment is based on studies demonstrating benefit of improved overall survival, disease-specific survival, prevention of major adverse clinical events, and restrained progression of metastatic disease in high-risk patients.[89–92] No such benefit has been demonstrated, however, for those patients with low risk of recurrence.[52,53] Current management guidelines offer congruent recommendations with respect to the degree of

TSH suppression for each risk stratification (**Table 3**).[3,4] Initial T4 dosing is weight based at 1.6 μg/kg/day and is titrated to achieve the goal TSH level within the first 6 to 12 postoperative weeks. Once a patient has maintained sustained appropriate levels, the TSH level should be monitored at least once in any give 12-month period.[3]

The consequences of sustained TSH suppression should not be ignored and this is especially true in older patients or those with ischemic heart disease. Supraphysiologic dosing of LT4 can potentiate cardiac arrhythmias and exacerbate angina symptoms, respectively.[3,93] Sustained elevation of serum thyroxine levels can lead to decreased bone density and is particularly pertinent in postmenopausal women; therefore, the concurrent use of calcium and vitamin D supplementation is advised, as is consideration of antiresorptive therapy when appropriate.[94,95]

POSTOPERATIVE ADJUNCTS FOR HIGH-RISK PATIENTS

Locally advanced WDTC with invasion into the aerodigestive tract or other vital structures of the head and neck, such as the carotid artery, is a surgical challenge even for high-volume thyroid surgeons. Every reasonable effort should be pursued to achieve a complete resection while preserving function. However, in those cases where complete resection is not possible and there is likely persistent aerodigestive tract invasion, treatment with external beam radiation should be considered as an adjunct to RAI treatment. This is especially true for tumors that lack iodine avidity on initial WBS.[3,4]

Conventional cytotoxic chemotherapeutic agents generally elicit a poor response for thyroid cancer and adjuvant systemic chemotherapy is enthusiastically not recommended in any circumstance for WDTC.[3,4,96] The future use of systemic treatment with targeted inhibitors to sensitize WDTC to RAI treatment is promising but its role in the routine care of more advanced cases is still uncertain.[97]

SURVEILLANCE

Following surgery and RAI when necessary, long-term surveillance entails a thorough physical examination of the surgical site and cervical lymph nodes, imaging, and laboratory values including degree of TSH suppression and Tg as a marker of tumor persistence/recurrence. This should be typically re-evaluated in the first 6 to 12 months

Table 3 TSH suppression range goal			
	ATA[b]	**[NCCN]**[c]	
Low risk	0.1–0.5 mU/L	—	Mild suppression[a]
Intermediate risk	<0.1 mU/L	Complete treatment response/remission Incomplete treatment response	Mild suppression[a] <0.1 mU/L
High risk	<0.1 mU/L	—	<0.1 mU/L

[a] Slightly below or above the laboratory lower level of normal reference (0.5 mU/L for most centers).
[b] Cooper DS, Doherty GM, Haugen BR, et al. American Thyroid Association (ATA) Guidelines Taskforce on Thyroid Nodules and Differentiated Thyroid Cancer Revised American Thyroid Association management guidelines for patients with thyroid nodules and differentiated thyroid cancer. Thyroid. 2009;19(11):1167–214. PMID: 19860577.
[c] Referenced with permission from the NCCN Clinical Practice Guidelines in Oncology (NCCN Guidelines®) for Thyroid Carcinoma V.2.2015 © National Comprehensive Cancer Network, Inc 2015. All rights reserved. Accessed September 14, 2015. To view the most recent and complete version of the guideline, go online to NCCN.org. NATIONAL COMPREHENSIVE CANCER NETWORK®, NCCN®, NCCN GUIDELINES®, and all other NCCN Content are trademarks owned by the National Comprehensive Cancer Network, Inc.

following initial treatment to establish a response to therapy and aid in the tempo of subsequent follow-up.[3,4]

Serum Tg is a highly sensitive and specific tumor marker in the context of WDTC. Tg measurement is integral in the long-term surveillance of patients with WDTC. Because Tg is a protein product exclusively of thyroid follicular origin, complete elimination of all normal and carcinoma-related thyroid cells from the body results in negligible or undetectable Tg levels. Tg is measured in most laboratories via immunometric assays and it is recommended that calibration be done against the CRM-457 international standard.[3,4] Furthermore, there is variability between different assays and has led to the recommendation that for a given patient the same assay be used consistently in the long-term follow-up to avoid clinical confusion regarding the real risk of persistent disease or the tempo of progression.[3,98,99] One key consideration in the use of Tg assays is the presence or absence of anti-Tg autoantibodies (TgAb) because these can dramatically interfere with conventional immunometric assays and provide for situations of falsely reported low Tg levels. Tg antibodies should be quantitatively measured every instance when Tg levels are assessed and with interpretation of the Tg level accordingly.[3,4] Furthermore, in the absence of TgAbs, the sensitivity of serum Tg assessment can be significantly enhanced with rhTSH stimulation and is used at pertinent times for assessing WDTC patients for their level of response to surgery and RAI treatment or the risk of persistent disease.[3,4,100]

When done well, high-resolution US (high frequency probe ≥10 MHz) is a sensitive imaging modality in the detection of cervical neck persistent/recurrent disease.[101] It is important that long-term follow-up neck US include all compartments of the neck with documentation of any enlarged or suspicious lymphadenopathy and thyroid bed remnant. Suspicious features on US include lymph nodes that demonstrate a loss of fatty hilum, rounded profile, cystic appearance, punctations concerning for microcalcifications, and a more chaotic vascular distribution.[102] Any suspicious lymph node identified in long-term follow-up with a suspected focus of thyroid cancer on shortest axis of 8 mm or greater in the central neck and 10 mm in the lateral neck should undergo cytologic evaluation with an US guided FNA.[103] To increase the sensitivity, all FNAs of potential recurrent cervical disease should be accompanied with a wash of a FNA pass into saline and quantified via routine Tg assay and consideration of levels greater than 10 ng/mL to be positive.[3,104,105]

It is the combination of serum Tg measurement and US that provides for the most sensitive assessment of WDTC in long-term cancer surveillance.[106] Interpretation of either result should rely on the other in the overall valuation of the data and the clinical judgment of whether a patient is tumor free or has recurrent disease. For example, a low detectable Tg level with a negative US may represent a patient with microscopic persistent cervical nodal disease that is of minimal long term morbidity, a high Tg level with a negative neck US may represent a patient with concern for persistent distant metastatic disease, and a low Tg level with a concerning neck US for bulky recurrent disease may represent a patient with a dedifferentiating process.

For patients managed with total thyroidectomy alone without RAI treatment, a negative US at the initial posttherapy assessment done at 6 to 12 months and a low unstimulated Tg level with undetectable TgAbs can be assured of a continued low risk of recurrence and surveyed further at 12 month or longer intervals. In the same subset of patients but with a detectable Tg level (TgAb negative), attention should be directed at the degree of thyroid remnant left from surgery and the Tg level judged accordingly. Long-term stability of the unstimulated Tg level without a rise and continued negative neck US is reassuring for low risk of recurrence. For patients with elevated TgAbs and a negative US, continued closer follow-up is warranted until there is resolution of TgAbs.

For patients managed with RAI ablative treatment, a negative US at the initial post-therapy assessment done at 6 to 12 months with an unstimulated Tg less than 1 ng/mL should be assessed then with a rhTSH-stimulated Tg level. If stimulated levels remain less than 1 ng/mL the patient is at low risk of recurrence and can be followed annually with unstimulated Tg levels and selective use of neck US. For this same subset of patients but with stimulated Tg levels of 1 to 2 ng/mL, closer follow-up is warranted following the trend of Tg over time and continued interval neck US interrogation. For patients with an initial stimulated Tg level greater than 2 ng/mL, the risk of recurrent disease is more significant and in the context of a negative neck US the patient should be considered for possible stimulated diagnostic RAI WBS to document sites of possible recurrent disease.[3,107]

For patients at high risk or recurrent disease and Tg greater than 10 ng/mL or concern for progressive recurrent disease with up-trending Tg levels over time and negative imaging by neck US and negative imaging on stimulated RAI WBS, consideration should be given to the addition of PET–computed tomography imaging. The use of ^{18}F-fluoro-deoxyglucose-based imaging has been shown to have an enhanced sensitivity and specificity in non-iodine-avid WDTC disease.[108] This is principally true in the context of more aggressive histologic subtypes, such as tall-cell PTC and HCC.[108]

TREATMENT OF RECURRENCE

After initial surgical treatment with or without RAI treatment, WDTC may exhibit locoregional recurrence in 15% to 30% of patients.[9,10,109] Because all of these disease recurrences can be considered persistent disease from the primary tumor and the initial surgery would have included this nascent cervical neck disease had it been detectable at the time of the original surgery, it is reasonable to consider that there is a clear role for surgery in the management of cervical neck recurrence. However, the surgical treatment of cervical recurrence needs to be tempered by weighing the risks of reoperation against the potential benefit of resecting what may be rather indolent disease. Studies have illustrated that most small-volume recurrent cervical nodal metastasis in the central compartment (91%) and lateral neck (71%) demonstrate minimal growth ($\leq$1 mm per year) over 3 to 5 years of observation and can be cautiously observed.[110,111] Moderate to large volume and locally invasive recurrent disease can portend long-term disease-specific adverse outcome.[112,113] Such locoregional recurrences are best managed surgically and should be considered when feasible with the understanding that it may not result in biochemical cure in most cases.[114]

The risks of operating in a previously dissected neck compartment are increased significantly compared with initial surgery and the challenge such surgery can entail is related to postoperative adhesive disease and the distortion of normal anatomy. In the case of development of structural disease in a previously undissected neck compartment, the risks are minimal and the benefit is significant and should be pursued in most cases exclusive of poor surgical candidates or evidence of persistent distant metastatic disease.[3,4] The pursuit of resection in a previously dissected compartment is more guarded and the threshold for surgery is set slightly higher. In general and when feasible, a reoperative surgery for persistent or recurrent disease should avoid "berry-picking" and proceed in a compartment-orientated dissection to include all tissue within the compartment with recurrence[3,4,103]; however, often some patients with WDTC have undergone several surgeries for neck recurrence and may present cases where a more focused dissection is warranted.[115] We find that this is best directed with surgeon-performed intraoperative US to plan and direct the approach and extend the dissection for recurrent disease.[115]

The angst for most thyroid surgeons relates to what qualifies as an actionable structural disease recurrence. An ATA taskforce has more recently provided some clarity for this issue with a synthesis of the available published data and expert opinion on appropriate management of recurrent cervical nodal WDTC disease.[103] In general, highly suspicious or biopsy-proved (inclusive of positive FNA Tg wash) neck recurrences of the central compartment (level VI) greater than or equal to 8 mm in the shortest axis measurement should be considered for reoperative compartment dissection, as should lateral neck compartments (levels I, II, III, IV, V) greater than or equal to 10 mm be considered.[103] A volume of disease below these limits should be observed.

RADIOACTIVE IODINE REFRACTORY DISEASE

For patients that demonstrate disease that is initially or becomes noniodine avid the treatment choices become significantly more limited. External beam radiation therapy is an option for patients with isolated unresectable cervical neck disease that has not responded to RAI. In the context of extracervical isolated or oligometastatic disease, directed stereotactic radiosurgery is considered. This is especially true for palliation if the lesions are symptomatic, present risk of pathologic fracture, risk of spinal cord compromise, or intracranial mass effect.[3,4] As a final option, systemic therapy with either a Food and Drug Administration–approved (for WDTC) kinase inhibitor or through a clinical trial should be considered for patients that have progressive disease despite all other treatment modalities.

SUMMARY

The postoperative management of WDTC requires a multidisciplinary approach and constant communication among all stakeholders including the patient. Most patients are going to have a long, uneventful clinical course and should be reassured of such when appropriate based on all available clinical data. It is fundamental to have rational clarity regarding what is and is not concerning. Long-term care should avoid situations of trying to treat the surgeons or endocrinologists and excessively pursue microscopic disease or a mild biochemical persistence of Tg. Instead, the focus needs to remain on treating the patient when it is going to serve a real benefit and avoid unnecessary surgery or radioactive treatment when it is unlikely to alter the disease course. The management guidelines will continue to evolve and it is essential that physicians and surgeons who treat WDTC maintain competency in this respect.

REFERENCES

1. Hundahl SA, Fleming ID, Fremgen AM, et al. A National Cancer Data Base report on 53,856 cases of thyroid carcinoma treated in the U.S., 1985-1995. Cancer 1998;83(12):2638–48.
2. Cooper DS, Doherty GM, Haugen BR, et al, American Thyroid Association Guidelines Taskforce. Management guidelines for patients with thyroid nodules and differentiated thyroid cancer. Thyroid 2006;16(2):109–42.
3. Cooper DS, Doherty GM, Haugen BR, et al. American Thyroid Association (ATA) Guidelines Taskforce on Thyroid Nodules and Differentiated Thyroid Cancer Revised American Thyroid Association management guidelines for patients

with thyroid nodules and differentiated thyroid cancer. Thyroid 2009;19(11): 1167–214.

4. Haddad RI, Lydiatt WM, Ball DW, et al. NCCN Clinical Practice Guidelines in Oncology (NCCN Guidelines®) Thyroid Carcinoma Version 2.2015. © 2015 National Comprehensive Cancer Network, Inc. Available at: NCCN.org. Accessed September 14, 2015.

5. Gharib H, Papini E, Paschke R, et al, AACE/AME/ETA Task Force on Thyroid Nodules. American Association of Clinical Endocrinologists, Associazione Medici Endocrinologi, and European Thyroid Association Medical guidelines for clinical practice for the diagnosis and management of thyroid nodules: executive summary of recommendations. Endocr Pract 2010;16(3):468–75.

6. Perros P, Boelaert K, Colley S, et al, British Thyroid Association. Guidelines for the management of thyroid cancer. Clin Endocrinol (Oxf) 2014;81(Suppl 1): 1–122.

7. Pacini F, Schlumberger M, Dralle H, et al, European Thyroid Cancer Taskforce. European consensus for the management of patients with differentiated thyroid carcinoma of the follicular epithelium. Eur J Endocrinol 2006;154(6):787–803.

8. Takami H, Ito Y, Okamoto T, et al. Revisiting the guidelines issued by the Japanese Society of Thyroid Surgeons and Japan Association of Endocrine Surgeons: a gradual move towards consensus between Japanese and western practice in the management of thyroid carcinoma. World J Surg 2014;38(8): 2002–10.

9. Mazzaferri EL, Jhiang SM. Long-term impact of initial surgical and medical therapy on papillary and follicular thyroid cancer. Am J Med 1994;97(5):418–28.

10. Mazzaferri EL, Kloos RT. Clinical review 128: current approaches to primary therapy for papillary and follicular thyroid cancer. J Clin Endocrinol Metab 2001; 86(4):1447–63.

11. Sanders LE, Cady B. Differentiated thyroid cancer: reexamination of risk groups and outcome of treatment. Arch Surg 1998;133(4):419–25.

12. Gilliland FD, Hunt WC, Morris DM, et al. Prognostic factors for thyroid carcinoma. A population-based study of 15,698 cases from the Surveillance, Epidemiology and End Results (SEER) program 1973-1991. Cancer 1997;79(3): 564–73.

13. Sherman SI, Brierley JD, Sperling M, et al. Prospective multicenter study of thyroid carcinoma treatment: initial analysis of staging and outcome. National Thyroid Cancer Treatment Cooperative Study Registry Group. Cancer 1998; 83(5):1012–21.

14. Tsang RW, Brierley JD, Simpson WJ, et al. The effects of surgery, radioiodine, and external radiation therapy on the clinical outcome of patients with differentiated thyroid carcinoma. Cancer 1998;82(2):375–88.

15. Ito Y, Kudo T, Kobayashi K, et al. Prognostic factors for recurrence of papillary thyroid carcinoma in the lymph nodes, lung, and bone: analysis of 5,768 patients with average 10-year follow-up. World J Surg 2012;36(6):1274–8.

16. Wenig BM, Thompson LD, Adair CF, et al. Thyroid papillary carcinoma of columnar cell type: a clinicopathologic study of 16 cases. Cancer 1998;82(4): 740–53.

17. Prendiville S, Burman KD, Ringel MD, et al. Tall cell variant: an aggressive form of papillary thyroid carcinoma. Otolaryngol Head Neck Surg 2000;122(3):352–7.

18. Akslen LA, LiVolsi VA. Prognostic significance of histologic grading compared with subclassification of papillary thyroid carcinoma. Cancer 2000;88(8): 1902–8.

19. Nikiforov YE, Erickson LA, Nikiforova MN, et al. Solid variant of papillary thyroid carcinoma: incidence, clinical-pathologic characteristics, molecular analysis, and biologic behavior. Am J Surg Pathol 2001;25(12):1478–84.

20. Regalbuto C, Malandrino P, Tumminia A, et al. A diffuse sclerosing variant of papillary thyroid carcinoma: clinical and pathologic features and outcomes of 34 consecutive cases. Thyroid 2011;21(4):383–9.

21. Tielens ET, Sherman SI, Hruban RH, et al. Follicular variant of papillary thyroid carcinoma. A clinicopathologic study. Cancer 1994;73(2):424–31.

22. Liu J, Singh B, Tallini G, et al. Follicular variant of papillary thyroid carcinoma: a clinicopathologic study of a problematic entity. Cancer 2006;107(6): 1255–64.

23. Herrera MF, Hay ID, Wu PS, et al. Hürthle cell (oxyphilic) papillary thyroid carcinoma: a variant with more aggressive biologic behavior. World J Surg 1992; 16(4):669–74 [discussion: 774–5].

24. Lopez-Penabad L, Chiu AC, Hoff AO, et al. Prognostic factors in patients with Hürthle cell neoplasms of the thyroid. Cancer 2003;97(5):1186–94.

25. Goffredo P, Roman SA, Sosa JA. Hurthle cell carcinoma: a population-level analysis of 3311 patients. Cancer 2013;119(3):504–11.

26. van Heerden JA, Hay ID, Goellner JR, et al. Follicular thyroid carcinoma with capsular invasion alone: a nonthreatening malignancy. Surgery 1992;112(6): 1130–6 [discussion: 1136–8].

27. Thompson LD, Wieneke JA, Paal E, et al. A clinicopathologic study of minimally invasive follicular carcinoma of the thyroid gland with a review of the English literature [review]. Cancer 2001;91(3):505–24.

28. Baek SK, Jung KY, Kang SM, et al. Clinical risk factors associated with cervical lymph node recurrence in papillary thyroid carcinoma. Thyroid 2010;20(2): 147–52.

29. Nixon IJ, Ganly I, Patel S, et al. The impact of microscopic extrathyroid extension on outcome in patients with clinical T1 and T2 well-differentiated thyroid cancer. Surgery 2011;150(6):1242–9.

30. Jukkola A, Bloigu R, Ebeling T, et al. Prognostic factors in differentiated thyroid carcinomas and their implications for current staging classifications. Endocr Relat Cancer 2004;11(3):571–9.

31. Ito Y, Tomoda C, Uruno T, et al. Prognostic significance of extrathyroid extension of papillary thyroid carcinoma: massive but not minimal extension affects the relapse-free survival. World J Surg 2006;30(5):780–6.

32. Radowsky JS, Howard RS, Burch HB, et al. Impact of degree of extrathyroidal extension of disease on papillary thyroid cancer outcome. Thyroid 2014;24(2): 241–4.

33. Fukushima M, Ito Y, Hirokawa M, et al. Prognostic impact of extrathyroid extension and clinical lymph node metastasis in papillary thyroid carcinoma depend on carcinoma size. World J Surg 2010;34(12):3007–14.

34. Gardner RE, Tuttle RM, Burman KD, et al. Prognostic importance of vascular invasion in papillary thyroid carcinoma. Arch Otolaryngol Head Neck Surg 2000; 126(3):309–12.

35. Nishida T, Katayama Si, Tsujimoto M. The clinicopathological significance of histologic vascular invasion in differentiated thyroid carcinoma. Am J Surg 2002;183(1):80–6.

36. Falvo L, Catania A, D'Andrea V, et al. Prognostic importance of histologic vascular invasion in papillary thyroid carcinoma. Ann Surg 2005;241(4): 640–6.

37. Mai KT, Khanna P, Yazdi HM, et al. Differentiated thyroid carcinomas with vascular invasion: a comparative study of follicular, Hürthle cell and papillary thyroid carcinoma. Pathology 2002;34(3):239–44.
38. Mete O, Asa SL. Pathological definition and clinical significance of vascular invasion in thyroid carcinomas of follicular epithelial derivation. Mod Pathol 2011;24(12):1545–52.
39. Noguchi S, Murakami N. The value of lymph-node dissection in patients with differentiated thyroid cancer. Surg Clin North Am 1987;67(2):251–61.
40. Gemsenjäger E, Perren A, Seifert B, et al. Lymph node surgery in papillary thyroid carcinoma. J Am Coll Surg 2003;197(2):182–90.
41. Bardet S, Malville E, Rame JP, et al. Macroscopic lymph-node involvement and neck dissection predict lymph-node recurrence in papillary thyroid carcinoma. Eur J Endocrinol 2008;158(4):551–60.
42. Hughes DT, White ML, Miller BS, et al. Influence of prophylactic central lymph node dissection on postoperative thyroglobulin levels and radioiodine treatment in papillary thyroid cancer. Surgery 2010;148(6):1100–6 [discussion: 1006–7].
43. Loh KC, Greenspan FS, Gee L, et al. Pathological tumor-node-metastasis (pTNM) staging for papillary and follicular thyroid carcinomas: a retrospective analysis of 700 patients. J Clin Endocrinol Metab 1997;82(11):3553–62.
44. Lee J, Song Y, Soh EY. Prognostic significance of the number of metastatic lymph nodes to stratify the risk of recurrence. World J Surg 2014;38(4):858–62.
45. Wada N, Duh QY, Sugino K, et al. Lymph node metastasis from 259 papillary thyroid microcarcinomas: frequency, pattern of occurrence and recurrence, and optimal strategy for neck dissection. Ann Surg 2003;237(3):399–407.
46. Lango M, Flieder D, Arrangoiz R, et al. Extranodal extension of metastatic papillary thyroid carcinoma: correlation with biochemical endpoints, nodal persistence, and systemic disease progression. Thyroid 2013;23(9):1099–105.
47. Randolph GW, Duh QY, Heller KS, et al, American Thyroid Association Surgical Affairs Committee's Taskforce on Thyroid Cancer Nodal Surgery. The prognostic significance of nodal metastases from papillary thyroid carcinoma can be stratified based on the size and number of metastatic lymph nodes, as well as the presence of extranodal extension. Thyroid 2012;22(11):1144–52.
48. Brierley JD, Panzarella T, Tsang RW, et al. A comparison of different staging systems predictability of patient outcome. Thyroid carcinoma as an example. Cancer 1997;79(12):2414–23.
49. Hay ID, Grant CS, Taylor WF, et al. Ipsilateral lobectomy versus bilateral lobar resection in papillary thyroid carcinoma: a retrospective analysis of surgical outcome using a novel prognostic scoring system. Surgery 1987;102(6): 1088–95.
50. Cady B, Rossi R. An expanded view of risk-group definition in differentiated thyroid carcinoma. Surgery 1988;104(6):947–53.
51. Hay ID, Bergstralh EJ, Goellner JR, et al. Predicting outcome in papillary thyroid carcinoma: development of a reliable prognostic scoring system in a cohort of 1779 patients surgically treated at one institution during 1940 through 1989. Surgery 1993;114(6):1050–7.
52. Byar DP, Green SB, Dor P, et al. A prognostic index for thyroid carcinoma. A study of the E.O.R.T.C. Thyroid Cancer Cooperative Group. Eur J Cancer 1979;15(8):1033–41.
53. Shaha AR, Loree TR, Shah JP. Prognostic factors and risk group analysis in follicular carcinoma of the thyroid. Surgery 1995;118(6):1131–6.

54. DeGroot LJ, Kaplan EL, Straus FH, et al. Does the method of management of papillary thyroid carcinoma make a difference in outcome? World J Surg 1994;18(1):123–30.
55. Lang BH, Lo CY, Chan WF, et al. Staging systems for papillary thyroid carcinoma: a review and comparison [review]. Ann Surg 2007;245(3):366–78.
56. Tuttle RM, Tala H, Shah J, et al. Estimating risk of recurrence in differentiated thyroid cancer after total thyroidectomy and radioactive iodine remnant ablation: using response to therapy variables to modify the initial risk estimates predicted by the new American Thyroid Association staging system. Thyroid 2010;20(12):1341–9.
57. Castagna MG, Maino F, Cipri C, et al. Delayed risk stratification, to include the response to initial treatment (surgery and radioiodine ablation), has better outcome predictivity in differentiated thyroid cancer patients. Eur J Endocrinol 2011;165(3):441–6.
58. Vaisman F, Momesso D, Bulzico DA, et al. Spontaneous remission in thyroid cancer patients after biochemical incomplete response to initial therapy. Clin Endocrinol (Oxf) 2012;77(1):132–8.
59. Pitoia F, Bueno F, Urciuoli C, et al. Outcomes of patients with differentiated thyroid cancer risk-stratified according to the American thyroid association and Latin American thyroid society risk of recurrence classification systems. Thyroid 2013;23(11):1401–7.
60. Davies L, Welch HG. Increasing incidence of thyroid cancer in the United States, 1973-2002. JAMA 2006;295(18):2164–7.
61. Baudin E, Travagli JP, Ropers J, et al. Microcarcinoma of the thyroid gland: the Gustave-Roussy Institute experience. Cancer 1998;83(3):553–9.
62. Roti E, degli Uberti EC, Bondanelli M, et al. Thyroid papillary microcarcinoma: a descriptive and meta-analysis study. Eur J Endocrinol 2008;159(6):659–73.
63. Sugino K, Ito K Jr, Ozaki O, et al. Papillary microcarcinoma of the thyroid. J Endocrinol Invest 1998;21(7):445–8.
64. Nixon IJ, Ganly I, Patel SG, et al. Thyroid lobectomy for treatment of well differentiated intrathyroid malignancy. Surgery 2012;151(4):571–9.
65. Hay ID, Hutchinson ME, Gonzalez-Losada T, et al. Papillary thyroid microcarcinoma: a study of 900 cases observed in a 60-year period. Surgery 2008;144(6):980–7.
66. Cibas ES, Ali SZ, NCI Thyroid FNA State of the Science Conference. The Bethesda system for reporting thyroid cytopathology. Am J Clin Pathol 2009;132(5):658–65.
67. Bilimoria KY, Bentrem DJ, Ko CY, et al. Extent of surgery affects survival for papillary thyroid cancer. Ann Surg 2007;246(3):375–81.
68. Matsuzu K, Sugino K, Masudo K, et al. Thyroid lobectomy for papillary thyroid cancer: long-term follow-up study of 1,088 cases. World J Surg 2014;38(1):68–79.
69. Barbesino G, Goldfarb M, Parangi S, et al. Thyroid lobe ablation with radioactive iodine as an alternative to completion thyroidectomy after hemithyroidectomy in patients with follicular thyroid carcinoma: long-term follow-up. Thyroid 2012;22(4):369–76.
70. Van Nostrand D, Atkins F, Yeganeh F, et al. Dosimetrically determined doses of radioiodine for the treatment of metastatic thyroid carcinoma. Thyroid 2002;12(2):121–34.
71. Holst JP, Burman KD, Atkins F, et al. Radioiodine therapy for thyroid cancer and hyperthyroidism in patients with end-stage renal disease on hemodialysis. Thyroid 2005;15(12):1321–31.

72. Nimmons GL, Funk GF, Graham MM, et al. Urinary iodine excretion after contrast computed tomography scan: implications for radioactive iodine use. JAMA Otolaryngol Head Neck Surg 2013;139(5):479–82.

73. Sawka AM, Ibrahim-Zada I, Galacgac P, et al. Dietary iodine restriction in preparation for radioactive iodine treatment or scanning in well-differentiated thyroid cancer: a systematic review. Thyroid 2010;20(10):1129–38.

74. Pacini F, Ladenson PW, Schlumberger M, et al. Radioiodine ablation of thyroid remnants after preparation with recombinant human thyrotropin in differentiated thyroid carcinoma: results of an international, randomized, controlled study. J Clin Endocrinol Metab 2006;91(3):926–32.

75. Chianelli M, Todino V, Graziano FM, et al. Low-activity (2.0 GBq; 54 mCi) radioiodine post-surgical remnant ablation in thyroid cancer: comparison between hormone withdrawal and use of rhTSH in low-risk patients. Eur J Endocrinol 2009;160(3):431–6.

76. Lee J, Yun MJ, Nam KH, et al. Quality of life and effectiveness comparisons of thyroxine withdrawal, triiodothyronine withdrawal, and recombinant thyroid-stimulating hormone administration for low-dose radioiodine remnant ablation of differentiated thyroid carcinoma. Thyroid 2010;20(2):173–9.

77. Schlumberger M, Catargi B, Borget I, et al, Tumeurs de la Thyroïde Refractaires Network for the Essai Stimulation Ablation Equivalence Trial. Strategies of radioiodine ablation in patients with low-risk thyroid cancer. N Engl J Med 2012;366(18):1663–73.

78. Mallick U, Harmer C, Yap B, et al. Ablation with low-dose radioiodine and thyrotropin alfa in thyroid cancer. N Engl J Med 2012;366(18):1674–85.

79. Robbins RJ, Schlumberger MJ. The evolving role of (131)I for the treatment of differentiated thyroid carcinoma. J Nucl Med 2005;46(Suppl 1):28S–37S.

80. Silberstein EB. Comparison of outcomes after (123)I versus (131)I pre-ablation imaging before radioiodine ablation in differentiated thyroid carcinoma. J Nucl Med 2007;48(7):1043–6.

81. Van Nostrand D, Aiken M, Atkins F, et al. The utility of radioiodine scans prior to iodine 131 ablation in patients with well-differentiated thyroid cancer. Thyroid 2009;19(8):849–55.

82. Schlumberger MJ, Pacini F. The low utility of pretherapy scans in thyroid cancer patients. Thyroid 2009;19(8):815–6.

83. Leger FA, Izembart M, Dagousset F, et al. Decreased uptake of therapeutic doses of iodine-131 after 185-MBq iodine-131 diagnostic imaging for thyroid remnants in differentiated thyroid carcinoma. Eur J Nucl Med 1998;25(3):242–6.

84. Hilditch TE, Dempsey MF, Bolster AA, et al. Self-stunning in thyroid ablation: evidence from comparative studies of diagnostic 131I and 123I. Eur J Nucl Med Mol Imaging 2002;29(6):783–8.

85. Robbins RJ, Tuttle RM, Sharaf RN, et al. Preparation by recombinant human thyrotropin or thyroid hormone withdrawal are comparable for the detection of residual differentiated thyroid carcinoma. J Clin Endocrinol Metab 2001;86(2):619–25.

86. Sherman SI, Tielens ET, Sostre S, et al. Clinical utility of posttreatment radioiodine scans in the management of patients with thyroid carcinoma. J Clin Endocrinol Metab 1994;78(3):629–34.

87. Fatourechi V, Hay ID, Mullan BP, et al. Are posttherapy radioiodine scans informative and do they influence subsequent therapy of patients with differentiated thyroid cancer? Thyroid 2000;10(7):573–7.

88. Haugen BR, Mandel SJ, Nikiforov Y, et al. 2014 American Thyroid Association (ATA) guidelines on thyroid nodules and differentiated thyroid cancer: highlights, consensus, and controversies. Paper presentation, 16th International Congress of Endocrinology. Chicago (IL), June 20, 2014.

89. Cooper DS, Specker B, Ho M, et al. Thyrotropin suppression and disease progression in patients with differentiated thyroid cancer: results from the National Thyroid Cancer Treatment Cooperative Registry. Thyroid 1998;8(9):737–44.

90. Jonklaas J, Sarlis NJ, Litofsky D, et al. Outcomes of patients with differentiated thyroid carcinoma following initial therapy. Thyroid 2006;16(12):1229–42.

91. Hovens GC, Stokkel MP, Kievit J, et al. Associations of serum thyrotropin concentrations with recurrence and death in differentiated thyroid cancer. J Clin Endocrinol Metab 2007;92(7):2610–5.

92. McGriff NJ, Csako G, Gourgiotis L, et al. Effects of thyroid hormone suppression therapy on adverse clinical outcomes in thyroid cancer. Ann Med 2002;34(7–8): 554–64.

93. Sawin CT, Geller A, Wolf PA, et al. Low serum thyrotropin concentrations as a risk factor for atrial fibrillation in older persons. N Engl J Med 1994;331(19): 1249–52.

94. Sugitani I, Fujimoto Y. Effect of postoperative thyrotropin suppressive therapy on bone mineral density in patients with papillary thyroid carcinoma: a prospective controlled study. Surgery 2011;150(6):1250–7.

95. Panico A, Lupoli GA, Fonderico F, et al. Osteoporosis and thyrotropin-suppressive therapy: reduced effectiveness of alendronate. Thyroid 2009; 19(5):437–42.

96. Sherman SI. Cytotoxic chemotherapy for differentiated thyroid carcinoma. Clin Oncol (R Coll Radiol) 2010;22(6):464–8.

97. Ho AL, Grewal RK, Leboeuf R, et al. Selumetinib-enhanced radioiodine uptake in advanced thyroid cancer. N Engl J Med 2013;368(7):623–32.

98. Spencer CA, Bergoglio LM, Kazarosyan M, et al. Clinical impact of thyroglobulin (Tg) and Tg autoantibody method differences on the management of patients with differentiated thyroid carcinomas. J Clin Endocrinol Metab 2005;90(10):5566–75.

99. Schlumberger M, Hitzel A, Toubert ME, et al. Comparison of seven serum thyroglobulin assays in the follow-up of papillary and follicular thyroid cancer patients. J Clin Endocrinol Metab 2007;92(7):2487–95.

100. Eustatia-Rutten CF, Smit JW, Romijn JA, et al. Diagnostic value of serum thyroglobulin measurements in the follow-up of differentiated thyroid carcinoma, a structured meta-analysis. Clin Endocrinol (Oxf) 2004;61(1):61–74.

101. Kouvaraki MA, Shapiro SE, Fornage BD, et al. Role of preoperative ultrasonography in the surgical management of patients with thyroid cancer. Surgery 2003; 134(6):946–54.

102. Leboulleux S, Girard E, Rose M, et al. Ultrasound criteria of malignancy for cervical lymph nodes in patients followed up for differentiated thyroid cancer. J Clin Endocrinol Metab 2007;92(9):3590–4.

103. Tufano RP, Clayman G, Heller KS, et al, American Thyroid Association Surgical Affairs Committee Writing Task Force. Management of recurrent/persistent nodal disease in patients with differentiated thyroid cancer: a critical review of the risks and benefits of surgical intervention versus active surveillance. Thyroid 2015; 25(1):15–27.

104. Torres MR, Nóbrega Neto SH, Rosas RJ, et al. Thyroglobulin in the washout fluid of lymph-node biopsy: what is its role in the follow-up of differentiated thyroid carcinoma? Thyroid 2014;24(1):7–18.

105. Grani G, Fumarola A. Thyroglobulin in lymph node fine-needle aspiration washout: a systematic review and meta-analysis of diagnostic accuracy. J Clin Endocrinol Metab 2014;99(6):1970–82.
106. Pacini F, Molinaro E, Castagna MG, et al. Recombinant human thyrotropin-stimulated serum thyroglobulin combined with neck ultrasonography has the highest sensitivity in monitoring differentiated thyroid carcinoma. J Clin Endocrinol Metab 2003;88(8):3668–73.
107. Mazzaferri EL, Robbins RJ, Spencer CA, et al. A consensus report of the role of serum thyroglobulin as a monitoring method for low-risk patients with papillary thyroid carcinoma. J Clin Endocrinol Metab 2003;88(4):1433–41.
108. Leboulleux S, Schroeder PR, Schlumberger M, et al. The role of PET in follow-up of patients treated for differentiated epithelial thyroid cancers. Nat Clin Pract Endocrinol Metab 2007;3(2):112–21.
109. Hay ID, Thompson GB, Grant CS, et al. Papillary thyroid carcinoma managed at the Mayo Clinic during six decades (1940-1999): temporal trends in initial therapy and long-term outcome in 2444 consecutively treated patients. World J Surg 2002;26(8):879–85.
110. Rondeau G, Fish S, Hann LE, et al. Ultrasonographically detected small thyroid bed nodules identified after total thyroidectomy for differentiated thyroid cancer seldom show clinically significant structural progression. Thyroid 2011;21(8):845–53.
111. Robenshtok E, Fish S, Bach A, et al. Suspicious cervical lymph nodes detected after thyroidectomy for papillary thyroid cancer usually remain stable over years in properly selected patients. J Clin Endocrinol Metab 2012;97(8):2706–13.
112. Grant CS, Hay ID, Gough IR, et al. Local recurrence in papillary thyroid carcinoma: is extent of surgical resection important? Surgery 1988;104(6):954–62.
113. Ito Y, Higashiyama T, Takamura Y, et al. Prognosis of patients with papillary thyroid carcinoma showing postoperative recurrence to the central neck. World J Surg 2011;35(4):767–72.
114. Uchida H, Imai T, Kikumori T, et al. Long-term results of surgery for papillary thyroid carcinoma with local recurrence. Surg Today 2013;43(8):848–53.
115. McCoy KL, Yim JH, Tublin ME, et al. Same-day ultrasound guidance in reoperation for locally recurrent papillary thyroid cancer. Surgery 2007;142(6):965–72.

Outpatient Thyroidectomy
Is it Safe?

Courtney J. Balentine, MD, MPH, Rebecca S. Sippel, MD*

KEYWORDS

- Outpatient thyroidectomy • Same day thyroidectomy • Short stay thyroidectomy
- Safety • Hematoma

KEY POINTS

- Safely performing outpatient thyroid surgery requires careful patient selection and preparation.
- It is important to identify both social and medical factors that place patients at higher risk for complications.
- Communication with patients is a key element of success because they must be able to identify postoperative complications and contact the surgical team.
- Choice of anesthetic agent and other medications can help to reduce postoperative nausea and vomiting to facilitate early discharge.

BACKGROUND

Thyroidectomy has traditionally been considered an inpatient procedure owing to concerns over the potential life-threatening consequences of a postoperative cervical hematoma. However, recent years have seen an increase in the volume of outpatient thyroidectomy because high-volume thyroid surgeons are frequently discharging patients on the same day or the morning after surgery.[1,2] Although outpatient thyroidectomy is becoming increasingly common, there remains considerable controversy over whether the best interests of patients are truly being served by anything less than a full inpatient admission after thyroid surgery.[3] Advocates for outpatient thyroidectomy point to low complication rates, decreased costs, and improved patient satisfaction as justifications for avoiding admission in carefully selected patients. Opponents of outpatient thyroid surgery generally cite concerns over missed hematomas as well as difficulty managing hypocalcemia as reasons for keeping patients

The authors have nothing to disclose.
Department of Surgery, University of Wisconsin, 600 Highland Avenue, K3/704 Clinical Science Center, Madison, WI 53792-7375, USA
* Corresponding author.
E-mail address: sippel@surgery.wisc.edu

in the hospital long enough to ensure that discharge is safe. Additionally, it is not entirely clear how to identify patients who can undergo outpatient thyroidectomy safely versus those who would benefit from additional supervision in the inpatient setting.

The American Thyroid Association (ATA) recently attempted to address the controversy over outpatient thyroidectomy by issuing a position paper that reviewed the evidence demonstrating safety and attempted to establish criteria for proper patient selection.[3] The final recommendation is that "outpatient thyroidectomy may be undertaken safely in a carefully selected patient population provided that certain precautionary measures are taken."[3] The present article expands on the ATA recommendations and attempts to offer practical advice for surgeons who wish to begin an outpatient thyroidectomy practice.

DEFINITION OF OUTPATIENT THYROIDECTOMY

One issue that has complicated analysis of outcomes for outpatient thyroidectomy is that the actual definition of "outpatient" surgery has been somewhat variable. Some groups categorize a thyroidectomy as an outpatient procedure only if performed at an ambulatory surgery center with discharge occurring the same day as surgery.[4–7] Others classify a patient admitted for a 23-hour observation period as an outpatient because the hospital does not categorize this as a full admission.[8] When analyzing national trends in outpatient thyroidectomy, it is important to remember that many datasets lack the ability to distinguish between these 2 definitions of outpatient surgery. A certain degree of caution is required when interpreting studies using datasets that merge same-day surgery and 23-hour observation. For the sake of completeness, we discuss data from papers using either definition, but we note (**Table 1**) which approach was taken in the individual studies.

BENEFITS OF OUTPATIENT THYROIDECTOMY
Cost

One of the main considerations prompting surgeons to perform outpatient thyroidectomy is the potential cost savings of avoiding a full inpatient admission. Mowschenson and colleagues[4] showed a $900 reduction in charges for outpatient versus inpatient thyroid surgery, whereas Terris and colleagues[9] showed charges of $10,288 for inpatient compared with $7814 for outpatient thyroidectomy. Although the 2 studies involve analysis of charges rather than actual costs, it does seem reasonable that fewer hospital resources are needed to care for a shorter rather than a longer stay. Because both studies defined outpatient surgery as a same-day discharge, it is less clear whether a 23-hour observation leads to substantially lower cost for the hospital or the patient. Stack and colleagues[8] evaluated both mean and median charges for a full inpatient admission compared with any stay less than 24 hours and found no difference in median charges, although analysis of mean charges did favor the outpatient approach.

Patient Satisfaction

Another argument for the value of outpatient thyroidectomy is that patients will be happier if they are able to avoid admission and can recover in the comfort of their own home. Although the notion that most individuals would rather be at home than in the hospital has considerable face validity, the supporting evidence is somewhat limited. Mowschenson and colleagues[4] surveyed patients undergoing outpatient thyroidectomy and found that 65% were satisfied with their care. As a control, they also surveyed patients undergoing laparoscopic cholecystectomy and found that 68% were satisfied. The authors concluded that outpatient thyroid surgery was just as acceptable to patients as other outpatient surgeries. Samson and colleagues[10] conducted a randomized trial of inpatient versus outpatient thyroid surgery in the Philippines as well as a separate analysis of patients treated after the trial. They found that 798 of 809 outpatients (99%) were "very pleased" with their care compared with only 25 of 369 (7%) in the inpatient group. Although it seems that the majority of patients who undergo outpatient thyroidectomy are reasonably satisfied with the experience, it is important to remember that a subset of patients are uncomfortable with the idea of going home right after having surgery. These individuals may gain more reassurance and ultimately be more satisfied with their perioperative experience by a full admission, even in the absence of any complications.

Other Benefits

In addition to cost savings and patient satisfaction, some have advocated for outpatient thyroidectomy as a way to minimize potential iatrogenic complications, including exposure to multidrug-resistant organisms and other nosocomial infections.[3] It does seem reasonable that shorter hospital stays result in less time exposed to hospital-based organisms, but the value of shortening that exposure time from 24 to 6 hours is not entirely clear. Other potential iatrogenic injuries include venous thrombosis or infection from maintaining peripheral intravenous lines as well as allergic reactions or other complications from medications administered in the hospital. Again, there is little evidence to quantify the benefits of outpatient over inpatient surgery with regard to avoiding iatrogenic complications, but it at least represents a theoretic benefit.

RISKS OF OUTPATIENT THYROIDECTOMY
Hematoma

The primary argument against performing thyroidectomy as an outpatient procedure is concern over missing a cervical hematoma that could lead to airway compromise and death. One of the original series of outpatient thyroidectomy was presented at the American Association of Endocrine Surgeons meeting in 1995 and one of the participants questioned whether the data should even have been presented at the meeting because "the true costs of observation in a safe setting are minimal; it would take a lot of patient days to match even one million-dollar lawsuit" if a patient were to die after developing a hematoma.[4] Anxiety over hematomas stems from several factors: the variable incidence reported in the literature, the potential for hematomas to develop hours to days after surgery, and the inability to accurately identify patients at high risk for hematomas.

The true incidence of postoperative hematoma is difficult to estimate given the absence of a universally accepted definition and variation in how the complication is identified. Additionally, because it is a relatively rare complication, smaller published series may have artificially low rates because the sample size is too small for reliable estimates. Larger series based on registries or administrative data may also underestimate the true incidence of hematoma because diagnostic codes are likely to be used only when some intervention is required. Given those limitations, **Table 1** shows the proportion of patients with hematomas in the most consistently cited studies on thyroid surgery. The incidence of cervical hematoma is generally around 1% or less. However, the reported rates are mostly from surgeons with considerable experience in endocrine surgery and may not accurately reflect the true risk for every patient.

Table 1
Studies assessing risk of postoperative cervical hematoma

Author	Total n	Hematoma (%)	Timing of Hematoma (Range)	Predictors	Mortality (%)	Exclusion for Outpatient
Bergamaschi et al,[16] 1998	1163	1.6	15 min–15 d	NR	0.08	NR
Bergenfelz et al,[13] 2008	3660	2.1	NR	Age, male	0	NR
Bononi et al,[32] 2010	562	0.53	<24 h–4 d	NR	0	NR
Burkey et al,[15] 2001	13,817	0.3	10 min–5 d	None found	0	NR
Champault et al,[25] 2009	95	1	2 h	NR	0	ASA ≥3, anticoagulation, OSA, >75 years old, >50 km from hospital, no phone, no one to stay with patient, toxic adenoma, indeterminate FNA, completion surgery
Chang et al,[33] 2011	1935	0.98	NR	NR	0.05	NR
Godballe et al,[11] 2009	5490	4.2	0–5 d	Age 50, male, drain, malignancy, consultant as surgeon, bilateral procedure	0	NR
Hessman,[34] 2011	148	1.3	3 and 5 d	NR	0	None
Inabnet et al,[28] 2008	224	1	1 h	NR	0	NR
Lang et al,[17] 2012	3086	0.7	<6–24 h	Reoperation, nodule size, male	0	NR
Leyre et al,[18] 2008	6830	1	<6–>24 h	Male, preoperative dyspnea	0	NR
Mazeh et al,[5] 2012	608	1	3–<24 h	NR	0	Patient preference, comorbidity needing monitoring, lymph node dissection, reoperation
Mowschenson et al,[4] 1995	100	0	NR	NR	0	None

Study			<1->24 h	Age, male, bilateral, extent of resection, reoperation		
Promberger et al,[19] 2012	30,142	1.7	NR	NR	0.01	NR
Rosato et al,[14] 2004	14,934	1.2	NR	NR	0	NR
Rosenbaum et al,[27] 2008	1050	0.6	<4 h–7 d	NR	0	NR
Samson et al,[10] 1997	1178	0	NR	NR	0.08	Elderly, comorbidity
Seybt et al,[6] 2010	418: 208 OP, 201 IP	0.24	20 d	NR	0	Comorbidity, anticoagulation or need for drain, concomitant procedures, lack of autonomy or social support
Snyder et al,[29] 2006	58	3.4	30 min–5 d	NR	0	NR
Snyder et al,[29] 2006	1242	0.4	2 h–2 d	NR	0.3	Lymph node dissection, sternotomy, other procedures normally on inpatient basis
Spanknebel et al,[7] 2005	1025	0.5	<6 h	NR	0	Anticoagulation, language barrier/cannot communicate, live in remote regions, living alone, difficult/extensive procedure, preference
Stack et al,[8] 2013	38,362	0.03	NR	NR	0	NR
Terris et al,[9] 2007	91: 52 OP, 26 observation, 13 IP	1.1	8 d	NR	0	Comorbidity, concomitant procedure, preference, drains
Thomusch et al,[12] 2000	7266	2.7	NR	NR	0.04	NR
Trottier et al,[26] 2009	232	0.4	2 d	NR	0	Lives in city or will stay within 1 h, adult around ×48 h, or done by 1 PM, total thyroidectomy as first procedure of the day only
Rios-Zambudio et al,[35] 2004	301	0.97	NR	NR	0	NR

Abbreviations: ASA, American Society of Anesthesiology; FNA, fine needle aspiration; IP, inpatient; NR, not reported; OP, outpatient; OR, operating room; OSA, obstructive sleep apnea.

Larger national registries, that include both high- and low-volume surgeons, tend to show higher rates of hematoma as well as a considerable difference in outcomes between high- and low-volume surgeons. Godballe and colleagues[11] examined 5490 patients using a national registry and found an overall hematoma rate of 4.2%, but when they analyzed the data at the level of the individual surgeon, rates ranged from 1.9% to 14.3%. Thomusch and colleagues[12] used a different national registry to analyze 7266 patients undergoing unilateral and bilateral thyroidectomy. They found that 2.7% of patients developed hematomas, but that the rate was 5.4% in hospitals performing fewer than 50 operations per year compared with 2.1% in hospitals performing 150 or more cases. Other large multiinstitutional cohort studies include work by Bergenfelz and colleagues,[13] where 3660 patients underwent thyroid surgery with 2.1% developing hematomas, and Rosato and colleagues[14] who looked at a cohort of 14,934 and found hematomas in 1.2% of patients. Although these large cohort studies tend to identify a higher incidence of hematoma compared with smaller institutional studies, 1 notable exception is the work of Stack and colleagues,[8] who used the University Health Collaborative data to assess 38,362 outpatient thyroidectomies and identified hematomas in only 13 patients (0.03%). The authors acknowledge, however, that the mechanism of data collection for their study likely means that this estimate is a significant underestimate of the true incidence and should be interpreted cautiously.

Another concern about hematomas is that the time interval from surgery to development of symptoms is unpredictable. Burkey and colleagues[15] studied 13,817 thyroidectomies and parathyroidectomies with 42 patients (0.3%) developing hematomas. The mean time for developing a hematoma was 17 hours and the range extended from 10 minutes to 5 days postoperatively. Notably, 18 hematomas developed within 6 hours of surgery, an additional 16 occurred between 7 and 24 hours, and only 8 developed after 24 hours. Other studies have also shown that hematomas can develop both early and late in the postoperative recovery. Bergamaschi and colleagues[16] found that hematomas developed anywhere from 15 minutes to 15 days after surgery with a median time of 240 minutes to detection. Godballe and colleagues[11] identified hematomas occurring up to 105 hours postoperatively with a median time of 3 hours and 97% developing within 24 hours of surgery. Lang and colleagues[17] found hematomas occurring at a median of 3 hours postoperatively with 73% discovered within 6 hours of surgery and the remaining 27% within 24 hours. Leyre and colleagues[18] saw 70 hematomas in 6830 patients with 53% occurring within 6 hours, 37% discovered 7 to 24 hours after surgery, and an additional 10% after 24 hours. Promberger and colleagues[19] reported that the vast majority of hematomas occurred within 24 hours, but 2.4% did still occur after that time. Overall, as shown in **Table 1**, the vast majority of hematomas occur within the first 24 hours after surgery, although a small percentage still develop after this time.

Because some hematomas develop after either a 6-hour or a 23-hour period of observation, it is unclear what the optimal time for observation after an outpatient thyroidectomy ought to be. Surgeons who prefer an overnight observation rather than a 6-hour stay at an outpatient center point out that a significant percentage of hematomas may be missed if observation is limited to only 6 hours. Surgeons arguing for performing thyroidectomy solely on an inpatient basis use a similar argument and note that even an overnight observation period still risks missing some early hematomas. Given that some studies show hematomas developing more than 1 week after surgery, it is clear that no duration of hospital stay will totally eliminate the possibility of a missed hematoma. Consequently, there needs to be some threshold of acceptable risk where discharge becomes reasonable; however, this threshold is quite difficult to define.

An important factor to consider when determining the balance between hematoma risk and duration of hospital stay is that not all hematomas are created equal. Some are clearly life threatening and require immediate intervention at the bedside or in the operating room, whereas others can be treated adequately with aspiration or even just observed. It seems logical that clinically significant and life-threatening hematomas would tend to develop earlier, whereas slower bleeding would tend to manifest later. If this assumption were true, then a period of observation after surgery would minimize the risk to the patient by identifying the bleeding most likely to be life threatening. Hematomas that developed after this time could then be identified by patients or family members while at home and they could return to the hospital or emergency room in time for effective treatment without a significant mortality risk. Unfortunately, it is difficult to verify this assumption based on retrospective data because the majority of hematomas that are identified tend to be symptomatic and low-grade bleeding may be missed entirely. It is also difficult to discern how quickly these hematomas developed and the urgency of their operative management. If they were not taken to the operating room until 24 hours after surgery, it is difficult to know if the hematoma was evident earlier, but not large enough or symptomatic enough to warrant operative management until later. It should also be pointed out that many of the hematomas developing after 24 hours are found in patients taking anticoagulation. The fact that these patients develop bleeding complications from surgery is not entirely surprising and should probably not invalidate the notion of outpatient surgery for those with normal coagulation profiles.

It might be possible to alleviate some concern over missing hematomas if there were an accurate way to distinguish patients who are at high or low risk of developing this complication. If hematoma risk could be determined before leaving the operating room, then surgeons might feel more comfortable discharging low-risk patients and keeping high-risk individuals for a longer period of observation. Several groups have attempted to identify predictors that could be used for risk stratification and have had mixed success in this endeavor because hematomas are such a rare event. Bergenfelz and colleagues[13] found that being older or male conferred a higher risk of hematoma, and Godballe and colleagues[11] had similar results, but added malignancy, use of drain, bilateral operations, and presence of a consultant as surgeon to the list of risk factors. Lang and colleagues[17] identified reoperative surgery and nodule size as predictors for developing hematoma requiring intervention, but found that male gender was associated with hematomas that did not require intervention. Leyre and colleagues[18] saw an association between hematoma and male gender or preoperative symptoms of dyspnea, although they were unable to find any factors that could predict the timing of hematoma. Promberger and colleagues[19] found a relationship between hematoma risk and several factors, including age, male gender, bilateral surgery, extent of resection, and reoperative surgery. Although these factors have been associated with a slightly greater risk of hematoma formation, the risk in most of these groups remains very low. None of these studies assessed the discrimination of their models or the ability to sort low- from high-risk patients, so the usefulness of the findings is somewhat limited, aside from providing a gestalt feeling about which patients might benefit from a longer period of postoperative observation. To place the conversation over bleeding risk in context, the probability of developing a hematoma after thyroid surgery is comparable to the risk after laparoscopic cholecystectomy.[20] The latter procedure is performed routinely on an outpatient basis with little controversy or discussion of requiring inpatient admission.

Hypoparathyroidism

Debate over bleeding and hematomas tends to dominate the discussion about the role of outpatient thyroidectomy, but there are other complications of the operation that also raise concern. Another complication that can cause difficulties in the postoperative management of thyroid surgery is hypoparathyroidism. Depending on the criteria used to diagnose hypoparathyroidism, it may occur in more than one-third of patients undergoing total or completion thyroidectomy.[21] Management with oral calcium supplementation is generally successful but some patients end up being readmitted for intravenous calcium in refractory cases. Considerable disagreement exists regarding the best approach to postoperative hypoparathyroidism with some groups routinely discharging all patients on calcium with or without calcitriol, whereas others take a more selective approach based on either parathyroid hormone (PTH) and/or calcium measured after the operation.[21,22] No combination of laboratory tests has proven to be 100% sensitive or specific for identifying patients with severe hypoparathyroidism, but our group and others have established protocols based on postoperative PTH levels that have proven largely successful in avoiding readmission for symptomatic hypocalcemia.[23,24] Because calcium levels tends to reach a nadir 2 to 3 days after surgery, it is unclear whether further observation in the hospital offers any benefit in the management of hypoparathyroidism because most patients would be at home by that point regardless of whether their operation was performed on an inpatient or an outpatient basis.

Recurrent Laryngeal Nerve Injury

This rare but significant complication generates considerable anxiety from patients but it is not clear whether any practical differences in either detection or management occur based on whether surgery is performed as an inpatient or outpatient. Especially with the use of recurrent laryngeal nerve monitors, surgeons are increasingly able to identify the possibility of nerve injury intraoperatively and can instruct patients appropriately immediately after surgery.

APPROPRIATE PATIENT SELECTION FOR OUTPATIENT THYROIDECTOMY

One area of agreement for both advocates and opponents of outpatient thyroidectomy is that not all patients are ideally suited for outpatient thyroid surgery. Careful patient selection is, therefore, a key element to avoiding complications and other problems with outpatient surgery. Unfortunately, selection criteria have not been tested rigorously and represent the opinions of individual authors or groups of experts. Patient preference is certainly an important factor, but other considerations involve both medical and social factors. In **Box 1**, we summarize information from the available studies to present a checklist that may be used to assess whether patients are reasonable candidates for outpatient thyroidectomy.

Champault and colleagues[25] only performed outpatient thyroidectomy on patients if they had someone to stay with and observe them overnight, lived within 50 km of the hospital and did not have any of the following medical risk factors: American Society of Anesthesiology score of 3 or greater, taking anticoagulation, obstructive sleep apnea, age 75 years or greater, toxic adenoma, indeterminate fine needle aspiration biopsy, and prior neck surgery. Mazeh and colleagues[5] were more liberal in the use of same-day surgery and their only exclusions were patient preference, comorbid conditions that required monitoring, concomitant lymph node dissection, and prior neck surgery. Seybt and colleagues[6] considered patients to be reasonable candidates for outpatient surgery unless they lacked the autonomy to make medical decisions, lacked social

Box 1
Checklist for outpatient thyroidectomy

Social support
- Reliable adult support at home for ≥24 hours
- Transportation home

Access to care and communication
- Lives within driving distance of medical facility
- Access to telephone
- No language barrier
- No medical condition that impairs communication

Medical
- No prohibitive comorbidities
- Not taking anticoagulation
- No previous problems with anesthesia

support including having an adult to observe them immediately after surgery, were on anticoagulation, had a drain placed in the operating room, or underwent a concomitant neck procedure. Spanknebel and colleagues[7] included patients unless they were taking anticoagulation, had a language barrier or medical condition that hindered communication with the surgical team, lived far away from medical care, lived alone or had no one to observe and assist after surgery, or if the surgery was difficult and the surgeon felt the patient would be better served by a full admission. Terris and colleagues[9] also excluded patients with significant comorbidity, concomitant procedures, or placement of drains. Finally, Trottier and colleagues[26] insisted that potential outpatients either lived in the same city as the hospital performing surgery or were willing to stay at a hotel or other venue within 1 hour of the hospital, and that the case was finished by 1 PM to allow sufficient time for observation. For total thyroidectomies, they also made sure that they were the first case of the day to allow for adequate observation time.

The range of selection criteria used in these studies reflects concerns over the medical fitness to handle surgery and the risk of bleeding. They also recognize that social support and the ability to communicate with the surgical team are important elements of successful outpatient surgery. From a medical standpoint, most groups made an effort to avoid outpatient thyroidectomy in patients with significant comorbidity or age that might increase the risk of complications. For most groups, use of any anticoagulation that increased bleeding risk was also a contraindication for outpatient surgery. Unfortunately, the exact threshold of age and comorbidity that constitutes prohibitive risk is somewhat subjective. Most surgeons would admit the proverbial patient "who would have trouble with a haircut," but clearly not all candidates for outpatient surgery need to be capable of running a marathon either. In the absence of specific guidelines for which comorbid conditions or ages constitute an absolute contraindication to outpatient thyroid surgery, it is up to the individual surgeon to assess patients and have an honest discussion about the potential risks of surgery.

There is also a significant social component required for successful outpatient thyroidectomy. Because patients will be tired and less than fully alert after surgery, it is important to have mechanisms in place to monitor them for the development of complications, and a capacity for notifying the surgical team when there is concern on the part of the patient or family. Several studies very appropriately insisted on adult supervision for at least the 24-hour period after the operation, and this role could be filled by spouses, family members, or friends who are willing to assist. Having someone physically available for assistance would seem to be a fairly straightforward requirement for safe surgery, because a rapidly developing hematoma could render the patients unable to help themselves. Similarly, it is important to make sure patients not only have a ride home arranged before completing the surgery, but that they have access to reliable transportation back to the hospital should a hematoma develop.

Some surgical groups insisted not only that patients have adequate social support for safe monitoring, but also offered outpatient thyroidectomy only to individuals who lived within close proximity to the hospital or were willing to stay at a hotel or other accommodation near the hospital for 24 hours after the operation. The argument for staying near the hospital is that returning in the event of a complication becomes more challenging the further the patient gets from the surgical team. Although this idea makes sense, there is no clear guideline regarding what constitutes an acceptable distance for the safe treatment of complications.

In addition to assessing the distance to the hospital, it is equally important to ensure that the patient has the ability to communicate effectively with the surgical team in the event that a complication occurs. Access to a phone as well as the absence of a language barrier or medical condition that impairs communication are important for rapidly identifying and appropriately triaging complications. At the same time, it is vital to make sure patients adequately understand the potential complications of thyroid surgery, how they manifest, and how to address problems that develop. Providing both written and verbal instructions to patients is important to reinforce the message and the written instructions should clearly illustrate warning signs of hematoma and hypocalcemia along with phone numbers where the surgeon can be reached (**Box 2**).

Careful patient selection is certainly important for outpatient surgery, but the extent of the planned procedure is also a key element in deciding whether to admit or discharge the patient. In particular, performing lymph node dissection represents a more comprehensive surgery that can potentially increase the risk of bleeding as well as lymphatic leak. The vast majority of studies evaluating complication risk after thyroidectomy (either inpatient or outpatient) focused solely on thyroid resection and did not include patients undergoing either central or lateral neck dissection. Rosenbaum and colleagues,[27] Stack and colleagues,[8] and Mowschenson and colleagues[4] did include lymph node dissection and the hematoma rate in these studies was not significantly different from the other groups in **Table 1**. That being said, a surgeon who is attempting outpatient thyroidectomy for the first time may be better served by starting with simpler surgeries first and only adding more complex operations and patients after a greater level of comfort has been reached.

A final component of building a successful outpatient thyroidectomy practice is preparing patients for the possibility of admission when the plan is for same-day discharge. Even the most straightforward surgery can be complicated by postoperative nausea, inadequate pain control, or difficulty maintaining adequate oxygenation or blood pressure. It is also difficult to predict what will be found at the time of the operation, which may influence surgeon comfort level with doing a case as an outpatient procedure. Having the conversation before the day of surgery can help patients to understand that the final discharge plan is flexible and contingent on what actually happens at the time of surgery. This planning may decrease unhappiness from patients who end up spending the night in the hospital instead of their own bed as expected.

Box 2
Instructions for outpatient thyroid surgery

Postoperative instructions
Contacting Your Surgeon

You can reach your surgeon at the following number: (999) 999-9999 If you are unable to reach your surgeon at this number, please call the hospital at (999) 999-9999 and ask for the surgeon on call to discuss your condition.

Complications and symptoms you need to watch for
Bleeding in Your Neck

Some bruising is normal but you should not have rapid or excess bruising and this may be owing to bleeding in your neck. This is rare, but if you are panicked owing to trouble breathing, sudden swelling in your throat, or are unable to swallow, call 911 immediately.

Low Calcium

If you develop numbness and tingling in your face, lips, fingertips, or toes take four 500-mg tablets of calcium carbonate (TUMS). The symptoms should go away in 15 to 30 minutes. If the symptoms persist, at 30 minutes you can repeat this. If the symptoms do still do not go away, call your doctor.

Infection

If you have a temperature above 100.4°F by mouth for 2 readings taken 4 hours apart, increased redness and/or warmth at the incision site, puslike drainage, or pain not relieved by pain pills, there may be an infection in your neck. Please call your doctor.

TECHNIQUES TO IMPROVE SUCCESS OF OUTPATIENT THYROIDECTOMY

Several techniques have been used to promote recovery and facilitate the use of outpatient thyroidectomy. These include the use of local rather than general anesthesia, dexamethasone to reduce nausea, intraoperative nerve monitoring, and the use of postoperative PTH testing to identify patients at risk for hypocalcemia.

Anesthesia Techniques and Antinausea Medication

In an effort to expedite recovery and avoid the side effects of general anesthesia, several groups have successfully performed thyroid surgery under local anesthesia. Inabnet and colleagues[28] published their experience with adopting local anesthesia for both unilateral and bilateral thyroidectomy and found that 88% of patients in the local anesthesia group were able to avoid inpatient admission, whereas only 45% of the general anesthesia cohort were successfully treated as outpatients. They also found that mean operative time was decreased from 101 to 71 minutes, although the mean thyroid weight in the local anesthesia group was less than 50% of the weight for the general anesthesia group. Snyder and colleagues[29] conducted a randomized trial comparing local with general anesthesia for thyroidectomy. The authors did not find a difference in operating time, but the overall total time spent in the postanesthesia care unit and surgical recovery area was nearly 1 hour less in the local anesthesia group. Although one of the presumed benefits of local anesthesia is decreased nausea and vomiting compared with general anesthesia, the authors did not find a difference in either nausea or vomiting within 24 hours of surgery.

Another study showed that the choice of anesthetic agent can significantly affect the rate of postoperative nausea and vomiting. Vari and colleagues[30] compared patient outcomes after the use of sevoflurane compared with propofol for maintenance of anesthesia and found that women had nearly a 30% reduction in nausea and vomiting when propofol rather than sevoflurane was used. This difference was not replicated in men; 47% in the sevoflurane group and 50% of the propofol group experienced postoperative nausea or vomiting. The use of antiemetic agents was also higher overall for patients receiving sevoflurane compared with propofol, and the only hematoma occurred in a patient after sevoflurane was used. A similar study by Sonner and colleagues[31] showed a 20% reduction in postoperative nausea and vomiting when patients received propofol compared with isoflurane for anesthesia maintenance. Once again, the benefit was limited to women, who experienced an approximately 30% decrease in nausea and vomiting.

Many medications are given to patients to try to minimize postoperative nausea because postoperative vomiting can not only delay discharge, but can increase cervical pressure and contribute to hematoma formation. Bononi and colleagues[32] conducted a randomized trial of 562 patients comparing the use of ondansetron versus ondansetron plus dexamethasone for high-risk cases. They found that the incidence of postoperative vomiting was reduced by a strategy combining ondansetron with dexamethasone, although the hematoma rate was equally low in both groups.

Nerve Monitoring

Intraoperative nerve monitoring is a potentially useful adjunct to facilitate safe outpatient surgery. The use of nerve monitors may not decrease the incidence of nerve injury, but it does provide a useful assessment of nerve function throughout the case. If the nerve signal is intact after the operation is complete, one can be reasonably comfortable that no injury has occurred. Conversely, signal loss can alert the surgeon to the possibility of nerve injury and patients can then be assessed postoperatively and either undergo further workup with a laryngoscopy or swallow evaluation, or at least be educated on techniques to minimize aspiration risk. Patients with suspected nerve injury could also be admitted overnight for further observation before discharge the next day to better assess the implications of nerve injury and determine the need for additional intervention. Regardless of how surgeons choose to use the information obtained from nerve monitoring, it can be used to adapt the discharge plan to minimize risk to the patient and avoid discovering complications only after discharge.

Postoperative Parathyroid Hormone

An unfortunate complication of total thyroidectomy is the risk of hypoparathyroidism with subsequent symptoms from hypocalcemia. Considerable effort has been devoted to predicting the risk of postoperative hypoparathyroidism so that patients who are at high risk can receive calcium with or without calcitriol after surgery. Several groups have attempted to use postoperative PTH levels to predict the risk of symptomatic hypocalcemia because PTH is a reflection of parathyroid function.[21] We developed a protocol that used a 4-hour postoperative PTH to stratify the risk for developing symptomatic hypocalcemia.[23,24] Patients in the highest risk group (PTH <10) were discharged with both calcitriol and calcium supplementation, moderate risk patients (PTH 10–20) received calcium alone, and all Graves' disease patients received calcium routinely. The protocol resulted in only 3.9% of patients having symptomatic hypocalcemia and only 0.1% of patients being readmitted. We have subsequently modified our protocol to use PTH levels drawn in the postanesthesia care unit immediately after surgery with similar results. We have also increased the dose of calcitriol given to patients with PTH levels that are less than 5 and have been able to further decrease the incidence of symptomatic hypocalcemia. For institutions without access to PTH testing, routine supplementation with calcium and calcitriol may be a cost-effective strategy to decrease symptoms and readmissions.

SUMMARY

Outpatient thyroid surgery is likely to remain controversial for the immediate future given concerns over the potential consequences of a neck hematoma. However, when performed by an experienced surgeon with adequate infrastructure and good patient selection, it should be possible to offer a safe outpatient operation with excellent patient satisfaction. Ongoing efforts to better define what constitutes a high-risk patient should continue to improve patient selection and minimize risk.

REFERENCES

1. Tuggle CT, Roman S, Udelsman R, et al. Same-day thyroidectomy: a review of practice patterns and outcomes for 1,168 procedures in New York State. Ann Surg Oncol 2011;18(4):1035–40.
2. Sun GH, DeMonner S, Davis MM. Epidemiological and economic trends in inpatient and outpatient thyroidectomy in the United States, 1996-2006. Thyroid 2013; 23(6):727–33.
3. Terris DJ, Snyder S, Carneiro-Pla D, et al. American Thyroid Association statement on outpatient thyroidectomy. Thyroid 2013;23(10):1193–202.
4. Mowschenson PM, Hodin RA. Outpatient thyroid and parathyroid surgery: a prospective study of feasibility, safety, and costs. Surgery 1995;118(6):1051–3 [discussion: 1053–4].
5. Mazeh H, Khan Q, Schneider DF, et al. Same-day thyroidectomy program: eligibility and safety evaluation. Surgery 2012;152(6):1133–41.
6. Seybt MW, Terris DJ. Outpatient thyroidectomy: experience in over 200 patients. Laryngoscope 2010;120(5):959–63.
7. Spanknebel K, Chabot JA, DiGiorgi M, et al. Thyroidectomy using local anesthesia: a report of 1,025 cases over 16 years. J Am Coll Surg 2005;201(3): 375–85.
8. Stack BC Jr, Moore E, Spencer H, et al. Outpatient thyroid surgery data from the University Health System (UHC) Consortium. Otolaryngol Head Neck Surg 2013; 148(5):740–5.
9. Terris DJ, Moister B, Seybt MW, et al. Outpatient thyroid surgery is safe and desirable. Otolaryngol Head Neck Surg 2007;136(4):556–9.
10. Samson PS, Reyes FR, Saludares WN, et al. Outpatient thyroidectomy. Am J Surg 1997;173(6):499–503.
11. Godballe C, Madsen AR, Pedersen HB, et al. Post-thyroidectomy hemorrhage: a national study of patients treated at the Danish departments of ENT Head and Neck Surgery. Eur Arch Otorhinolaryngol 2009;266(12):1945–52.
12. Thomusch O, Machens A, Sekulla C, et al. Multivariate analysis of risk factors for postoperative complications in benign goiter surgery: prospective multicenter study in Germany. World J Surg 2000;24(11):1335–41.
13. Bergenfelz A, Jansson S, Kristoffersson A, et al. Complications to thyroid surgery: results as reported in a database from a multicenter audit comprising 3,660 patients. Langenbecks Arch Surg 2008;393(5):667–73.
14. Rosato L, Avenia N, Bernante P, et al. Complications of thyroid surgery: analysis of a multicentric study on 14,934 patients operated on in Italy over 5 years. World J Surg 2004;28(3):271–6.

15. Burkey SH, van Heerden JA, Thompson GB, et al. Reexploration for symptomatic hematomas after cervical exploration. Surgery 2001;130(6):914–20.

16. Bergamaschi R, Becouarn G, Ronceray J, et al. Morbidity of thyroid surgery. Am J Surg 1998;176(1):71–5.

17. Lang BH, Yih PC, Lo CY. A review of risk factors and timing for postoperative hematoma after thyroidectomy: is outpatient thyroidectomy really safe? World J Surg 2012;36(10):2497–502.

18. Leyre P, Desurmont T, Lacoste L, et al. Does the risk of compressive hematoma after thyroidectomy authorize 1-day surgery? Langenbecks Arch Surg 2008; 393(5):733–7.

19. Promberger R, Ott J, Kober F, et al. Risk factors for postoperative bleeding after thyroid surgery. Br J Surg 2012;99(3):373–9.

20. Kaushik R. Bleeding complications in laparoscopic cholecystectomy: Incidence, mechanisms, prevention and management. J Minim Access Surg 2010;6(3): 59–65.

21. Grodski S, Serpell J. Evidence for the role of perioperative PTH measurement after total thyroidectomy as a predictor of hypocalcemia. World J Surg 2008;32(7): 1367–73.

22. Wang TS, Cheung K, Roman SA, et al. To supplement or not to supplement: a cost-utility analysis of calcium and vitamin D repletion in patients after thyroidectomy. Ann Surg Oncol 2011;18(5):1293–9.

23. Carter Y, Chen H, Sippel RS. An intact parathyroid hormone-based protocol for the prevention and treatment of symptomatic hypocalcemia after thyroidectomy. J Surg Res 2014;186(1):23–8.

24. Youngwirth L, Benavidez J, Sippel R, et al. Postoperative parathyroid hormone testing decreases symptomatic hypocalcemia and associated emergency room visits after total thyroidectomy. Surgery 2010;148(4):841–4 [discussion: 844–6].

25. Champault A, Vons C, Zilberman S, et al. How to perform a thyroidectomy in an outpatient setting. Langenbecks Arch Surg 2009;394(5):897–902.

26. Trottier DC, Barron P, Moonje V, et al. Outpatient thyroid surgery: should patients be discharged on the day of their procedures? Can J Surg 2009;52(3):182–6.

27. Rosenbaum MA, Haridas M, McHenry CR. Life-threatening neck hematoma complicating thyroid and parathyroid surgery. Am J Surg 2008;195(3):339–43 [discussion: 343].

28. Inabnet WB, Shifrin A, Ahmed L, et al. Safety of same day discharge in patients undergoing sutureless thyroidectomy: a comparison of local and general anesthesia. Thyroid 2008;18(1):57–61.

29. Snyder SK, Roberson CR, Cummings CC, et al. Local anesthesia with monitored anesthesia care vs general anesthesia in thyroidectomy: a randomized study. Arch Surg 2006;141(2):167–73.

30. Vari A, Gazzanelli S, Cavallaro G, et al. Post-operative nausea and vomiting (PONV) after thyroid surgery: a prospective, randomized study comparing totally intravenous versus inhalational anesthetics. Am Surg 2010;76(3):325–8.

31. Sonner JM, Hynson JM, Clark O, et al. Nausea and vomiting following thyroid and parathyroid surgery. J Clin Anesth 1997;9(5):398–402.

32. Bononi M, Amore Bonapasta S, Vari A, et al. Incidence and circumstances of cervical hematoma complicating thyroidectomy and its relationship to postoperative vomiting. Head Neck 2010;32(9):1173–7.

33. Chang LY, O'Neill C, Suliburk J, et al. Sutureless total thyroidectomy: a safe and cost-effective alternative. ANZ J Surg 2011;81(7-8):510–4.

34. Hessman C, Fields J, Schuman E. Outpatient thyroidectomy: is it a safe and reasonable option? Am J Surg 2011;201(5):565–8.
35. Zambudio AR, Rodriguez J, Riquelme J, et al. Prospective study of postoperative complications after total thyroidectomy for multinodular goiters by surgeons with experience in endocrine surgery. Ann Surg 2004;240(1):18–25.

Asymptomatic Primary Hyperparathyroidism

Diagnostic Pitfalls and Surgical Intervention

James X. Wu, MD*, Michael W. Yeh, MD

KEYWORDS

- Asymptomatic primary hyperparathyroidism • Parathyroid hormone
- Parathyroidectomy • Hypercalcemia • Nonclassic primary hyperparathyroidism

KEY POINTS

- In most cases, primary hyperparathyroidism can be diagnosed by measuring serum calcium and parathyroid hormone.
- Nearly half of cases of primary hyperparathyroidism have a "nonclassic" presentation, with hypercalcemia and inappropriately normal parathyroid hormone levels.
- Parathyroidectomy has become a more commonplace and safe procedure, but many patients, especially elderly patients, are not appropriately referred for surgical consultation.

INTRODUCTION

Primary hyperparathyroidism (PHPT) is a disease caused by the excess production of parathyroid hormone (PTH), resulting in the dysregulation of calcium metabolism. The current estimated prevalence of PHPT is as high as 1 in every 400 women, and 1 in 1000 men.[1] Symptoms caused by hypercalcemia and elevated PTH levels manifest insidiously over an extended period of time; most patients with PHPT are asymptomatic, with only a small fraction exhibiting classic signs and symptoms. Patients with asymptomatic disease were largely undiagnosed until the advent of the multichannel autoanalyzer in the 1970s, which subsequently led to the adoption of routine serum calcium measurements. Detection of hypercalcemia on routine serum calcium screening has greatly facilitated the diagnosis of PHPT: from 1995 to 2010, the

The authors have nothing to disclose.

Section of Endocrine Surgery, UCLA David Geffen School of Medicine, 10833 Le Conte Avenue, Los Angeles, CA 90095, USA

* Corresponding author. UCLA David Geffen School of Medicine, 10833 Le Conte Avenue, 72-228 CHS, Los Angeles, CA 90095.

E-mail address: JamesWu@mednet.ucla.edu

http://dx.doi.org/10.1016/j.soc.2015.08.004
1055-3207/16/$ – see front matter
surgonc.theclinics.com

incidence of PHPT tripled.[1] This article addresses the diagnosis and surgical management of asymptomatic PHPT.

BIOCHEMICAL DIAGNOSIS OF PRIMARY HYPERPARATHYROIDISM

Our standard biochemical panel for the initial workup of suspected PHPT is shown in **Box 1**. Most ambulatory patients have normal serum phosphorus, creatinine, and albumin. Hence, the diagnosis can be determined by serum calcium and serum PTH in most cases. We routinely measure the serum 25-hydroxy (25-OH) vitamin D level to clarify the diagnosis in borderline cases, and to help differentiate between primary and secondary hyperparathyroidism.

Calcium

Suspicion of asymptomatic hyperparathyroidism typically begins with incidental detection of elevated serum calcium. A single elevation of the serum calcium is frequently spurious. Therefore, repeat testing of the serum calcium is recommended before proceeding further in the diagnostic workup of PHPT. Because 40% to 45% of serum calcium is protein-bound, total serum calcium should be corrected for serum albumin. Corrected serum calcium is calculated by the following: measured total serum calcium (mg/dL) + 0.8 (4.0 − measured serum albumin [g/dL]). Per the recent 2013 guidelines established by the Fourth International Workshop on the Management of Asymptomatic Primary Hyperparathyroidism, total serum calcium should be used to establish the diagnosis and not ionized calcium, because ionized calcium testing is not widely available.[2]

Ionized calcium directly measures the bioactive (free) fraction of serum calcium, which more accurately reflects patients' true calcium status than albumin-corrected total calcium, particularly for patients with hyperparathyroidism.[3] Among patients with histologically confirmed PHPT, up to 24% have elevated ionized calcium levels despite normal total calcium levels.[4,5] Additionally, ionized calcium may be informative in hypoalbuminemic patients (ie, patients with cirrhosis or nephrotic syndrome) with suspected PHPT. However, we have noted greater intra-assay variability when

---

Box 1
Initial diagnostic workup of hyperparathyroidism

Routine tests

Serum calcium

Parathyroid hormone

Serum phosphorus

Serum creatinine

Serum albumin

Optional tests

Ionized calcium (hypoalbuminemic patients, borderline diagnoses)

25-OH vitamin D (nonclassic presentation or suspected vitamin D deficiency)

Urinary calcium excretion (suggestive family history for FHH)

Abbreviation: FHH, familial hypocalciuric hypercalcemia.

measuring ionized calcium compared with total calcium, which may be attributed to the pH-dependence of ionized calcium.

Parathyroid Hormone

Excess production of PTH can be easily determined by measuring serum PTH. Serum PTH should be interpreted in the context of serum calcium. In patients with hypercalcemia or calcium levels near the upper limit of the reference range, an elevated serum PTH is diagnostic of PHPT. However, a normal PTH level does not rule out PHPT; up to half of patients with PHPT have hypercalcemia with inappropriately normal levels of PTH.[1,6]

PTH assay has undergone evolution over the past 53 years.[7] First-generation PTH assays are obsolete, now replaced by second-generation and third-generation assays. The second-generation PTH assays cross-react with large degradation products of PTH, whereas third-generation assays are more specific for biologically active PTH. Nonetheless, the diagnostic sensitivity of second-generation and third-generation PTH assays are similar for PHPT.[8] In patients with chronic kidney disease, impaired clearance of degradation products of PTH will result in much higher readings with second-generation assays compared with third-generation assays. Third-generation PTH assays also have greater utility as intraoperative PTH assays.[9] Today, most commercial PTH assays are second-generation assays, but also include third-generation assays. Significant variability has been demonstrated between commercially available assays, even between tests of the same generation, so it is important to remain consistent and to interpret results using test-specific reference ranges.[10,11]

Hypercalcemia with Inappropriately Normal Parathyroid Hormone: Nonclassic Primary Hyperparathyroidism

In some patients with PHPT, serum PTH is not elevated above the 95% reference range. An inappropriately normal (nonsuppressed) PTH level despite hypercalcemia is still indicative of disrupted negative feedback, and confirms the diagnosis of nonclassic PHPT. Nonclassic PHPT simply refers to PHPT that presents with elevated serum calcium but inappropriately normal PTH (PTH 21–65 pg/mL). In a study of 3.5 million patients within a vertically integrated health care organization, we found that the number of patients with nonclassic PHPT nearly equaled the number with classic PHPT (**Fig. 1**).[1] Patients with nonclassic PHPT were not regularly monitored, infrequently underwent bone densitometry measurement, and were rarely referred for surgery, reflecting missed or delayed recognition of the diagnosis. In our practice, we

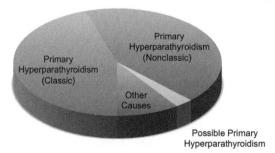

Fig. 1. Causes of hypercalcemia. Classic primary hyperparathyroidism: hypercalcemia and PTH; Nonclassic primary hyperparathyroidism: hypercalcemia with inappropriately normal (nonsuppressed) parathyroid hormone.

have noted considerable confusion on the part of general practitioners and even endocrinologists with regard to establishing the diagnosis nonclassic PHPT.

Vitamin D

Although vitamin D levels are not required to establish the diagnosis of PHPT in patients with "classic" PHPT, serum 25-OH vitamin D levels can clarify the diagnosis in challenging or borderline cases. Because adequate levels of vitamin D can suppress PTH secretion, the Endocrine Society and Institute of Medicine both agree that the reference range of PTH values for vitamin D–replete patients should be lower than for patients who are vitamin D deficient. The strict definition of "vitamin D replete" is controversial, as the Institute of Medicine and 2013 International Workshop both recommend a threshold of 50 nmol/L to be considered "vitamin D replete," whereas the Endocrine Society has recommended a more stringent threshold of 75 nmol/L.[12] Reference ranges for PTH for vitamin D replete versus vitamin D deficient have not been well characterized, and remain an area for future research. Nonetheless, clinicians should have a higher degree of suspicion for PHPT in hypercalcemic patients with inappropriately normal serum PTH who are vitamin D replete.

Vitamin D measurements are also important in patients who have elevated serum PTH but normal or high-normal serum calcium to rule out secondary hyperparathyroidism due to vitamin D deficiency. Vitamin D deficiency is quite commonplace, and may account for normal or high-normal PTH values in patients with PHPT. The estimated prevalence of vitamin D deficiency in adults is as high as 41.6%, and more common among individuals with pigmented skin, obesity, or poor milk intake.[13] Among internal medicine housestaff, 51.4% of residents were found to be vitamin D deficient at some point over the course of a year, more so during winter months.[14] Significant vitamin D deficiency can cause a physiologic increase in PTH secretion, mimicking incipient (normocalcemic) PHPT. PHPT and secondary hyperparathyroidism due to vitamin D deficiency can be distinguished by measuring serum 25-OH vitamin D.

Patients who have undergone malabsorptive bariatric surgery (ie, Roux-en-Y gastric bypass, biliopancreatic diversion with duodenal switch) frequently experience postoperative fat-soluble vitamin deficiencies, including vitamin D deficiency.[15] This does not include purely restrictive bariatric procedures, such as vertical banded gastroplasty or sleeve gastrectomy. Vitamin D deficiency and elevated PTH following malabsorptive bariatric surgery are not only long-term, but may also worsen over time.[16–18] Furthermore, patients who have undergone bariatric surgery have been shown to have impaired calcium absorption despite normal 25-OH vitamin D levels.[19] In our practice, patients who have undergone malabsorptive bariatric surgery are assumed to have secondary hyperparathyroidism due to vitamin D deficiency unless hypercalcemia has been confirmed with laboratory testing.

Urinary Calcium Excretion

Urinary calcium excretion can help distinguish PHPT from familial hypocalciuric hypercalcemia, where patients also experience hypercalcemia and have elevated levels of serum PTH. However, familial hypocalciuric hypercalcemia (FHH) is rare, with an estimated prevalence of 1 in 78,000 in the general population.[20,21] Thus, we only obtain urinary calcium excretion in patients with a suggestive family history. Patients with familial hypocalciuric hypercalcemia will have 24-hour urine calcium excretion less than 100 mg. Of note, patients with vitamin D deficiency superimposed on PHPT can have low 24-hour urinary calcium excretion, although generally closer to low-normal levels of approximately 200 mg.

CONSIDERATIONS FOR DIFFERENTIAL DIAGNOSIS
Familial Hypocalciuric Hypercalcemia

FHH is a disorder caused by a mutation in the calcium-sensing receptor (CaSR) found in a number of organs, including the parathyroid glands and kidneys. The parathyroid glands are unable to sense changes in serum calcium, and do not inhibit secretion of PTH in response to elevated serum calcium. More importantly, CaSR regulates renal excretion of calcium; the CaSR mutation in patients with FHH inhibits renal calcium excretion, leading to hypercalcemia. Patients with familial hypocalciuric hypercalcemia have elevated serum calcium, and up to 20% also have mild elevations in serum PTH, mimicking PHPT. As stated previously, the main distinguishing feature of FHH is low urinary calcium excretion, whereas urinary calcium excretion is normal or high in PHPT. Patients with FHH also typically exhibit hypercalcemia in childhood, and do not show signs and symptoms of hypercalcemia.

Malignancy

Malignancy is the second most common cause of hypercalcemia after PHPT, and the most common cause of hypercalcemia among inpatients. Hypercalcemia of malignancy can occur via a number of different mechanisms: humoral hypercalcemia of malignancy caused by secretion of PTH-related protein (PTHrP), osteoclast-mediated osteolysis typically caused by bony metastatic disease, or, in rare cases, ectopic secretion of 1,25-OH vitamin D or PTH (**Fig. 2**).[22] In most cases, hypercalcemia of malignancy occurs after malignancy is clinically evident. Hypercalcemia of malignancy should lead to suppression of endogenous PTH, so it can easily be distinguished from PHPT by measuring serum PTH and/or serum PTHrP. In rare cases, there can be concomitant hyperparathyroidism where PTH will be elevated as well as parathyroid-related peptide.

Thiazides

Thiazide diuretics act on the distal convoluted tubule of the kidney, reducing calcium excretion, and can cause a mild hypercalcemia. Patients with mild hypercalcemia with normal or high-normal PTH should discontinue thiazide medications and have calcium and PTH reassessed after 3 months. Elevated serum calcium despite withdrawal of thiazides supports the diagnosis of PHPT.

Lithium

The exact mechanism of action of lithium on calcium metabolism is unknown, although it is hypothesized to act downstream of the calcium-sensing receptor.

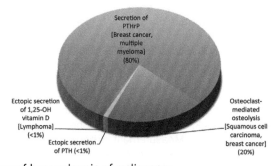

Fig. 2. Mechanisms of hypercalcemia of malignancy.

Lithium appears to interfere with CaSR activity in the parathyroid gland and kidneys, leading to elevated PTH levels, hypercalcemia, and hypocalciuria. If possible, patients with hypercalcemia should be switched to an alternative medication and have their calcium retested.

INDICATIONS, RISKS, AND BENEFITS OF PARATHYROIDECTOMY FOR PRIMARY HYPERPARATHYROIDISM

Surgery is the only curative therapy for PHPT, and is clearly indicated in all symptomatic patients. Even for asymptomatic patients, parathyroidectomy halts, or even reverses, the classic negative effects of this disease: parathyroidectomy decreases the risk of nephrolithiasis and improves bone mineral density (BMD).[23–27] There is also additional evidence that parathyroidectomy may also improve quality of life in "asymptomatic" patients, possibly by alleviating nonspecific or atypical symptoms.[26–29] Finally, there may still be unrecognized effects of asymptomatic PHPT: a large population-based study examining 2299 patients with untreated asymptomatic PHPT found an increased risk of nonfatal and fatal cardiovascular disease and all-cause mortality.[30]

In the past decade, the safety of parathyroidectomy has improved: the overall complication rate following 17,082 patients who underwent parathyroidectomy fell from 8.7% to 3.8% from 1999 to 2008.[31] The most common surgical complication was hypocalcemia, and vocal cord paresis accounts for only 3.7% of all complications.[31]

The indications for surgery in asymptomatic hyperparathyroidism have been an area of intense research and debate. The first official guidelines for surgery for asymptomatic hyperparathyroidism were established in 1990, at a consensus conference sponsored by the National Institutes of Health.[32] These guidelines have undergone several revisions by conferences convened in 2002 and 2008, and most recently during the 2013 Fourth International Workshop on the Management of Asymptomatic Primary Hyperparathyroidism.[2,33–35] The surgical criteria for parathyroidectomy are listed, by year of consensus statement, in **Table 1**. Analyses of the individual components of surgical criteria for PHPT are as follows.

SURGICAL CRITERIA FOR ASYMPTOMATIC PRIMARY HYPERPARATHYROIDISM
Serum Calcium

The most recent 2013 guidelines maintained that surgery is recommended for patients with serum calcium 1.0 mg/dL above the upper limit of the reference range. No recommendations based on ionized serum calcium were made, because the test is not yet widely available. The current recommendation has been in place since 2002, and is based on the consensus that hypercalcemia above this threshold increases the risk of disease progression to symptomatic PHPT. Patients below this threshold who are managed nonoperatively should undergo annual serum calcium testing. Tests for initial evaluation and observation of patients with asymptomatic PHPT are listed in **Table 2**.

Skeletal Criteria

The 2013 Workshop recommends surgery for patients with a T-score less than −2.5 at the lumbar spine, femoral neck, total hip, or distal one-third of the radius on dual-energy X-ray densitometry (DXA). Measurement of bone density at the distal forearm is the most important, but often omitted, part of DXA for patients with PHPT. Bone loss in PHPT occurs more rapidly in cortical bone than trabecular bone; thus, bone loss will

Table 1
Surgical criteria for parathyroidectomy in asymptomatic primary hyperparathyroidism, by year of consensus guidelines

	1990	2002	2009	2013
Serum calcium	1–1.6 mg/dL above reference range	1.0 mg/dL above reference range	1.0 mg/dL above reference range	1.0 mg/dL above reference range
Skeletal criteria	DXA: Z-score <−2	DXA: T-score <−2.5 at any site	DXA: T-score <−2.5 at any site	DXA: T-score <−2.5 at lumbar spine, total hip, femoral neck, or distal one-third radius Vertebral fracture by spinal imaging or vertebral fracture assessment
Renal criteria	eGFR reduction >30% from expected 24-h urine calcium excretion >400 mg	eGFR reduction >30% from expected 24-h urine calcium excretion >400 mg	eGFR <60 mL/min	Creatinine clearance <60 mL/min 24-h urine calcium excretion >400 mg AND High-risk urinary biochemical stone risk analysis Nephrocalcinosis or nephrolithiasis
Age	Age <50	Age <50	Age <50	Age <50

Abbreviations: DXA, dual-energy X-ray absorptiometry; eGFR, estimated glomerular filtration rate.
Adapted from Bilezikian JP, Brandi ML, Eastell R, et al. Guidelines for the management of asymptomatic primary hyperparathyroidism: summary statement from the Fourth International Workshop. J Clin Endocrinol Metab 2014;99(10):3562.

likely first be evident at the distal forearm, which is mostly composed of cortical bone.[36] Despite this, only 45% of patients with PHPT who receive DXA testing undergo testing of the distal radius.[37] DXA testing reports 2 scores: a Z-score, which reports BMD compared with patients of the same age, gender, and race, as well as a T-score, which is BMD compared with a healthy 30-year-old. Starting in 2002, the consensus conferences have recommended exclusively using the T-score, which is more reflective of absolute changes in BMD over time in the same individual.

This focus on preserving BMD is meant to identify patients who have an elevated fracture risk, and to reduce that risk through surgery. It is clear that patients with asymptomatic PHPT experience progressive bone loss that can be prevented with surgical intervention.[23–27,38] It is currently unknown whether this loss of BMD in asymptomatic PHPT also increases fracture risk. Retrospective studies of patients with PHPT of varying severity have an increased fracture risk compared with age-matched and sex-matched controls, which normalizes after parathyroidectomy.[39,40] Further studies are needed to determine whether parathyroidectomy reduces fracture risk in asymptomatic PHPT.

A new recommendation is to evaluate patients with asymptomatic PHPT for vertebral fractures using radiographs, computed tomography (CT), MRI, or vertebral fracture assessment (VFA). Compared with 4% in age-matched controls, patients with asymptomatic PHPT who meet surgical criteria have a 28% risk of vertebral fracture,

Table 2
Tests for initial evaluation and observation of asymptomatic primary hyperparathyroidism

Initial Evaluation of Asymptomatic Primary Hyperparathyroidism	Observation of Asymptomatic Primary Hyperparathyroidism
Laboratory testing (serum calcium, phosphate, creatinine, albumin, 25-OH vitamin D)	Annual serum calcium
DXA	DXA every 1–2 y
Vertebral spine assessment (radiograph, CT, MRI, or VFA)	Radiograph, CT, MRI, or VFA if patients develop back pain or height loss
24-h urine stone risk profile	Annual estimated glomerular filtration rate, serum creatinine
Renal imaging (radiograph, ultrasound, CT)	24-h biochemical stone profile, renal imaging (radiograph, ultrasound, CT) if suspected nephrolithiasis

Abbreviations: CT, computed tomography; DXA, dual-energy X-ray absorptiometry; VFA, vertebral fracture assessment.

and those who do not meet surgical criteria have an 11% risk.[41] A recent study of 140 patients with PHPT diagnosed in 2009 to 2013 found that 34.7% of patients with asymptomatic PHPT had evidence of vertebral fracture on spinal radiograph.[42] VFA is a particular radiographic methodology using DXA to detect vertebral fractures, but has been found to be less predictive than trabecular bone score in nonosteoporotic patients.[43] Trabecular bone score (TBS) is an emerging technology that better detects and predicts vertebral fracture than BMD determined by DXA. TBS is generated by using computer software to apply a gray-level textural analysis to existing DXA images and should be easily available to institutions able to perform DXA scans.[44] A TBS score of less than 1.2 has an area-under-the-curve of 0.716 for detecting vertebral fractures within in a population that otherwise had similar BMD.[45] Last, TBS has been shown to improve after parathyroidectomy.[45]

Patients with asymptomatic PHPT are recommended to undergo DXA every 1 to 2 years, which must include measurement of 3 different sites, including the distal radius, and imaging or VFA of the spine if they are experiencing height loss or back pain.

Renal Criteria

The 2013 Workshop identified 3 renal criteria for parathyroidectomy: (1) Creatinine clearance less than 60 mL/min, (2) 24-hour urine calcium greater than 400 mg AND increased risk by urinary biochemical stone risk analysis, and (3) nephrolithiasis or nephrocalcinosis seen on radiograph, ultrasound, or CT.

The first criterion, creatinine clearance less than 60 mL/min, represents the onset of stage 3 or greater chronic kidney disease (CKD).[46] This recommendation was made, in part, based on the assumption that serum calcium and PTH levels rise with progressive kidney disease, which may lead to worse disease sequelae of PHPT. However, recent studies have shown that serum calcium is not significantly elevated in stage 3 or 4 CKD, and PTH is only significantly elevated in patients with creatinine clearance less than 30 mL/min.[47,48] Nonetheless, creatinine clearance less than 60 mL/min is associated with altered bone remodeling, suggesting that impaired renal function may negatively impact bone health in a manner unrelated to PTH and calcium in patients with PHPT.[47,48]

Second, surgery is recommended for patients with urinary calcium excretion of greater than 400 mg, and if the patient is determined to be at high risk by urinary biochemical stone risk analysis. Urinary biochemical kidney stone risk panels are widely available through commercial laboratories, and involve testing of calcium, creatinine, uric acid, citric acid, and oxalate levels in urine collected over 24 hours. Although the 1990 Panel had initially recommended surgery for high urinary calcium excretion alone, the 2008 Committee determined that there was no evidence that high urine calcium excretion alone predicts formation of kidney stones.

Finally, the 2013 guidelines recommend patients diagnosed with asymptomatic PHPT should undergo renal imaging to detect subclinical nephrolithiasis or nephrocalcinosis. Renal ultrasound performed on 141 patients with PHPT without a history of nephrolithiasis found silent nephrolithiasis in 11% of patients, compared with 2% in controls.[49] Another recent study found that 35.5% of patients with asymptomatic PHPT were found to have kidney stones on renal ultrasound.[42] Any abnormal findings on renal imaging would be an indication for parathyroidectomy.

Patients who do not undergo surgery should be encouraged to maintain adequate hydration at all times, possibly with above-average fluid intake. These patients should receive annual laboratory testing of estimated glomerular filtration rate and creatinine. If patients have signs and symptoms of possible kidney stones, repeat urine biochemical stone risk profile and/or renal imaging should be obtained.

Age

The 2013 guidelines continue to support age younger than 50 as a criterion for surgery. The rationale is that younger patients have sufficient life expectancy to derive benefit from surgical resection, regardless of disease severity. Among patients younger than 50 who do not meet surgical criteria (aside from age), 27% to 62% will progress to meet surgical criteria in 9 to 10 years.[50,51] None of these patients developed fractures or renal stones during the study period. Moreover, the percentage of disease progression was overestimated: these studies included the development of urinary calcium excretion greater than 400 mg per day as a surgical indication, which was the sole reason nearly half of the patients defined as having progression of disease. Urinary calcium excretion alone was eliminated as a criterion in 2009, and the 2013 Workshop now recommends surgery for urinary calcium excretion of 400 mg per day and high-risk urinary biochemical stone risk profile.

The focus on younger patients should not deter clinicians from recommending surgery in elderly patients who meet surgical criteria. Most patients with PHPT are older than 60, but many older patients who meet surgical criteria are not offered parathyroidectomy.[52] Only 24% of patients older than 70 who meet surgical criteria undergo parathyroidectomy.[52] Even for patients with PHPT who are older than 70 or 80, parathyroidectomy is associated with minimal morbidity, no mortality, high cure rate, and improvement in quality of life.[53,54] In our practice, we assess each patient according to their perioperative risk and "physiologic age" regardless of their chronologic age. Surgery should be offered to all patients with minimal perioperative risk and sufficient life expectancy.

Atypical Symptoms

Cardiovascular

No clear relationship has been established between asymptomatic PHPT and adverse cardiovascular outcomes. A study of 2097 patients with nonoperatively managed PHPT found that mild PHPT is associated with increased cardiovascular mortality, and that baseline PTH levels correlated with all-cause mortality as well as fatal and nonfatal cardiovascular disease.[55] Although these findings have yet to be confirmed with prospective studies, mild PHPT has been linked to elevated systolic blood pressure, lower 25-OH vitamin D levels, increased carotid artery stiffness, and increased carotid-intima thickness.[56,57] Conversely, a randomized controlled trial of surgery versus observation found no difference in blood pressure, biomarkers of endothelial function, or C-reactive protein 2 years after parathyroidectomy.[58] Several studies also have shown that parathyroidectomy has minimal or no effect on cardiac structure or function at 2 years.[59–61] Currently, there are insufficient data to include cardiovascular factors as criteria for parathyroidectomy. Prospective studies are needed to better characterize the effect of asymptomatic PHPT on cardiovascular outcomes.

Neuropsychiatric and cognitive

Despite being referred to as "asymptomatic" PHPT, many patients who do not exhibit typical signs and symptoms of PHPT do experience nonspecific neuropsychiatric symptoms. Following parathyroidectomy, patients with asymptomatic PHPT have reported improvements in overall quality of life, sleep disturbances, fatigue, aches and pains, weakness, constipation, and memory loss.[26–29] A prospective study of 24 patients with asymptomatic PHPT demonstrated improvement in the Hospital Depression and Mood Rating Scales after parathyroidectomy, using patients undergoing thyroid lobectomy for benign nodules as controls.[62–64] Despite these findings, the 2013 Workshop concluded that improvements in neuropsychiatric symptoms are not consistent between studies, and that there was no reliable method to predict which patients would benefit from surgery; therefore, neuropsychiatric dysfunction should not yet be considered in the decision to perform parathyroidectomy.[2]

SUMMARY

PHPT is a common disease, and the vast majority of patients with PHPT are asymptomatic. Classic PHPT can be easily diagnosed by elevated total calcium and PTH. However, one-half of cases of PHPT are nonclassic, and exhibit hypercalcemia with inappropriately normal (nonsuppressed) levels of PTH. For patients with asymptomatic PHPT, parathyroidectomy has been shown to increase BMD and improve quality of life, and may even decrease risk of fracture and adverse cardiovascular outcomes. It is our belief that surgery should be considered in all patients with asymptomatic PHPT who have minimal perioperative risk and sufficient life expectancy, regardless of chronologic age.

REFERENCES

1. Yeh MW, Ituarte PHG, Zhou HC, et al. Incidence and prevalence of primary hyperparathyroidism in a racially mixed population. J Clin Endocrinol Metab 2013;98: 1122–9.
2. Silverberg SJ, Clarke BL, Peacock M, et al. Current issues in the presentation of asymptomatic primary hyperparathyroidism: proceedings of the fourth international workshop. J Clin Endocrinol Metab 2014;99:3580–94.
3. Ladenson JH, Lewis JW, McDonald JM, et al. Relationship of free and total calcium in hypercalcemic conditions. J Clin Endocrinol Metab 1979;48:393–7.
4. Ong GS, Walsh JP, Stuckey BG, et al. The importance of measuring ionized calcium in characterizing calcium status and diagnosing primary hyperparathyroidism. J Clin Endocrinol Metab 2012;97:3138–45.

5. Glendenning P, Gutteridge DH, Retallack RW, et al. High prevalence of normal to-tal calcium and intact PTH in 60 patients with proven primary hyperparathyroid-ism: a challenge to current diagnostic criteria. Aust N Z J Med 1998;28:173–8.
6. Nussbaum SR, Zahradnik RJ, Lavigne JR, et al. Highly sensitive two-site immu-noradiometric assay of parathyrin, and its clinical utility in evaluating patients with hypercalcemia. Clin Chem 1987;33:1364–7.
7. Berson SA, Yalow RS, Aurbach GD, et al. Immunoassay of bovine and human parathyroid hormone. Proc Natl Acad Sci U S A 1963;49:613.
8. Boudou P, Ibrahim F, Cormier C, et al. Third- or second-generation parathyroid hormone assays: a remaining debate in the diagnosis of primary hyperparathy-roidism. J Clin Endocrinol Metab 2005;90:6370–2.
9. Cavalier E, Daly AF, Betea D, et al. The ratio of parathyroid hormone as measured by third- and second-generation assays as a marker for parathyroid carcinoma. J Clin Endocrinol Metab 2010;95:3745–9.
10. Tan K, Ong L, Sethi SK, et al. Comparison of the Elecsys PTH (1–84) assay with four contemporary second generation intact PTH assays and association with other biomarkers in chronic kidney disease patients. Clin Biochem 2013;46: 781–6.
11. Souberbielle JC, Boutten A, Carlier MC, et al. Inter-method variability in PTH mea-surement: implication for the care of CKD patients. Kidney Int 2006;70:345–50.
12. Eastell R, Brandi ML, Costa AG, et al. Diagnosis of asymptomatic primary hyper-parathyroidism: proceedings of the Fourth International Workshop. J Clin Endo-crinol Metab 2014;99:3570–9.
13. Forrest KY, Stuhldreher WL. Prevalence and correlates of vitamin D deficiency in US adults. Nutr Res 2011;31:48–54.
14. Haney EM, Stadler D, Bliziotes MM. Vitamin D insufficiency in internal medicine residents. Calcif Tissue Int 2005;76:11–6.
15. Slater GH, Ren CJ, Siegel N, et al. Serum fat-soluble vitamin deficiency and abnormal calcium metabolism after malabsorptive bariatric surgery. J Gastrointest Surg 2004;8:48–55.
16. Johnson JM, Maher JW, DeMaria EJ, et al. The long-term effects of gastric bypass on vitamin D metabolism. Ann Surg 2006;243:701.
17. Beckman LM, Earthman CP, Thomas W, et al. Serum 25 (OH) vitamin D concen-tration changes after Roux-en-Y gastric bypass surgery. Obesity (Silver Spring) 2013;21:E599–606.
18. Karefylakis C, Näslund I, Edholm D, et al. Vitamin D status 10 years after primary gastric bypass: gravely high prevalence of hypovitaminosis D and raised PTH levels. Obes Surg 2014;24:343–8.
19. Schafer AL, Weaver CM, Black DM, et al. Intestinal calcium absorption decreases dramatically after gastric bypass surgery despite optimization of vitamin D status. J Bone Miner Res 2015;30(8):1377–85.
20. Hinnie J, Bell E, McKillop E, et al. The prevalence of familial hypocalciuric hyper-calcemia. Calcif Tissue Int 2001;68:216–8.
21. Marx SJ. Familial hypocalciuric hypercalcemia. Clin Endocrinol 2013;2:217–32.
22. Stewart AF. Hypercalcemia associated with cancer. N Engl J Med 2005;352: 373–9.
23. Dy BM, Grant CS, Wermers RA, et al. Changes in bone mineral density after sur-gical intervention for primary hyperparathyroidism. Surgery 2012;152:1051–8.
24. VanderWalde LH, Liu IL, Haigh PI. Effect of bone mineral density and parathyroid-ectomy on fracture risk in primary hyperparathyroidism. World J Surg 2009;33: 406–11.

25. Bollerslev J, Jansson S, Mollerup CL, et al. Medical observation, compared with parathyroidectomy, for asymptomatic primary hyperparathyroidism: a prospective, randomized trial. J Clin Endocrinol Metab 2007;92:1687–92.

26. Ambrogini E, Cetani F, Cianferotti L, et al. Surgery or surveillance for mild asymptomatic primary hyperparathyroidism: a prospective, randomized clinical trial. J Clin Endocrinol Metab 2007;92:3114–21.

27. Rao DS, Phillips ER, Divine GW, et al. Randomized controlled clinical trial of surgery versus no surgery in patients with mild asymptomatic primary hyperparathyroidism. J Clin Endocrinol Metab 2004;89:5415–22.

28. Eigelberger MS, Cheah WK, Ituarte PHG, et al. The NIH criteria for parathyroidectomy in asymptomatic primary hyperparathyroidism: are they too limited? Ann Surg 2004;239:528.

29. Perrier ND, Balachandran D, Wefel JS, et al. Prospective, randomized, controlled trial of parathyroidectomy versus observation in patients with "asymptomatic" primary hyperparathyroidism. Surgery 2009;146:1116–22.

30. Yu N, Donnan PT, Leese GP. A record linkage study of outcomes in patients with mild primary hyperparathyroidism: the Parathyroid Epidemiology and Audit Research Study (PEARS). Clin Endocrinol 2011;75:169–76.

31. Abdulla AG, Ituarte PH, Harari A, et al. Trends in the frequency and quality of parathyroid surgery: analysis of 17,082 cases over 10 years. Ann Surg 2015; 261:746–50.

32. Potts JT. NIH conference-diagnosis and management of asymptomatic primary hyperparathyroidism—consenus development conference statement. Ann Intern Med 1991;114:593–7.

33. Bilezikian JP, Potts JT Jr, Fuleihan GE-H, et al. Summary statement from a workshop on asymptomatic primary hyperparathyroidism: a perspective for the 21st century. J Clin Endocrinol Metab 2002;87:5353–61.

34. Consensus development conference statement. J Bone Miner Res 1991;6(Suppl 2):S9–13.

35. Bilezikian JP, Khan AA, Potts JT Jr. Guidelines for the management of asymptomatic primary hyperparathyroidism: summary statement from the third international workshop. J Clin Endocrinol Metab 2009;94:335–9.

36. Silverberg SJ, Shane E, de la Cruz L, et al. Skeletal disease in primary hyperparathyroidism. J Bone Miner Res 1989;4:283–91.

37. Wood K, Dhital S, Chen H, et al. What is the utility of distal forearm DXA in primary hyperparathyroidism? Oncologist 2012;17:322–5.

38. Rubin MR, Bilezikian JP, McMahon DJ, et al. The natural history of primary hyperparathyroidism with or without parathyroid surgery after 15 years. J Clin Endocrinol Metab 2008;93:3462–70.

39. Vestergaard P, Mollerup CL, Frøkjær VG, et al. Cohort study of risk of fracture before and after surgery for primary hyperparathyroidism. BMJ 2000;321:598–602.

40. Khosla S, Melton LJ, Wermers RA, et al. Primary hyperparathyroidism and the risk of fracture: a population-based study. J Bone Miner Res 1999;14:1700–7.

41. Vignali E, Viccica G, Diacinti D, et al. Morphometric vertebral fractures in postmenopausal women with primary hyperparathyroidism. J Clin Endocrinol Metab 2009;94:2306–12.

42. Cipriani C, Biamonte F, Costa AG, et al. Prevalence of kidney stones and vertebral fractures in primary hyperparathyroidism using imaging technology. J Clin Endocrinol Metab 2015;100(4):1309–15.

43. Nassar K, Paternotte S, Kolta S, et al. Added value of trabecular bone score over bone mineral density for identification of vertebral fractures in patients with areal

bone mineral density in the non-osteoporotic range. Osteoporos Int 2014;25: 243–9.

44. Silva BC, Boutroy S, Zhang C, et al. Trabecular bone score (TBS)–a novel method to evaluate bone microarchitectural texture in patients with primary hyperparathyroidism. J Clin Endocrinol Metab 2013;98:1963–70.

45. Eller-Vainicher C, Filopanti M, Palmieri S, et al. Bone quality, as measured by trabecular bone score, in patients with primary hyperparathyroidism. Eur J Endocrinol 2013;169:155–62.

46. Johnson CA, Levey AS, Coresh J, et al. Clinical practice guidelines for chronic kidney disease in adults: part I. Definition, disease stages, evaluation, treatment, and risk factors. Am Fam Physician 2004;70:869–76.

47. Tassone F, Gianotti L, Emmolo I, et al. Glomerular filtration rate and parathyroid hormone secretion in primary hyperparathyroidism. J Clin Endocrinol Metab 2009;94:4458–61.

48. Walker MD, Dempster DW, McMahon DJ, et al. Effect of renal function on skeletal health in primary hyperparathyroidism. J Clin Endocrinol Metab 2012;97:1501–7.

49. Cassibba S, Pellegrino M, Gianotti L, et al. Silent renal stones in primary hyperparathyroidism: prevalence and clinical features. Endocr Pract 2014;20:1137–42.

50. Silverberg SJ, Brown I, Bilezikian JP. Age as a criterion for surgery in primary hyperparathyroidism. Am J Med 2002;113:681–4.

51. Silverberg SJ, Shane E, Jacobs TP, et al. A 10-year prospective study of primary hyperparathyroidism with or without parathyroid surgery. N Engl J Med 1999;341: 1249–55.

52. Wu B, Haigh PI, Hwang R, et al. Underutilization of parathyroidectomy in elderly patients with primary hyperparathyroidism. J Clin Endocrinol Metab 2010;95:4324–30.

53. Chen H, Parkerson S, Udelsman R. Parathyroidectomy in the elderly: do the benefits outweigh the risks? World J Surg 1998;22:531–6.

54. Egan KR, Adler JT, Olson JE, et al. Parathyroidectomy for primary hyperparathyroidism in octogenarians and nonagenarians: a risk–benefit analysis. J Surg Res 2007;140:194–8.

55. Yu N, Leese GP, Donnan PT. What predicts adverse outcomes in untreated primary hyperparathyroidism? The Parathyroid Epidemiology and Audit Research Study (PEARS). Clin Endocrinol 2013;79:27–34.

56. Walker MD, Fleischer J, Rundek T, et al. Carotid vascular abnormalities in primary hyperparathyroidism. J Clin Endocrinol Metab 2009;94:3849–56.

57. Farahnak P, Lärfars G, Sten-Linder M, et al. Mild primary hyperparathyroidism: vitamin D deficiency and cardiovascular risk markers. J Clin Endocrinol Metab 2011;96:2112–8.

58. Bollerslev J, Rosen T, Mollerup CL, et al. Effect of surgery on cardiovascular risk factors in mild primary hyperparathyroidism. J Clin Endocrinol Metab 2009;94: 2255–61.

59. Persson A, Bollerslev J, Rosen T, et al. Effect of surgery on cardiac structure and function in mild primary hyperparathyroidism. Clin Endocrinol 2011;74:174–80.

60. Walker MD, Fleischer JB, Di Tullio MR, et al. Cardiac structure and diastolic function in mild primary hyperparathyroidism. J Clin Endocrinol Metab 2010;95:2172–9.

61. Walker MD, Rundek T, Homma S, et al. Effect of parathyroidectomy on subclinical cardiovascular disease in mild primary hyperparathyroidism. Eur J Endocrinol 2012;167:277–85.

62. Kahal H, Aye M, Rigby AS, et al. The effect of parathyroidectomy on neuropsychological symptoms and biochemical parameters in patients with asymptomatic primary hyperparathyroidism. Clin Endocrinol 2012;76:196–200.

63. Espiritu RP, Kearns AE, Vickers KS, et al. Depression in primary hyperparathyroidism: prevalence and benefit of surgery. J Clin Endocrinol Metab 2011;96: E1737–45.
64. Coker LH, Rorie K, Cantley L, et al. Primary hyperparathyroidism, cognition, and health-related quality of life. Ann Surg 2005;242:642.

Intraoperative Parathyroid Hormone Monitoring
Optimal Utilization

Kepal N. Patel, MD[a,b,c],*, Raul Caso, BS[d]

KEYWORDS

- Primary hyperparathyroidism • PTH • Intraoperative PTH monitoring
- Minimally invasive parathyroidectomy

KEY POINTS

- Advances in preoperative localizing studies and surgical adjuncts, such as the introduction of intraoperative parathyroid hormone (IOPTH) monitoring, have shifted the traditional bilateral operative approach for primary hyperparathyroidism to a focused surgery or minimally invasive parathyroidectomy.
- Focused parathyroidectomy guided by IOPTH monitoring makes this procedure safer, less invasive, and highly successful.
- The utilization of IOPTH interpretation criteria can predict operative success, minimize unnecessary bilateral exploration, decrease the likelihood of resecting parathyroid glands that are not hypersecreting, and prevent recurrence.

INTRODUCTION

With an annual incidence of 21.6 per 100,000 persons in the United States,[1] primary hyperparathyroidism (PHPT) is the most common cause of hypercalcemia due to hypersecretion of parathyroid hormone (PTH) from one or more parathyroid glands. The incidence of PHPT is similar in men and women before the age of 45 but peaks in the seventh decade with most cases occurring in women (74%).[2] With the increasing utilization of calcium screening in the developed world, the clinical profile of PHPT, typically characterized by hypercalcemic symptoms, nephrolithiasis, bone disease, and neuromuscular symptoms, has shifted from symptomatic hyperparathyroidism to one with subtle or no specific symptoms.[3] After ruling out other causes of hypercalcemia, the diagnosis of PHPT is made via biochemical confirmation of an inappropriately

Disclosure: The authors have nothing to disclose.
[a] Division of Endocrine Surgery, Department of Surgery, NYU Langone Medical Center, New York, NY, USA; [b] Department of Biochemistry and Molecular Pharmacology, NYU Langone Medical Center, New York, NY, USA; [c] Department of Otolaryngology, NYU Langone Medical Center, New York, NY, USA; [d] NYU School of Medicine, New York, NY, USA
* Corresponding author. 530 First Avenue, Suite 6H, New York, NY 10016.
E-mail address: kepal.patel@nyumc.org

Surg Oncol Clin N Am 25 (2016) 91–101
http://dx.doi.org/10.1016/j.soc.2015.08.005
1055-3207/16/$ – see front matter © 2016 Elsevier Inc. All rights reserved.

normal or elevated serum PTH concentration in the setting of normal renal function. Most patients with PHPT present with a single adenoma (70%–95%), whereas close to 4% have double adenomas, 15% have parathyroid hyperplasia, and very few cases are due to parathyroid carcinoma.[4]

Surgery is the mainstay of treatment for PHPT, resulting in long-term cure and reversal of symptoms. Although medical therapy for secondary hyperparathyroidism is well established, its role in PHPT is limited to refractory disease and nonsurgical candidates.[5] Bilateral exploration (BE) is the traditional surgical approach, allowing the surgeon to visualize all parathyroid glands and remove one or more grossly enlarged glands. Although this approach has a high cure rate,[6] most patients with PHPT have one causative lesion, and a unilateral approach is feasible in most cases. The introduction of highly accurate parathyroid imaging techniques, such as sesta-mibi scintigraphy and high-resolution ultrasonography of the neck, and the implementation of surgical adjuncts such as intraoperative PTH (IOPTH) monitoring have heralded the idea of minimally invasive parathyroidectomy (MIP), with focused neck exploration and excision of only hypersecreting glands.[7–11] Focused parathyroidectomy has a lower incidence of postoperative hypocalcemia and decreased risk of recurrent nerve damage. By limiting the dissection, a favorable operative field is preserved in the event of reexploration. Focused surgery guided by IOPTH monitoring allows the surgeon to confirm the removal of all hypersecreting parathyroid glands, and to predict operative success and long-term cure from PHPT.

INTRAOPERATIVE PARATHYROID HORMONE: HISTORICAL PERSPECTIVE

Focused parathyroidectomy relies on accurate preoperative localization of all abnormal parathyroid glands; however, many preoperative parathyroid imaging technologies are subject to missing double adenomas, parathyroid hyperplasia, and ectopically located glands. In these cases, focused parathyroidectomy guided by imaging studies alone would fail in a significant subset of patients. To overcome this deficit, in 1988 Nuss-baum and colleagues[12] introduced postresection measurement of PTH as an adjunct to show cure. In 1991, Irvin and colleagues[13] introduced a rapid IOPTH assay to assess adequacy of resection. For the first time, a series of 21 patients had their parathyroid surgery guided by IOPTH using an immunoradiometric method. The short half-life of PTH (2–4 minutes)[14] makes it ideal for intraoperative use. In 1996, this rapid assay method was further developed to an immunochemiluminescence method, and the "quick" IOPTH assay became commercially available for intraoperative use.[15] The assay allowed surgeons to verify resection of hyperfunctioning parathyroid glands with a 15-minute turnaround and, after noting an appropriate decline in serum PTH, the surgeon could forgo visual inspection of the remaining glands. In contrast, a persistently elevated serum PTH prompted further exploration. The use of IOPTH monitoring to confirm cure as a practical adjunct of focused parathyroidectomy has since been validated.[15–17]

OPERATIVE SUCCESS WITH INTRAOPERATIVE PARATHYROID HORMONE MONITORING

The utilization of IOPTH monitoring to determine the extent of surgery in the setting of PHPT is highly accurate, resulting in excellent outcomes when preoperative localization studies are implemented.[18–24] Patients with concordant preoperative localization studies represent the easiest to treat group of patients, as image-guided focused surgery results in cure rates exceeding 95% even in operations without IOPTH. When patients undergo focused surgery guided by IOPTH monitoring, this leads to similar or in some cases higher operative success rates ranging from 97% to 99% compared with the operative success of BE, which exceeds 94%.[23–25] In a large series of patients with PHPT, focused resection led to a 99% cure rate compared to 97% with BE.[26] Numerous studies have reported decreased operative time, shorter incisional length, and shorter hospital stay with focused surgery or MIP.[9,26,27] Equivalence in long-term outcome has also been observed between focused surgery guided by IOPTH monitoring and BE.[28–31]

Higher estimated rates of unrecognized multiglandular disease (MGD) have been reported with focused surgery guided by IOPTH monitoring compared with BE.[32] In a series of 15,000 patients with a mean follow-up of 6 years, Norman and colleagues[33] examined the ongoing differences between unilateral and bilateral surgical techniques for 10-year recurrence, multigland removal, operative times, and length of hospital stay. Recurrence was 11 times more likely for unilateral explorations, causing gradual increases in BEs in their practice. Ten-year cure rates were unchanged for bilateral operations, and unilateral operations showed continued slow recurrence rates of 5%. Removal of more than one gland occurred 16 times more frequently with a bilateral operation, increasing cure rates to their current 99.4%. Of 1060 reoperations performed for recurrence, IOPTH levels fell greater than 50% in 22% of patients, yet a second adenoma was subsequently found. The investigators conclude that regardless of surgical adjuncts, unilateral parathyroidectomy carries a 1-year failure rate of 3% to 5% and a 10-year recurrence rate of 4% to 6%. They postulate that the only way to achieve 10-year cure rates greater than 94.5% is to examine all 4 parathyroid glands. Allowing rapid analysis of all 4 glands through the same 1-inch incision has caused this group to abandon unilateral parathyroidectomy. However, another 10-year follow-up study highlighted the successful utility of IOPTH monitoring during focused surgery to predict complete resection and recognize other hypersecreting glands, thus sparing normally secreting glands.[34] Additionally, randomized trials, in which patients with positive sestamibi scans had MIP versus BE with and without IOPTH guidance, have described a lower incidence of MGD with focused surgery when compared with patients who underwent BE and excision based on gland size.[35,36] This suggests that not all enlarged glands observed in BE are hypersecreting and contributing to hypercalcemia.[37]

APPLICATION OF INTRAOPERATIVE PARATHYROID HORMONE MONITORING

Greater than 90% of high-volume parathyroid surgeons use IOPTH to guide extent of parathyroidectomy.[38] IOPTH monitoring aids the surgeon by (1) confirming that all hypersecreting parathyroid glands have been excised without the need for visual confirmation of normally functioning glands, (2) indicating additional hyperfunctioning glands by an insufficient IOPTH drop, thus requiring further neck exploration to achieve operative success, (3) differentiating parathyroid tissue from nonparathyroid tissue, and (4) identifying the side of the neck containing the hypersecreting parathyroid gland(s) with the use of differential jugular venous sampling.[39] Importantly, IOPTH monitoring value-adds to surgical decision-making in patients with discordant preoperative imaging.[40]

INTRAOPERATIVE PARATHYROID HORMONE SAMPLING PROTOCOL

The timing of blood sample collection is critical for the success of focused surgery, which essentially takes advantage of PTH clearance rates to guide the extent of dissection. Therefore, it is essential that the surgeon has an understanding of PTH dynamics. Throughout the procedure, whole blood is collected at specific times: in the operating room before induction of anesthesia or skin incision (baseline), and at variable intervals after parathyroid gland excision. The authors also obtain an IOPTH sample immediately after gland excision (at-excision IOPTH). It is known that approximately 20% of patients will experience a spike in IOPTH levels during surgery. In the absence of an at-excision IOPTH, a spike in the hormone level may be missed, thus prompting unnecessary BE. While waiting for PTH results to be reported, the surgeon normally proceeds with closure of the incision site, while avoiding manipulation of the remaining parathyroid glands, to minimize the chance that a false elevation in the PTH level occurs.[41] Importantly, it is the successful interpretation of changes in PTH levels that is essential for using this technique in a way to optimize cure. To reduce complications, the IOPTH criterion used to predict cure should minimize unnecessary BE and decrease the likelihood of resecting parathyroid glands that are not hypersecreting.

INTRAOPERATIVE PARATHYROID HORMONE CRITERIA FOR PREDICTING OPERATIVE SUCCESS

The goal of parathyroidectomy guided by IOPTH monitoring is to achieve operative success, defined as eucalcemia for at least 6 months postoperatively. Alternatively, operative failure or persistent hyperparathyroidism is defined as hypercalcemia and elevated serum PTH levels within 6 months after surgery. When preoperative localization studies are concordant for single gland involvement, IOPTH monitoring may not significantly contribute to surgical success. In patients in whom the preoperative localization studies are discordant, the incidence of MGD is higher and thus the surgeon must carefully choose the protocol and IOPTH interpretation criteria that will result in complete cure.[40]

In 1993, Irvin and colleagues[42] first established that a 50% decline from a preexcision IOPTH level best predicted postoperative normocalcemia. The "Miami criterion" was later refined to be a drop of 50% or more from the highest PTH level, from either the preincision or preexcision level, occurring 10 minutes after the suspected gland is excised.[43] If the 10-minute PTH sample decreases sufficiently, then the procedure can be terminated; however, if the criterion is not met at this point, then the neck is reexplored and the protocol for blood sampling is once again repeated for each additional excised gland until all abnormal tissue is removed as indicated by an appropriate drop in serum PTH. The Miami criterion predicts postoperative normal or low calcium levels with an accuracy of 97% to 98%.[44–48]

A retrospective review of 260 patients with sporadic PHPT and concordant preoperative imaging evaluated the predictive values of the Miami, Halle, Rome, and Vienna IOPTH interpretation criteria.[49] Barczynski and colleagues[49] reported 97% accuracy in intraoperative prediction of cure using the Miami criterion followed by the Vienna criterion (92%). The Rome criterion followed by the Halle criterion performed better at detecting MGD. However, given their low negative predictive value, their application in patients qualified for MIP and concordant imaging studies would result in a significantly higher number of unnecessary conversions to BE, with only a marginal improvement in the success rate of the primary procedure. In another retrospective study, the Vienna and Halle criteria were better predictors of MGD than the Miami criterion.[50] Riss and colleagues attributed the success of the Vienna criterion to its defined baseline, a factor that can lead to inaccurate interpretation of the PTH curve. Similar findings have been supported elsewhere.[51]

The choice of IOPTH criteria to predict operative success remains controversial. There is a lack of standardization regarding baseline PTH samples, percent decline used as a cutoff, sampling times, and sampling frequency. There is a need for objective IOPTH criteria that accurately predict operative success, obviating the need for further surgical exploration. It is worth noting that as IOPTH criteria become stricter, BE is performed more frequently and a greater number of enlarged but normally functioning glands are excised without improving operative success.[50–52] The most commonly used criteria for predicting the outcome of focused parathyroid surgery are summarized in **Table 1**.

PREDICTING RECURRENCE WITH INTRAOPERATIVE PARATHYROID HORMONE

Based on a retrospective analysis of 194 patients who underwent focused surgery for PHPT guided by IOPTH,[56] the author currently uses a modified version of the Miami criterion: (1) a drop in PTH greater than 50% from baseline and a return to normal range (<65 pg/mL) of the final PTH sample and (2) an absolute final PTH level less than 40 pg/mL. Heller and Blumberg[56] have shown that patients with a final IOPTH less than 40 pg/mL had no disease recurrence at a median follow-up of 5 months. Wharry and colleagues,[57] who analyzed 1108 cases of sporadic PHPT using IOPTH monitoring, found that a final IOPTH that was within the normal range and dropped by greater than 50% from baseline was a strong predictor of operative success. Moreover, patients with a final IOPTH between 41 and 65 pg/mL had greater long-term recurrence. This observation was also recently confirmed by Rajaei and colleagues[58] in a retrospective review of 1371 patients with PHPT, grouped based on final IOPTH of less than 40, 40 to 59, and greater than 60 pg/mL with 2 years of follow-up. Patients with a final IOPTH less than 40 pg/mL experienced less hypercalcemia at 6-month follow-up and the lowest recurrence rate beyond 6 months postoperatively. Disease-free status was also greatest in patients with a final IOPTH less than 40 pg/mL beyond 2 years postoperatively. Thus, patients with a final IOPTH remaining above 40 pg/mL may be at an increased risk of having persistent PHPT and should be followed closely and indefinitely following surgery.

Table 1
Commonly used intraoperative parathyroid hormone monitoring criteria for predicting outcomes of parathyroid surgery

Criterion	Definition	Sensitivity, %	Specificity, %	Accuracy, %
Miami[53]	Decay ≥50% from highest baseline value within 10 min after resection	98	94	97
Halle[50]	Decay into the low normal range (≤35 pg/L) within 15 min after resection	70	87	72
Rome[54]	Decay ≥50% from highest baseline value, and/or 20 min postexcision value within reference range, and/or ≤7.5 ng/L lower than 10 min postexcision value	83	90	84
Vienna[50]	Decay ≥50% from the preincision value within 10 min after resection	92	89	92
Charleston[55]	Decay >50% from highest baseline value 10 min after resection and return to normal range or decay >65%, or decay >50% and return to normal range within 20 min after resection	97	98	97

In a retrospective review of 2185 patients who underwent surgery for PHPT guided by IOPTH monitoring, Wachtel and colleagues[59] performed multivariate and univariate analyses to determine factors associated with intraoperative failure. The intraoperative failure group had patients with more multigland disease and smaller glands. On multivariate analysis, PTH level was statistically, but not clinically, associated with intraoperative failure. Median IOPTH decrease was lower in patients with persistent disease. The investigators concluded that intraoperative failure is associated with higher rates of multigland disease and smaller parathyroid glands. Additionally, patients with persistent disease had significantly lower decreases in IOPTH, but half of patients who experienced failure by IOPTH criteria were eucalcemic 6 months postoperatively.

Schneider and colleagues[60] reported long-term results of 1368 parathyroid operations for PHPT guided by IOPTH monitoring, including 1006 MIP and 380 BE. There were no differences in recurrence between the MIP and BE groups, and the operative approach did not predict recurrent disease in a multivariate analysis. However, the percentage decrease in IOPTH was protective against recurrence for the entire cohort of patients. A higher postoperative IOPTH also independently predicted disease recurrence. This provides evidence that the percentage decrease in IOPTH is one of the many pieces of data a surgeon can use to decide whether to terminate the operation or undertake a BE, whereas the postoperative PTH level can guide patient follow-up.

COST-EFFECTIVENESS OF INTRAOPERATIVE PARATHYROID HORMONE MONITORING

The added value of IOPTH monitoring has been debated in the context of adequate preoperative localization.[61] It remains a contested issue because its ability to prevent failed parathyroid surgery due to unrecognized MGD must be balanced against assay-related costs. To address this issue, Morris and colleagues[62] performed a literature review identifying 17 studies involving 4280 patients, permitting estimation of base case costs and probabilities by using a decision tree and cost analysis model. The base case assumption was that in well-localized PHPT, IOPTH monitoring would increase the success rate of MIP from 96.3% to 98.8%. The cost of IOPTH varied with operating room time used. The investigators found that IOPTH reduced overall treatment costs only when total assay-related costs fell below $110 per case. Inaccurate localization and high reoperation cost both independently increased the value of IOPTH monitoring. However, the IOPTH strategy was cost saving when the rate of unrecognized MGD exceeded 6% or if the cost of reoperation exceeded $12,000 (compared with the initial MIP cost of $3733). Setting the positive predictive value of IOPTH at 100% and reducing the false-negative rate to 0% did not significantly alter their findings. The investigators concluded that factors influencing the added value of IOPTH are institution-specific. In their model, IOPTH increased the cure rate marginally while incurring approximately 4% additional cost.[62]

The extent of IOPTH sampling in the setting of preoperative single gland involvement has also been questioned.[63] Gupta and colleagues[63] found that in 79% of their patients, with a preoperative diagnosis of a solitary adenoma, the procedure may have been successfully terminated following a 5-minute IOPTH drop by more than 50% from baseline. In this group, histopathology confirmed the preoperative diagnosis, and no recurrences and no failed resections were reported. Using the 23 patients who had 5-minute IOPTH levels drop greater than 50% but not into the normal range, the investigators estimated a total savings of $18,100 if the procedures had been terminated after the initial 5-minute sample. The estimated costs included the cost of running a PTH sample at their institution and additional intraoperative time.

Using the previously mentioned at-excision IOPTH, the investigators conducted a retrospective analysis of their institutional patient database to determine the utility of an at-excision IOPTH at predicting completion of surgery after parathyroid gland excision for PHPT. Importantly, all patients had preoperative localization studies confirming single gland involvement and were candidates for focused surgery. When the at-excision IOPTH declined by greater than 50% but not into the normal range, the surgeon obtained a success rate of 97%. Implementing the stricter criterion of a decline in the at-excision IOPTH level greater than 50% and into the normal range (<65 pg/mL) achieved a success rate of 98% and a failure rate of 2%. There were no recurrences at 6 months of follow-up. Had the procedure been terminated when the at-excision IOPTH declined by more than 50% from baseline, the surgeon would have achieved acceptable success rates. Thereby, when preoperative localization studies are concordant for single gland disease, adequate cure rates can be achieved using an at-excision IOPTH value alone, thus resulting in an overall time, risk, and potential cost benefit.

SUMMARY

More than 80% of patients with sporadic PHPT have a single hyperactive parathyroid gland. Advances in preoperative localizing studies and surgical adjuncts, such as IOPTH, have shifted the traditional bilateral operative approach to a focused surgery or MIP. Focused surgery guided by IOPTH monitoring allows confirmation of cure and absence of MGD without intraoperative visualization of all parathyroid glands. The utilization of IOPTH during focused surgery makes this procedure safer, less invasive, and highly successful. It is imperative that the surgeon has an understanding of hormone dynamics and carefully chooses the appropriate IOPTH protocol and interpretation criteria that will best predict operative success and prevent recurrence. Focused parathyroidectomy guided by IOPTH monitoring may improve the success rate and low morbidity associated with BE, and may result in higher long-term cure rates when used as the procedure of choice for sporadic PHPT.

REFERENCES

1. Wermers RA, Khosla S, Atkinson EJ, et al. Incidence of primary hyperparathyroidism in Rochester, Minnesota, 1993-2001: an update on the changing epidemiology of the disease. J Bone Miner Res 2006;21(1):171-7.
2. Marcocci C, Cetani F. Clinical practice. Primary hyperparathyroidism. N Engl J Med 2011;365(25):2389-97.
3. Silverberg SJ, Lewiecki EM, Mosekilde L, et al. Presentation of asymptomatic primary hyperparathyroidism: proceedings of the third international workshop. J Clin Endocrinol Metab 2009;94(2):351-65.
4. Fraker DL, Harsono H, Lewis R. Minimally invasive parathyroidectomy: benefits and requirements of localization, diagnosis, and intraoperative PTH monitoring. Long-term results. World J Surg 2009;33(11):2256-65.
5. Rothe HM, Liangos O, Biggar P, et al. Cinacalcet treatment of primary hyperparathyroidism. Int J Endocrinol 2011;2011:415719.
6. Allendorf J, DiGorgi M, Spanknebel K, et al. 1112 consecutive bilateral neck explorations for primary hyperparathyroidism. World J Surg 2007;31(11):2075-80.
7. Chen H, Sokoll LJ, Udelsman R. Outpatient minimally invasive parathyroidectomy: a combination of sestamibi-SPECT localization, cervical block anesthesia, and intraoperative parathyroid hormone assay. Surgery 1999;126(6):1016-21.
8. Udelsman R. Six hundred fifty-six consecutive explorations for primary hyperparathyroidism. Ann Surg 2002;235(5):665-70.

9. Norman J, Chheda H, Farrell C. Minimally invasive parathyroidectomy for primary hyperparathyroidism: decreasing operative time and potential complications while improving cosmetic results. Am Surg 1998;64(5):391–5 [discussion: 395–6].

10. Ypsilantis E, Charfare H, Wassif WS. Intraoperative PTH assay during minimally invasive parathyroidectomy may be helpful in the detection of double adenomas and may minimise the risk of recurrent surgery. Int J Endocrinol 2010;2010: 178671.

11. Kunstman JW, Udelsman R. Superiority of minimally invasive parathyroidectomy. Adv Surg 2012;46:171–89.

12. Nussbaum SR, Thompson AR, Hutcheson KA, et al. Intraoperative measurement of parathyroid hormone in the surgical management of hyperparathyroidism. Surgery 1988;104(6):1121–7.

13. Irvin GL 3rd, Dembrow VD, Prudhomme DL. Operative monitoring of parathyroid gland hyperfunction. Am J Surg 1991;162(4):299–302.

14. Libutti SK, Alexander HR, Bartlett DL, et al. Kinetic analysis of the rapid intraoperative parathyroid hormone assay in patients during operation for hyperparathyroidism. Surgery 1999;126(6):1145–50.

15. Boggs JE, Irvin GL 3rd, Molinari AS, et al. Intraoperative parathyroid hormone monitoring as an adjunct to parathyroidectomy. Surgery 1996;120(6):954–8.

16. Irvin GL 3rd, Deriso GT 3rd. A new, practical intraoperative parathyroid hormone assay. Am J Surg 1994;168(5):466–8.

17. Gordon LL, Snyder WH, Wians F, et al. The validity of quick intraoperative parathyroid hormone assay: an evaluation in seventy-two patients based on gross morphologic criteria. Surgery 1999;126:1030–5.

18. Carneiro DM, Solorzano CC, Irvin GL 3rd. Recurrent disease after limited parathyroidectomy for sporadic primary hyperparathyroidism. J Am Coll Surg 2004; 199(6):849–53 [discussion: 853–5].

19. Miccoli P, Berti P, Materazzi G, et al. Results of video-assisted parathyroidectomy: single institution's six-year experience. World J Surg 2004;28(12):1216–8.

20. Johnson LR, Doherty G, Lairmore T, et al. Evaluation of the performance and clinical impact of a rapid intraoperative parathyroid hormone assay in conjunction with preoperative imaging and concise parathyroidectomy. Clin Chem 2001; 47(5):919–25.

21. Inabnet WB 3rd, Dakin GF, Haber RS, et al. Targeted parathyroidectomy in the era of intraoperative parathormone monitoring. World J Surg 2002;26(8): 921–5.

22. Burkey SH, Van Heerden JA, Farley DR, et al. Will directed parathyroidectomy utilizing the gamma probe or intraoperative parathyroid hormone assay replace bilateral cervical exploration as the preferred operation for primary hyperparathyroidism? World J Surg 2002;26(8):914–20.

23. Irvin GL, Carneiro DM, Solorzano CC. Progress in the operative management of sporadic primary hyperparathyroidism over 34 years. Ann Surg 2004;239(5): 704–8.

24. Sokoll LJ, Drew H, Udelsman R. Intraoperative parathyroid hormone analysis: a study of 200 consecutive cases. Clin Chem 2000;46(10):1662–8.

25. Grant CS, Thompson G, Farley D, et al. Primary hyperparathyroidism surgical management since the introduction of minimally invasive parathyroidectomy— Mayo Clinic experience. Arch Surg 2005;140(5):472–8.

26. Udelsman R, Lin Z, Donovan P. The superiority of minimally invasive parathyroidectomy based on 1650 consecutive patients with primary hyperparathyroidism. Ann Surg 2011;253(3):585–91.

27. Slepavicius A, Beisa V, Janusonis V, et al. Focused versus conventional parathyroidectomy for primary hyperparathyroidism: a prospective, randomized, blinded trial. Langenbecks Arch Surg 2008;393(5):659–66.
28. Bergenfelz A, Lindblom P, Tibblin S, et al. Unilateral versus bilateral neck exploration for primary hyperparathyroidism—a prospective randomized controlled trial. Ann Surg 2002;236(5):543–51.
29. Westerdahl J, Bergenfelz A. Unilateral versus bilateral neck exploration for primary hyperparathyroidism: five-year follow-up of a randomized controlled trial. Ann Surg 2007;246(6):976–80 [discussion: 980–1].
30. Schneider DF, Mazeh H, Sippel RS, et al. Is minimally invasive parathyroidectomy associated with greater recurrence compared to bilateral exploration? Analysis of more than 1,000 cases. Surgery 2012;152(6):1008–15.
31. Beyer TD, Solorzano CC, Starr F, et al. Parathyroidectomy outcomes according to operative approach. Am J Surg 2007;193(3):368–72 [discussion: 372–3].
32. Siperstein A, Berber E, Barbosa GF, et al. Predicting the success of limited exploration for primary hyperparathyroidism using ultrasound, sestamibi, and intraoperative parathyroid hormone: analysis of 1158 cases. Ann Surg 2008;248(3):420–8.
33. Norman J, Lopez J, Politz D. Abandoning unilateral parathyroidectomy: why we reversed our position after 15,000 parathyroid operations. J Am Coll Surg 2012;214(3):260–9.
34. Lew JI, Irvin GL 3rd. Focused parathyroidectomy guided by intra-operative parathormone monitoring does not miss multiglandular disease in patients with sporadic primary hyperparathyroidism: a 10-year outcome. Surgery 2009;146(6):1021–7.
35. Bergenfelz A, Kanngiesser V, Zielke A, et al. Conventional bilateral cervical exploration versus open minimally invasive parathyroidectomy under local anaesthesia for primary hyperparathyroidism. Br J Surg 2005;92(2):190–7.
36. Russell CF, Dolan SJ, Laird JD. Randomized clinical trial comparing scan-directed unilateral versus bilateral cervical exploration for primary hyperparathyroidism due to solitary adenoma. Br J Surg 2006;93(4):418–21.
37. Genc H, Morita E, Perrier ND, et al. Differing histologic findings after bilateral and focused parathyroidectomy. J Am Coll Surg 2003;196(4):535–40.
38. Greene AB, Butler RS, McIntyre S, et al. National trends in parathyroid surgery from 1998 to 2008: a decade of change. J Am Coll Surg 2009;209(3):332–43.
39. Carneiro-Pla D. Contemporary and practical uses of intraoperative parathyroid hormone. Endocr Pract 2011;17:44–53.
40. Barczynski M, Konturek A, Cichon S, et al. Intraoperative parathyroid hormone assay improves outcomes of minimally invasive parathyroidectomy mainly in patients with a presumed solitary parathyroid adenoma and missing concordance of preoperative imaging. Clin Endocrinol 2007;66(6):878–85.
41. Yang GP, Levine S, Weigel RJ. A spike in parathyroid hormone during neck exploration may cause a false-negative intraoperative assay result. Arch Surg 2001;136(8):945–9.
42. Irvin GL 3rd, Dembrow VD, Prudhomme DL. Clinical usefulness of an intraoperative "quick parathyroid hormone" assay. Surgery 1993;114(6):1019–22 [discussion: 1022–3].
43. Irvin GL, Solorzano CC, Carneiro DA. Quick intraoperative parathyroid hormone assay: Surgical adjunct to allow limited parathyroidectomy, improve success rate, and predict outcome. World J Surg 2004;28(12):1287–92.

44. Carneiro DM, Solorzano CC, Nader MC, et al. Comparison of intraoperative iPTH assay (QPTH) criteria in guiding parathyroidectomy: which criterion is the most accurate? Surgery 2003;134(6):973–9 [discussion: 979–1].
45. Vignali E, Picone A, Materazzi G, et al. A quick intraoperative parathyroid hormone assay in the surgical management of patients with primary hyperparathyroidism: a study of 206 consecutive cases. Eur J Endocrinol 2002;146(6): 783–8.
46. Chen H, Pruhs Z, Starling JR, et al. Intraoperative parathyroid hormone testing improves cure rates in patients undergoing minimally invasive parathyroidectomy. Surgery 2005;138(4):583–7.
47. Miccoli P, Berti P, Materazzi G, et al. Endoscopic bilateral neck exploration versus quick intraoperative parathormone assay (qPTHa) during endoscopic parathyroidectomy: a prospective randomized trial. Surg Endosc 2008;22(2): 398–400.
48. Garner SC, Leight GS Jr. Initial experience with intraoperative PTH determinations in the surgical management of 130 consecutive cases of primary hyperparathyroidism. Surgery 1999;126(6):1132–7 [discussion: 1137–8].
49. Barczynski M, Konturek A, Hubalewska-Dydejczyk A, et al. Evaluation of Halle, Miami, Rome, and Vienna intraoperative iPTH assay criteria in guiding minimally invasive parathyroidectomy. Langenbecks Arch Surg 2009;394(5):843–9.
50. Riss P, Kaczirek K, Heinz G, et al. A "defined baseline" in PTH monitoring increases surgical success in patients with multiple gland disease. Surgery 2007;142(3):398–404.
51. Chiu B, Sturgeon C, Angelos P. Which intraoperative parathyroid hormone assay criterion best predicts operative success? A study of 352 consecutive patients. Arch Surg 2006;141:483–7.
52. Karakousis GC, Han D, Kelz RR, et al. Interpretation of intra-operative PTH changes in patients with multi-glandular primary hyperparathyroidism (pHPT). Surgery 2007;142(6):845–50 [discussion: 850.e1–2].
53. Irvin GL, Carneiro DM. Rapid parathyroid hormone assay guided exploration. Oper Tech Gen Surg 1999;1(1):18–27.
54. Lombardi C, Raffaelli M, Traini E, et al. Intraoperative PTH monitoring during parathyroidectomy: the need for stricter criteria to detect multiglandular disease. Langenbecks Arch Surg 2008;393(5):639–45.
55. Carneiro-Pla D, Irvin GL. Intraoperative PTH criterion can be highly specific without leading to unnecessary bilateral neck explorations: what have we learned in 16 years? J Am Coll Surg 2010;211(3):S86–7.
56. Heller KS, Blumberg SN. Relation of final intraoperative parathyroid hormone level and outcome following parathyroidectomy. Arch Otolaryngol Head Neck Surg 2009;135(11):1103–7.
57. Wharry LI, Yip L, Armstrong MJ, et al. The final intraoperative parathyroid hormone level: how low should it go? World J Surg 2014;38(3):558–63.
58. Rajaei MH, Bentz AM, Schneider DF, et al. Justified follow-up: a final intraoperative parathyroid hormone (IOPTH) over 40 pg/ml is associated with an increased risk of persistence and recurrence in primary hyperparathyroidism. Ann Surg Oncol 2015;22(2):454–9.
59. Wachtel H, Cerullo I, Bartlett EK, et al. What can we learn from intraoperative parathyroid hormone levels that do not drop appropriately? Ann Surg Oncol 2014;22(6): 1781–8.
60. Schneider DF, Mazeh H, Chen H, et al. Predictors of recurrence in primary hyperparathyroidism: an analysis of 1386 cases. Ann Surg 2014;259(3):563–8.

61. Stalberg P, Sidhu S, Sywak M, et al. Intraoperative parathyroid hormone measurement during minimally invasive parathyroidectomy: does it "value-add" to decision-making? J Am Coll Surg 2006;203(1):1–6.
62. Morris LF, Zanocco K, Ituarte PH, et al. The value of intraoperative parathyroid hormone monitoring in localized primary hyperparathyroidism: a cost analysis. Ann Surg Oncol 2010;17(3):679–85.
63. Gupta A, Unawane A, Subhas G, et al. Parathyroidectomies using intraoperative parathormone monitoring: when should we stop measuring intraoperative parathormone levels? Am Surg 2012;78(8):844–50.

Minimally Invasive Parathyroidectomy Versus Bilateral Neck Exploration for Primary Hyperparathyroidism

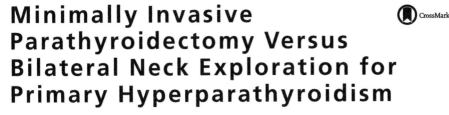

Amanda M. Laird, MD*, Steven K. Libutti, MD

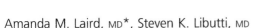

KEYWORDS

- Primary hyperparathyroidism • Parathyroidectomy
- Intraoperative parathyroid hormone • Surgery
- Minimally invasive parathyroidectomy

KEY POINTS

- The gold-standard surgical management of primary hyperparathyroidism (1⁰HPT) is cervical exploration and identification of all 4 parathyroid glands.
- Imaging techniques, including ultrasound, sestamibi scans, and 4D-CT scans, have made identification of single parathyroid adenomas possible.
- Intraoperative parathyroid hormone (PTH) monitoring is a method to confirm biochemical cure before a patient leaves the operating room.
- There is some debate surrounding optimal surgical management of 1⁰HPT because cure rates between minimally invasive parathyroidectomy (MIP) and bilateral neck exploration (BNE) are equivalent.
- Advantages of MIP include reduced operative time, reduced recovery time, less postoperative pain, and lower complication rate with respect to injury to parathyroid glands and recurrent laryngeal nerves.

INTRODUCTION

1⁰HPT is a common disease, with a prevalence as high as 3%.[1] Many advances in the surgical management of 1⁰HPT have been made since the first parathyroidectomy was performed by Felix Mandl in 1925.[2] Traditional surgical management consists of identification of all 4 parathyroid glands through a transverse cervical incision.[3] Better understanding of the disease, interest in the practice of endocrine neck surgery,

The authors have nothing to disclose.
Montefiore Medical Center/Albert Einstein College of Medicine, Greene Medical Arts Pavilion, 3400 Bainbridge Avenue, 4th Floor, Bronx, NY 10467, USA
* Corresponding author.
E-mail address: alaird@montefiore.org

surgonc.theclinics.com

and operative experience increased cure rates to greater than 95%.[4–6] Surgery remains the only cure for 1°HPT because medical management ultimately fails.[7]

As in other areas of surgery, there has been a shift from the standard 4-gland exploration to a more minimally invasive approach. The success rate of MIP rivals that of BNE.[8,9] Questions remain as to which approach is better. This primarily depends on proved benefit of each operation over its shortcomings. With MIP, incisions are smaller and recovery time is improved, but these may be achieved at the cost of higher rates of persistence or recurrence. BNE may be less advantageous because MIP may achieve a similar outcome with fewer complications. This article seeks to define MIP and BNE and to compare them for advantages and disadvantages.

PATIENT EVALUATION

A diagnosis of 1°HPT is made when the serum calcium level is elevated in the setting of an inappropriately nonsuppressed PTH level. This results from overproduction of PTH by 1 or more of the parathyroid glands. The incidence of 1°HPT is increasing overall as the population in the United States has aged, with incidence rates ranging from 0.7% in the general population up to 3% in postmenopausal women.[1,10,11] 1°HPT occurs at a higher rate in women, at a 2:1 ratio,[12] and is the most common cause of hypercalcemia in the outpatient population. Overall rates of hypercalcemia have also increased as a result of a change in the calcium assay in the 1970s, leading to earlier diagnosis of hypercalcemia.[13] Thus, the presentation of symptomatic 1°HPT changed from a disease that was typically associated with kidney stones and skeletal disease to one that is asymptomatic.[14] Associated symptoms may include fatigue, polydipsia, polyuria, depression, generalize muscle weakness, joint pain, memory loss, nausea, and loss of appetite,[4,15,16] although these subtle symptoms are often found in the general population as well.

Hypercalcemia may occur as a result of other conditions, such as malignancy, sarcoidosis, hyperthyroidism, and use of thiazide diuretics,[17] and the diagnosis of 1°HPT involves a comprehensive evaluation to eliminate these conditions as a cause for hypercalcemia. 1°HPT results in an overproduction of PTH, which stimulates bone reabsorption, stimulates the production of vitamin D, inhibits renal excretion of calcium, and stimulates intestinal reabsorption.[18] Typically, PTH and its relationship to serum calcium levels function in a negative feedback loop, where, once the calcium-sensing receptor in the parathyroid gland perceives adequate levels of PTH, hormone production ends. In 1°HPT, both serum calcium and PTH are elevated, or PTH is abnormally elevated relative to serum calcium level. This then differentiates it from other conditions, such as malignancy, benign familial hypocalciuric hypercalcemia, vitamin D deficiency, and sarcoidosis, where either calcium or PTH may be elevated independently. Careful interpretation of calcium levels relative to PTH levels is necessary because the laboratory findings may be subtle as in cases of normocalcemic hyperparathyroidism and normohormonal hyperparathyroidism.[19,20]

Indications for surgical management of 1°HPT are outlined in consensus group guidelines written originally in 1990 and updated most recently in 2013.[21–24]

The most current international consensus guidelines recommend surgery if any of the following criteria are met: age less than 50; calcium elevated to greater than 1 mg/dL above the upper limit of the normal range; reduced bone mineral density with T-score less than −2.5 at lumbar spine, total hip, femoral neck, or distal radius; creatinine clearance less than 60 mL/min; 24-hour urine calcium greater than 400 mg/d and increased stone risk by biochemical stone analysis; and presence of nephrolithiasis or nephrocalcinosis by imaging[24] (**Table 1**). Additionally, patients

Table 1
Summary of the most recent international consensus guidelines for the management of asymptomatic primary hyperparathyroidism, 2013

Criterion	Indication for Surgery
Age	<50
Calcium	>1 mg/dL above upper limit of normal range
BMD	1. T-score $\leq$ −2.5 at any site (osteoporosis) 2. Vertebral fracture on imaging
Renal	1. Creatinine clearance <60 mL/min 2. 24-h Urine calcium >400 mg/dL + increased stone risk 3. Nephrolithiasis or nephrocalcinosis by imaging

Abbreviation: BMD, bone mineral density.

who prefer surgery or are unable or unwilling to commit to follow-up should undergo parathyroidectomy.

SURGICAL TREATMENT OPTIONS
Minimally Invasive Parathyroidectomy

Like many other surgical techniques, the approach to parathyroidectomy has evolved. Although traditional parathyroidectomy includes a transverse cervical incision and identification of all 4 parathyroid glands, a minimally invasive approach is performed through a limited incision with the goal of removing the preoperatively localized abnormal gland. A high degree of success is achieved as a result of both careful preoperative planning and because 85% of patients have a single parathyroid adenoma. MIP may have more than 1 meaning, however. MIP is most traditionally thought of as a parathyroidectomy done as a unilateral or focused neck exploration (FNE). Through a 2.5-cm transverse cervical incision, the preoperatively localized parathyroid adenoma is removed. Dissection is focused at the anatomically localized site. The procedure may be done under local or general anesthesia and is typically done as outpatient surgery. Success of surgery is confirmed biochemically by intraoperative PTH (IOPTH) monitoring. MIP may also mean minimally invasive video-assisted parathyroidectomy (MIVAP) or robotic-assisted parathyroidectomy, although FNE is the most widely applied technique.[25] The majority of this discussion thus focuses on FNE. I⁰PTH monitoring and application of imaging techniques in patients with 1⁰HPT have made FNE possible.

The short half-life of PTH, ranging from 3 to 5 minutes, has made IOPTH monitoring a useful adjunct to parathyroid surgery, confirming a biochemical cure during operation. A rapid immunoradiometric assay was developed in 1987[26] and was successfully applied during parathyroidectomy in a small series of patients.[27] These investigators suggested that a more limited approach might be taken in the surgical management of 1⁰HPT. Other groups applied the rapid assay routinely, and the FNE became a more widely accepted operation.[28,29] Subsequently, criteria for interpretation of IOPTH results were developed. A PTH level is sampled at the outset of parathyroidectomy; levels are then obtained at timed intervals after removal of the adenoma. Initially implemented at the University of Miami,[30] other criteria have been used by different groups.[31–33] Biochemical cure is established when PTH falls by at least 50% of the highest pre-excision level and into the normal PTH range[34]; failure to do so may miss multigland disease. The critically important step of application of IOPTH is to use the same technique at each operation; use of a varied technique makes interpretation of results difficult and may lead to persistent disease. In cases of IOPTH not falling appropriately, the operation is converted to a BNE.

Imaging studies are used in the operative planning of FNE and are not used to make or confirm the diagnosis of 1^0HPT. Instead, a decision is made to operate and subsequently localization studies are obtained. As the interventional radiologist John Doppman stated, "The only localization that a patient needs who has 1^0HPT is the localization f an experienced surgeon."[35] There are multiple imaging modalities, however, available to the surgeon who plans FNE.

Sestamibi scintigraphy was the earliest routinely applied imaging modality in operative planning of FNE. Technetium 99m sestamibi is thought to be retained in the mitochondria of parathyroid adenomas, making visualization possible.[36] Sestamibi localizes parathyroid adenomas in up to 90% of patients[37–39] but may be unrevealing in patients with multigland disease or with small adenomas.[40–42] Multidimensional imaging with the addition of single-photon emission CT (SPECT) to sestamibi scintigraphy improves sensitivity[43] (**Fig. 1**). False-positive studies may be a result of concomitant thyroid nodules or lymphadenopathy, and the addition of a second imaging tool, such as ultrasound, may improve identification of abnormal glands. Sestamibi-SPECT may be most useful in the identification of ectopic adenomas, such as those in the mediastinum.

Ultrasound is commonly used for localization of adenomas. Ultrasounds are portable, often available in a surgeon's or endocrinologist's office, do not expose patients to radiation, and cost less than nuclear medicine or multidimensional studies. The accuracy is similar to that of sestamibi-SPECT, at 70% to 80%.[44,45] Concomitant thyroid pathology, including benign nodules and thyroid cancer, is identified on ultrasound in 30% to 50% of patients with 1^0HPT,[46–48] and ultrasound-guided fine-needle aspiration also may be used to aspirate suspected adenomas for PTH. When combined with sestamibi-SPECT, accuracy of localization of an adenoma increases to approximately 90%.[49–51] Series demonstrate that concordant sestamibi-SPECT and ultrasound have operative cure rates of 98% to 99%,[52,53] suggesting that this may be an alternative to IOPTH monitoring. The typical appearance of a parathyroid adenoma is shown in **Fig. 2**.

High-resolution CT with and without intravenous contrast (4D-CT) and MRI can demonstrate parathyroid adenomas due to their contrast washout (**Fig. 3**). 4D-CT is more sensitive than both ultrasound and sestamibi-SPECT for identification of adenomas and may be useful to detect multigland disease.[54,55] MRI is an option for localization, although it is the least commonly used; this modality is best used in cases of reoperative parathyroidectomy.

Additional techniques for MIP include radioguided parathyroidectomy (RP), MIVAP, and robotic-assisted parathroidectomy. Like FNE, RP is an ambulatory procedure. Preoperatively patients are injected with technetium 99m sestamibi approximately 2 hours before the procedure, and a scan is performed the day of surgery. In the operating room, a gamma probe is used to measure activity of the excised tumor compared with the central neck. IOPTH may be additionally used to confirm biochemical success.[56,57] MIVAP uses a small scope that is inserted through the primary incision or a separate trochar to remove the preoperatively localized adenoma. There is more than 1 described technique to this approach with similar success rates.[58–60] Robotic assistance may be added to an endoscopic technique or used alone.[61,62] Compared with FNE, MIVAP and robotic procedures add operative time and complexity as well as an increased cost.[46,63,64] Although groups have achieved outcomes comparable to FNE, they are done in high-volume centers with a focus on these endoscopic and robotic

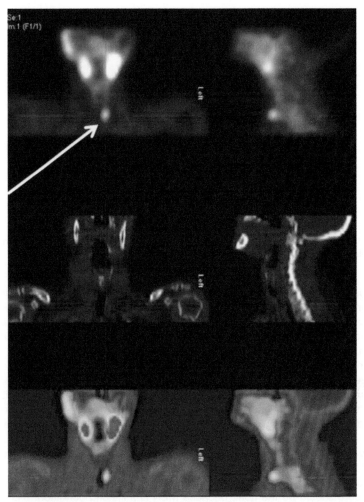

Fig. 1. Sestamibi-SPECT scan of a left inferior parathyroid adenoma. The *arrow* indicates the parathyroid adenoma. the three panels are coronal (L) and sagittal (R) images. Each panel represents the same anatomic site.

procedures.[65] The authors prefer FNE because it is a procedure applicable across different practice types.

Bilateral Neck Exploration

BNE is the traditional operation for 1^0HPT and was the only option prior to the development of IOPTH testing and reliable of imaging studies. The surgical technique is essentially the same as MIP, although the operation is typically done through a larger incision, at a minimum of 3 cm. Parathyroid glands are identified by the operating surgeon as abnormal if they are either larger than typical size of 30 to 50 mg or have abnormal morphology. Most glands are identified in the expected anatomic location[66]; if not, the gland may be ectopic. The exploration then continues in the typical locations for ectopic parathyroid glands, including the thymus, anterior mediastinum, the

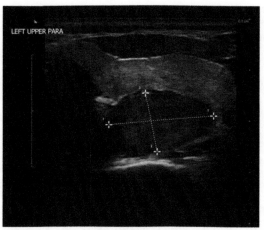

Fig. 2. Ultrasound of left superior parathyroid adenoma. The parathyroid is oval and hypo-echoic relative to the thyroid.

tracheoesophageal groove and retroesophageal space extending into the posterior mediastinum, the carotid sheaths, and lastly the thyroid gland. All glands should be identified before any are removed. Excision may involve removal 1 to 3.5 glands, as described previously. IOPTH may be used as an adjunct to BNE and levels are interpreted in the same manner as in MIP to confirm biochemical cure.

BNE may be indicated rather than FNE in specific situations. Patients in whom FNE is intended but have negative imaging studies need to undergo 4-gland exploration. The risk of multigland disease is as high as 25% in these patients.[67–69] Additionally, patients who have conditions in which multigland disease or multiple adenomas are expected should have BNE.[70] These include multiple endocrine neoplasia (MEN) types 1 and 2a, familial 1°HPT, and lithium-induced hyperparathyroidism. Up to 90% of patients with MEN1 and 30% of patients with MEN2a have multiple adenomas in any of the 4 parathyroid glands and thus benefit from BNE.[71–73] In patients predisposed to multigland disease, debulking abnormal glands rather than resection to achieve cure should be the goal, because MEN is a lifelong condition.[74] Long-term lithium therapy may cause hyperparathyroidism; because it is a systemic therapy it may affect all 4 glands.[75] Series demonstrate that more than half of patients treated with lithium have 1°HPT and benefit from BNE if treated operatively.[76–78]

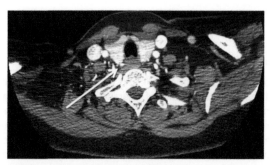

Fig. 3. 4D-CT scan of right superior parathyroid adenoma on arterial phase. The *arrow* indicates the parathyroid adenoma imaged on arterial phase.

Surgeon preference may dictate the choice of BNE over FNE. This is a result of some published evidence that there is a higher failure rate of FNE, and that unilateral exploration may fail to identify multigland disease even with the addition of IOPTH.[79] Some have reversed their preference of FNE versus BNE, stating that the rates of persistence and recurrence are unacceptably high; however, IOPTH was not used in this cohort.[80] Furthermore, data suggest that BNE is more time-efficient in patients who do not localize preoperatively.[81]

COMPARISON OF FOCUSED NECK EXPLORATION TO BILATERAL NECK EXPLORATION

In the United States, there is a trend toward the performance of FNE.[25] Moreover, there is a trend in surgical training programs toward surgeon-performed ultrasound, use of IOPTH, and FNE.[82] Thus, it is important to understand the differences in and outcomes of FNE and BNE.

Outcomes

Generally, both FNE and BNE are low-risk procedures associated with good outcomes. Complication rates overall are similar, likely because large published series are performed by high-volume surgeons.[83] In a series of 184 patients who underwent FNE, the rate of persistent disease was 1.6%, permanent hypocalcemia 0.5%, and permanent vocal cord paralysis 1%.[84] This is similar to other groups, with reported persistence rate of 1.5%, recurrence 6%, and permanent hypocalcemia 0.02%.[85,86] In comparison, traditional BNE outcomes are also good, with rate of persistent disease of 6%. The rates of multigland disease in these reports were higher in patients who underwent BNE versus FNE (10% vs 3%) due to surgeon evaluation of abnormal-appearing glands.[87] Similarly, other series have reported overall complication rates of up to 3%, including recurrent laryngeal nerve injury, postoperative hypocalcemia, and neck hematoma.[88,89] Data from the endocrine surgery group at Yale University reveal that cure rates are improved with FNE versus BNE at 1.45% versus 3.1% with similar low rates of permanent hypocalcemia and recurrent laryngeal nerve injury.[8] Additional series have compared these techniques through either randomized or retrospective data with similar findings.[5,8,90–93] These results are compared from selected series in **Table 2**.

Cost

Variability exists between the costs of FNE versus BNE. Contributing to this are the expenses related to anesthesia, hospitalization, use of IOPTH, and preoperative localization studies. FNE may be performed under local rather than general anesthesia, lowering treatment costs. Hospital admission adds to expenses; those patients undergoing BNE are more likely to be observed rather than discharged postoperatively.[94] FNE requires preoperative localization with ultrasound and/or sestamibi scan or 4D-CT as well as IOPTH to confirm success intraoperatively. There are mixed data regarding application of imaging and IOPTH to FNE and their contributing costs. In a large series of patients, overall cost was reduced by performing FNE by $1471.[8] This same group reported a savings of almost $2700 in a prior series.[88] Furthermore, a cost-benefit analysis of FNE compared with BNE revealed that use of any localizing study reduced cost of the procedure given the risk-reduction of recurrent laryngeal nerve injury, permanent hypoparathyroidism, rate of persistent disease, and need for reoperation.[95] In addition, the preoperative localization strategy may be modified to a less costly method; the most cost-effective tools are ultrasound alone or ultrasound along with 4D-CT.[96,97] FNE may save time, thereby reducing expenses;

Table 2
Randomized and retrospective series comparing focused neck exploration and bilateral neck exploration

Series	Study Type	Outcome
Westerdahl & Bergenfelz,[90] 2007	Randomized	= Cure rate at 5 y
Bergenfelz et al,[5] 2002	Randomized	= Cure rate; increased cost and operative time in FNE; increased postoperative hypocalcemia with BNE
Slepavicius et al,[91] 2008	Randomized	= OR time and cure rate; increased cost with FNE; increased postoperative hypocalcemia with BNE
Aarum et al,[93] 2007	Randomized	= Cure rate; = complication rate; increased cost with FNE
Grant et al,[92] 2005	Retrospective	= Cure rate; = complication rate
Udelsman et al,[8] 2011	Retrospective	Increased cure rate and lower complication rate with FNE

Note that studies do not compare all similar outcome measures.
Abbreviations: =, equivalent; OR, operating room.

operative time for FNE has been reported lower than BNE.[8,98] This reduction in operative time may further reduce expenses.[99]

There are conflicting data, however, that demonstrate cost reduction with BNE rather than FNE. Preoperative localization studies are not necessarily required for surgical planning for BNE.[81] Initial operations for 1°HPT did not use localization because imaging techniques were not available.[100] In a series of patients who were randomized to localization with 2 studies versus no localization, there was a 21% cost reduction if BNE rather than FNE with localization was performed.[93] Similarly, in a retrospective study, BNE without localization significantly reduced cost over FNE with localization, despite a reduced operating time.[101] Other groups have similar findings in their patient populations.[102] IOPTH adds cost to the surgical management of 1°HPT, and it may not be necessary in BNE. In a cost-analysis model evaluating IOPTH use versus BNE without IOPTH, success was marginally increased and thought not statistically significant while increasing overall cost of care by 4%.[103]

Consensus Guidelines

Recent consensus guidelines have made recommendations regarding optimal surgical approach. Both the European Society of Endocrine Surgeons and the Fourth International Workshop on the Management of Asymptomatic Primary Hyperparathyroidism that convened in 2013 have published recommendations regarding the ideal surgical management of 1°HPT.[104,105] Both groups favor FNE in patients who have parathyroid adenomas localized by preoperative imaging by 1 or more studies who have not had previous neck surgery. Imaging may include ultrasound or sestamibi scan. IOPTH monitoring must be used to ensure a successful outcome of the operation. Patients with negative preoperative imaging studies, a familial syndrome, or a condition predisposing to multigland disease should undergo BNE without the need for further imaging.

Box 1
Comparison of advantages of focused neck exploration versus bilateral neck exploration

Advantages of FNE

Smaller incision

Shorter operative time

Reduced cost compared with BNE

Outpatient surgery

Lower complication rate compared with BNE

Reduced postoperative pain

Cure rate equals BNE

Advantages of BNE

May be done through small incision

Shorter operative time

Reduced cost compared with FNE

May be done in outpatient setting

Detects multigland disease better than FNE

Does not require localization or IOPTH

Advantages and Disadvantages of Focused Neck Exploration Versus Bilateral Neck Exploration

There are advantages and disadvantages to each surgical approach for the management of 1^0HPT, and the operation must be tailored to the individual patient. Given equivalent cure rates and variable data regarding cost, the argument in favor of one technique versus the other depends on complication rates, impact on potential reoperative surgery, and patient satisfaction. First, complication rates with respect to permanent hypoparathyroidism and permanent recurrent laryngeal nerve injury are lower with FNE[106,107] with equivalent cure rates. The small number of patients who require reoperation for recurrent or persistent disease has a higher number of complications if the primary operation is BNE.[108] Patients who undergo FNE report significantly less postoperative pain.[109] Furthermore, FNE may be performed under local rather than general anesthesia; patients who have local anesthetic only have less postoperative nausea and are less likely to require antiemetic drugs.[110] These advantages are summarized in **Box 1**. Most patients (85%) have single-gland disease. Patients with concordant imaging studies have a single adenoma 96% to 98% of the time.[52,111] Despite increased identification of multigland disease with BNE, only a small percentage of patients subjected to this technique have any benefit, with an increase in injury rates to uninvolved parathyroid glands and to both recurrent laryngeal nerves. Thus, the authors believe that FNE is the appropriate choice for most patients.

SUMMARY

Many advances have shaped the surgical management of 1^0HPT. With the development of imaging techniques, application of the PTH assay as a key part of the operative management of the disease, and the overall predominance of single-gland disease, surgical management has shifted toward a minimally invasive approach. There are questions that remain, however. Which is the ideal preoperative imaging study? If a surgeon prefers BNE, are imaging studies necessary, and do these studies contribute unnecessary cost? If imaging studies are concordant or if the operation is BNE, is use of IOPTH mandatory? Advantages of FNE include a smaller incision, a potentially lower cost, shorter hospital stay, and reduced patient discomfort. With the application of endoscopic technology, both video-assisted and robot-assisted techniques are being developed in high-volume groups as an alternative to FNE. Some debate continues regarding the ideal approach: should FNE replace traditional BNE? While research continues to address this question, improved outcomes are clearly achieved with high-volume surgeons and experience.

REFERENCES

1. Sivula A, Ronni-Sivula H. The changing picture of primary hyperparathyroidism in the years 1956-1979. Ann Chir Gynaecol 1984;73(6):319–24.
2. Mandl F. Chirurgie der spertanfalle, ein leitfaden für stucherende und arzte 1925.
3. Cope O. The study of hyperparathyroidism at the Massachusetts General Hospital. N Engl J Med 1966;274(21):1174–82.
4. Uden P, Chan A, Duh QY, et al. Primary hyperparathyroidism in younger and older patients: symptoms and outcome of surgery. World J Surg 1992;16(4):791–7 [discussion: 798].
5. Bergenfelz A, Lindblom P, Tibblin S, et al. Unilateral versus bilateral neck exploration for primary hyperparathyroidism: a prospective randomized controlled trial. Ann Surg 2002;236(5):543–51.
6. McGill J, Sturgeon C, Kaplan SP, et al. How does the operative strategy for primary hyperparathyroidism impact the findings and cure rate? A comparison of 800 parathyroidectomies. J Am Coll Surg 2008;207(2):246–9.
7. Rubin MR, Bilezikian JP, McMahon DJ, et al. The natural history of primary hyperparathyroidism with or without parathyroid surgery after 15 years. J Clin Endocrinol Metab 2008;93(9):3462–70.
8. Udelsman R, Lin Z, Donovan P. The superiority of minimally invasive parathyroidectomy based on 1650 consecutive patients with primary hyperparathyroidism. Ann Surg 2011;253(3):585–91.
9. Bergenfelz A, Kanngiesser V, Zielke A, et al. Conventional bilateral cervical exploration versus open minimally invasive parathyroidectomy under local anaesthesia for primary hyperparathyroidism. Br J Surg 2005;92(2):190–7.
10. Jorde R, Bonaa KH, Sundsfjord J. Primary hyperparathyroidism detected in a health screening. The Tromso study. J Clin Epidemiol 2000;53(11):1164–9.
11. Wermers RA, Khosla S, Atkinson EJ, et al. Incidence of primary hyperparathyroidism in Rochester, Minnesota, 1993-2001: an update on the changing epidemiology of the disease. J Bone Miner Res 2006;21(1):171–7.
12. Heath H 3rd, Hodgson SF, Kennedy MA. Primary hyperparathyroidism. Incidence, morbidity, and potential economic impact in a community. N Engl J Med 1980;302(4):189–93.
13. Haff RC, Black WC, Ballinger WF. Primary hyperparathyroidism: changing clinical, surgical and pathologic aspects. Ann Surg 1970;171(1):85–92.
14. Bilezikian JP, Potts JT Jr. Asymptomatic primary hyperparathyroidism: new issues and new questions–bridging the past with the future. J Bone Miner Res 2002;17(Suppl 2):N57–67.

15. Pyrah LN, Hodgkinson A, Anderson CK. Primary hyperparathyroidism. Br J Surg 1966;53(4):245–316.

16. Wells SA Jr. Surgical therapy of patients with primary hyperparathyroidism: long-term benefits. J Bone Miner Res 1991;6(Suppl 2):S143–9 [discussion: S151–2].

17. Goldsmith RS. Differential diagnosis of hypercalcemia. N Engl J Med 1966; 274(12):674–7.

18. Spiegel AM. Pathophysiology of primary hyperparathyroidism. J Bone Miner Res 1991;6(Suppl 2):S15–7 [discussion: S31–2].

19. Koumakis E, Souberbielle JC, Sarfati E, et al. Bone mineral density evolution after successful parathyroidectomy in patients with normocalcemic primary hyperparathyroidism. J Clin Endocrinol Metab 2013;98(8):3213–20.

20. Wallace LB, Parikh RT, Ross LV, et al. The phenotype of primary hyperparathyroidism with normal parathyroid hormone levels: how low can parathyroid hormone go? Surgery 2011;150(6):1102–12.

21. Diagnosis and management of asymptomatic primary hyperparathyroidism. National Institutes of Health Consensus Development Conference. October 29-31, 1990. Consens Statement 1990;8(7):1–18.

22. Bilezikian JP, Potts JT Jr, Fuleihan Gel H, et al. Summary statement from a workshop on asymptomatic primary hyperparathyroidism: a perspective for the 21st century. J Bone Miner Res 2002;17(Suppl 2):N2–11.

23. Bilezikian JP, Khan AA, Potts JT Jr, et al. Guidelines for the management of asymptomatic primary hyperparathyroidism: summary statement from the third international workshop. J Clin Endocrinol Metab 2009;94(2):335–9.

24. Bilezikian JP, Brandi ML, Eastell R, et al. Guidelines for the management of asymptomatic primary hyperparathyroidism: summary statement from the Fourth International Workshop. J Clin Endocrinol Metab 2014;99(10):3561–9.

25. Greene AB, Butler RS, McIntyre S, et al. National trends in parathyroid surgery from 1998 to 2008: a decade of change. J Am Coll Surg 2009;209(3):332–43.

26. Nussbaum SR, Zahradnik RJ, Lavigne JR, et al. Highly sensitive two-site immunoradiometric assay of parathyrin, and its clinical utility in evaluating patients with hypercalcemia. Clin Chem 1987;33(8):1364–7.

27. Nussbaum SR, Thompson AR, Hutcheson KA, et al. Intraoperative measurement of parathyroid hormone in the surgical management of hyperparathyroidism. Surgery 1988;104(6):1121–7.

28. Irvin GL 3rd, Prudhomme DL, Deriso GT, et al. A new approach to parathyroidectomy. Ann Surg 1994;219(5):574–9 [discussion: 579–1].

29. Bergenfelz A, Algotsson L, Ahren B. Surgery for primary hyperparathyroidism performed under local anaesthesia. Br J Surg 1992;79(9):931–4.

30. Irvin GL 3rd, Dembrow VD, Prudhomme DL. Operative monitoring of parathyroid gland hyperfunction. Am J Surg 1991;162(4):299–302.

31. Richards ML, Thompson GB, Farley DR, et al. An optimal algorithm for intraoperative parathyroid hormone monitoring. Arch Surg 2011;146(3):280–5.

32. Gauger PG, Mullan MH, Thompson NW, et al. An alternative analysis of intraoperative parathyroid hormone data may improve the ability to detect multiglandular disease. Arch Surg 2004;139(2):164–9.

33. Wharry LI, Yip L, Armstrong MJ, et al. The final intraoperative parathyroid hormone level: how low should it go? World J Surg 2014;38(3):558–63.

34. Irvin GL 3rd, Sfakianakis G, Yeung L, et al. Ambulatory parathyroidectomy for primary hyperparathyroidism. Arch Surg 1996;131(10):1074–8.

35. Brennan MF. Lessons learned. Ann Surg Oncol 2006;13(10):1322–8.

36. Chiu ML, Kronauge JF, Piwnica-Worms D. Effect of mitochondrial and plasma membrane potentials on accumulation of hexakis (2-methoxyisobutylisonitrile) technetium(I) in cultured mouse fibroblasts. J Nucl Med 1990;31(10):1646–53.

37. Taillefer R, Boucher Y, Potvin C, et al. Detection and localization of parathyroid adenomas in patients with hyperparathyroidism using a single radionuclide imaging procedure with technetium-99m-sestamibi (double-phase study). J Nucl Med 1992;33(10):1801–7.

38. Wei JP, Burke GJ, Mansberger AR Jr. Prospective evaluation of the efficacy of technetium 99m sestamibi and iodine 123 radionuclide imaging of abnormal parathyroid glands. Surgery 1992;112(6):1111–6 [discussion: 1116–7].

39. Thule P, Thakore K, Vansant J, et al. Preoperative localization of parathyroid tissue with technetium-99m sestamibi 123I subtraction scanning. J Clin Endocrinol Metab 1994;78(1):77–82.

40. Johnston LB, Carroll MJ, Britton KE, et al. The accuracy of parathyroid gland localization in primary hyperparathyroidism using sestamibi radionuclide imaging. J Clin Endocrinol Metab 1996;81(1):346–52.

41. Hindie E, Melliere D, Simon D, et al. Primary hyperparathyroidism: is technetium 99m-Sestamibi/iodine-123 subtraction scanning the best procedure to locate enlarged glands before surgery? J Clin Endocrinol Metab 1995; 80(1):302–7.

42. McHenry CR, Lee K, Saadey J, et al. Parathyroid localization with technetium-99m-sestamibi: a prospective evaluation. J Am Coll Surg 1996;183(1):25–30.

43. Perez-Monte JE, Brown ML, Shah AN, et al. Parathyroid adenomas: accurate detection and localization with Tc-99m sestamibi SPECT. Radiology 1996; 201(1):85–91.

44. Light VL, McHenry CR, Jarjoura D, et al. Prospective comparison of dual-phase technetium-99m-sestamibi scintigraphy and high resolution ultrasonography in the evaluation of abnormal parathyroid glands. Am Surg 1996;62(7):562–7 [discussion: 567–8].

45. Solorzano CC, Carneiro-Pla DM, Irvin GL 3rd. Surgeon-performed ultrasonography as the initial and only localizing study in sporadic primary hyperparathyroidism. J Am Coll Surg 2006;202(1):18–24.

46. Levy JM, Kandil E, Yau LC, et al. Can ultrasound be used as the primary screening modality for the localization of parathyroid disease prior to surgery for primary hyperparathyroidism? A review of 440 cases. ORL J Otorhinolaryngol Relat Spec 2011;73(2):116–20.

47. Milas M, Stephen A, Berber E, et al. Ultrasonography for the endocrine surgeon: a valuable clinical tool that enhances diagnostic and therapeutic outcomes. Surgery 2005;138(6):1193–200 [discussion: 1200–1].

48. Morita SY, Somervell H, Umbricht CB, et al. Evaluation for concomitant thyroid nodules and primary hyperparathyroidism in patients undergoing parathyroidectomy or thyroidectomy. Surgery 2008;144(6):862–6 [discussion: 866–8].

49. De Feo ML, Colagrande S, Biagini C, et al. Parathyroid glands: combination of (99m)Tc MIBI scintigraphy and US for demonstration of parathyroid glands and nodules. Radiology 2000;214(2):393–402.

50. Scheiner JD, Dupuy DE, Monchik JM, et al. Pre-operative localization of parathyroid adenomas: a comparison of power and colour Doppler ultrasonography with nuclear medicine scintigraphy. Clin Radiol 2001;56(12):984–8.

51. Barczynski M, Golkowski F, Konturek A, et al. Technetium-99m-sestamibi subtraction scintigraphy vs. ultrasonography combined with a rapid parathyroid hormone assay in parathyroid aspirates in preoperative localization of

parathyroid adenomas and in directing surgical approach. Clin Endocrinol (Oxf) 2006;65(1):106–13.

52. Suliburk JW, Sywak MS, Sidhu SB, et al. 1000 minimally invasive parathyroidectomies without intra-operative parathyroid hormone measurement: lessons learned. ANZ J Surg 2011;81(5):362–5.

53. Gawande AA, Monchik JM, Abbruzzese TA, et al. Reassessment of parathyroid hormone monitoring during parathyroidectomy for primary hyperparathyroidism after 2 preoperative localization studies. Arch Surg 2006;141(4):381–4 [discussion: 384].

54. Hunter GJ, Schellingerhout D, Vu TH, et al. Accuracy of four-dimensional CT for the localization of abnormal parathyroid glands in patients with primary hyperparathyroidism. Radiology 2012;264(3):789–95.

55. Starker LF, Mahajan A, Bjorklund P, et al. 4D parathyroid CT as the initial localization study for patients with de novo primary hyperparathyroidism. Ann Surg Oncol 2011;18(6):1723–8.

56. Chen H, Mack E, Starling JR. Radioguided parathyroidectomy is equally effective for both adenomatous and hyperplastic glands. Ann Surg 2003;238(3):332–7 [discussion: 337–8].

57. Chen H, Mack E, Starling JR. A comprehensive evaluation of perioperative adjuncts during minimally invasive parathyroidectomy: which is most reliable? Ann Surg 2005;242(3):375–80 [discussion: 380–3].

58. Naitoh T, Gagner M, Garcia-Ruiz A, et al. Endoscopic endocrine surgery in the neck. An initial report of endoscopic subtotal parathyroidectomy. Surg Endosc 1998;12(3):202–5 [discussion: 206].

59. Henry JF, Defechereux T, Gramatica L, et al. Minimally invasive videoscopic parathyroidectomy by lateral approach. Langenbecks Arch Surg 1999;384(3):298–301.

60. Miccoli P, Bendinelli C, Conte M, et al. Endoscopic parathyroidectomy by a gasless approach. J Laparoendosc Adv Surg Tech A 1998;8(4):189–94.

61. Landry CS, Grubbs EG, Morris GS, et al. Robot assisted transaxillary surgery (RATS) for the removal of thyroid and parathyroid glands. Surgery 2011; 149(4):549–55.

62. Noureldine SI, Lewing N, Tufano RP, et al. The role of the robotic-assisted transaxillary gasless approach for the removal of parathyroid adenomas. ORL J Otorhinolaryngol Relat Spec 2014;76(1):19–24.

63. Tolley N, Garas G, Palazzo F, et al. A long-term prospective evaluation comparing robotic parathyroidectomy with minimally invasive open parathyroidectomy for primary hyperparathyroidism. Head Neck 2014. [Epub ahead of print].

64. Fouquet T, Germain A, Zarnegar R, et al. Totally endoscopic lateral parathyroidectomy: prospective evaluation of 200 patients. ESES 2010 Vienna presentation. Langenbecks Arch Surg 2010;395(7):935–40.

65. Stang MT, Perrier ND. Robotic thyroidectomy: do it well or don't do it. JAMA Surg 2013;148(9):806–8.

66. Perrier ND, Edeiken B, Nunez R, et al. A novel nomenclature to classify parathyroid adenomas. World J Surg 2009;33(3):412–6.

67. Chiu B, Sturgeon C, Angelos P. What is the link between nonlocalizing sestamibi scans, multigland disease, and persistent hypercalcemia? A study of 401 consecutive patients undergoing parathyroidectomy. Surgery 2006;140(3):418–22.

68. Dy BM, Richards ML, Vazquez BJ, et al. Primary hyperparathyroidism and negative Tc99 sestamibi imaging: to operate or not? Ann Surg Oncol 2012;19(7):2272–8.

69. Perrier ND, Ituarte PH, Morita E, et al. Parathyroid surgery: separating promise from reality. J Clin Endocrinol Metab 2002;87(3):1024–9.
70. Ogilvie JB, Clark OH. Parathyroid surgery: we still need traditional and selective approaches. J Endocrinol Invest 2005;28(6):566–9.
71. Wells SA Jr, Pacini F, Robinson BG, et al. Multiple endocrine neoplasia type 2 and familial medullary thyroid carcinoma: an update. J Clin Endocrinol Metab 2013;98(8):3149–64.
72. Thakker RV. Multiple endocrine neoplasia type 1. Indian J Endocrinol Metab 2012;16(Suppl 2):S272–4.
73. Thakker RV, Newey PJ, Walls GV, et al. Clinical practice guidelines for multiple endocrine neoplasia type 1 (MEN1). J Clin Endocrinol Metab 2012;97(9): 2990–3011.
74. Carling T, Udelsman R. Parathyroid surgery in familial hyperparathyroid disorders. J Intern Med 2005;257(1):27–37.
75. Awad SS, Miskulin J, Thompson N. Parathyroid adenomas versus four-gland hyperplasia as the cause of primary hyperparathyroidism in patients with prolonged lithium therapy. World J Surg 2003;27(4):486–8.
76. Hundley JC, Woodrum DT, Saunders BD, et al. Revisiting lithium-associated hyperparathyroidism in the era of intraoperative parathyroid hormone monitoring. Surgery 2005;138(6):1027–31 [discussion: 1031–2].
77. Norlen O, Sidhu S, Sywak M, et al. Long-term outcome after parathyroidectomy for lithium-induced hyperparathyroidism. Br J Surg 2014;101(10):1252–6.
78. Marti JL, Yang CS, Carling T, et al. Surgical approach and outcomes in patients with lithium-associated hyperparathyroidism. Ann Surg Oncol 2012;19(11):3465–71.
79. Siperstein A, Berber E, Barbosa GF, et al. Predicting the success of limited exploration for primary hyperparathyroidism using ultrasound, sestamibi, and intraoperative parathyroid hormone: analysis of 1158 cases. Ann Surg 2008; 248(3):420–8.
80. Norman J, Lopez J, Politz D. Abandoning unilateral parathyroidectomy: why we reversed our position after 15,000 parathyroid operations. J Am Coll Surg 2012; 214(3):260–9.
81. Nehs MA, Ruan DT, Gawande AA, et al. Bilateral neck exploration decreases operative time compared to minimally invasive parathyroidectomy in patients with discordant imaging. World J Surg 2013;37(7):1614–7.
82. Wang TS, Pasieka JL, Carty SE. Techniques of parathyroid exploration at North American endocrine surgery fellowship programs: what the next generation is being taught. Am J Surg 2014;207(4):527–32.
83. Abdulla AG, Ituarte PH, Harari A, et al. Trends in the frequency and quality of parathyroid surgery: analysis of 17,082 cases over 10 years. Ann Surg 2015; 261(4):746–50.
84. Sidhu S, Neill AK, Russell CF. Long-term outcome of unilateral parathyroid exploration for primary hyperparathyroidism due to presumed solitary adenoma. World J Surg 2003;27(3):339–42.
85. Robertson GS, Johnson PR, Bolia A, et al. Long-term results of unilateral neck exploration for preoperatively localized nonfamilial parathyroid adenomas. Am J Surg 1996;172(4):311–4.
86. Boggs JE, Irvin GL 3rd, Carneiro DM, et al. The evolution of parathyroidectomy failures. Surgery 1999;126(6):998–1002 [discussion: 1002–3].
87. Irvin GL 3rd, Carneiro DM, Solorzano CC. Progress in the operative management of sporadic primary hyperparathyroidism over 34 years. Ann Surg 2004; 239(5):704–8 [discussion; 708–1].

88. Udelsman R. Six hundred fifty-six consecutive explorations for primary hyper-parathyroidism. Ann Surg 2002;235(5):665–70 [discussion: 670–2].
89. van Heerden JA, Grant CS. Surgical treatment of primary hyperparathyroidism: an institutional perspective. World J Surg 1991;15(6):688–92.
90. Westerdahl J, Bergenfelz A. Unilateral versus bilateral neck exploration for pri-mary hyperparathyroidism: five-year follow-up of a randomized controlled trial. Ann Surg 2007;246(6):976–80 [discussion: 980–1].
91. Slepavicius A, Beisa V, Janusonis V, et al. Focused versus conventional parathy-roidectomy for primary hyperparathyroidism: a prospective, randomized, blinded trial. Langenbecks Arch Surg 2008;393(5):659–66.
92. Grant CS, Thompson G, Farley D, et al. Primary hyperparathyroidism surgical management since the introduction of minimally invasive parathyroidectomy: Mayo Clinic experience. Arch Surg 2005;140(5):472–8 [discussion: 478–9].
93. Aarum S, Nordenstrom J, Reihner E, et al. Operation for primary hyperparathy-roidism: the new versus the old order. A randomised controlled trial of preoper-ative localisation. Scand J Surg 2007;96(1):26–30.
94. Goldstein RE, Blevins L, Delbeke D, et al. Effect of minimally invasive radioguided parathyroidectomy on efficacy, length of stay, and costs in the management of primary hyperparathyroidism. Ann Surg 2000;231(5): 732–42.
95. Fahy BN, Bold RJ, Beckett L, et al. Modern parathyroid surgery: a cost-benefit analysis of localizing strategies. Arch Surg 2002;137(8):917–22 [discussion: 922–3].
96. Lubitz CC, Stephen AE, Hodin RA, et al. Preoperative localization strategies for primary hyperparathyroidism: an economic analysis. Ann Surg Oncol 2012; 19(13):4202–9.
97. Wang TS, Cheung K, Farrokhyar F, et al. Would scan, but which scan? A cost-utility analysis to optimize preoperative imaging for primary hyperparathyroid-ism. Surgery 2011;150(6):1286–94.
98. Harari A, Allendorf J, Shifrin A, et al. Negative preoperative localization leads to greater resource use in the era of minimally invasive parathyroidectomy. Am J Surg 2009;197(6):769–73.
99. Lowney JK, Weber B, Johnson S, et al. Minimal incision parathyroidectomy: cure, cosmesis, and cost. World J Surg 2000;24(11):1442–5.
100. Doppman JL, Miller DL. Localization of parathyroid tumors in patients with asymptomatic hyperparathyroidism and no previous surgery. J Bone Miner Res 1991;6(Suppl 2):S153–8 [discussion: S159].
101. Roe SM, Brown PW, Pate LM, et al. Initial cervical exploration for parathyroidec-tomy is not benefited by preoperative localization studies. Am Surg 1998;64(6): 503–7 [discussion: 507–8].
102. Mihai R, Weisters M, Stechman MJ, et al. Cost-effectiveness of scan-directed parathyroidectomy. Langenbecks Arch Surg 2008;393(5):739–43.
103. Morris LF, Zanocco K, Ituarte PH, et al. The value of intraoperative parathyroid hormone monitoring in localized primary hyperparathyroidism: a cost analysis. Ann Surg Oncol 2010;17(3):679–85.
104. Udelsman R, Akerstrom G, Biagini C, et al. The surgical management of asymp-tomatic primary hyperparathyroidism: proceedings of the Fourth International Workshop. J Clin Endocrinol Metab 2014;99(10):3595–606.
105. Bergenfelz AO, Hellman P, Harrison B, et al. Positional statement of the Euro-pean Society of Endocrine Surgeons (ESES) on modern techniques in pHPT sur-gery. Langenbecks Arch Surg 2009;394(5):761–4.

106. Mihai R, Barczynski M, Iacobone M, et al. Surgical strategy for sporadic primary hyperparathyroidism an evidence-based approach to surgical strategy, patient selection, surgical access, and reoperations. Langenbecks Arch Surg 2009; 394(5):785–98.
107. Vogel LM, Lucas R, Czako P. Unilateral parathyroid exploration. Am Surg 1998; 64(7):693–6 [discussion: 696–7].
108. Morris LF, Lee S, Warneke CL, et al. Fewer adverse events after reoperative parathyroidectomy associated with initial minimally invasive parathyroidectomy. Am J Surg 2014;208(5):850–5.
109. Miccoli P, Barellini L, Monchik JM, et al. Randomized clinical trial comparing regional and general anaesthesia in minimally invasive video-assisted parathyroidectomy. Br J Surg 2005;92(7):814–8.
110. Monchik JM, Barellini L, Langer P, et al. Minimally invasive parathyroid surgery in 103 patients with local/regional anesthesia, without exclusion criteria. Surgery 2002;131(5):502–8.
111. Powell AC, Alexander HR, Chang R, et al. Reoperation for parathyroid adenoma: a contemporary experience. Surgery 2009;146(6):1144–55.

Pheochromocytoma and Paraganglioma
Diagnosis, Genetics, and Treatment

Colleen M. Kiernan, MD, MPH*, Carmen C. Solórzano, MD[1]

KEYWORDS

- Neuroendocrine tumor • Pheochromocytoma • Paraganglioma
- Biochemical evaluation • Genetics • Imaging • Perioperative management • Surgery

KEY POINTS

- Pheochromocytomas and paragangliomas (Pheo/PGL) are rare neuroendocrine tumors that are being discovered incidentally at an increasing rate.
- At least one-quarter of patients with Pheo/PGL display germline mutations; genetic testing plays an increasingly important role in the evaluation and management of these patients.
- Plasma-free metanephrines and urinary fractionated metanephrine levels are highly sensitive in the diagnosis of Pheo/PGL.
- Selective or nonselective alpha blocking agents and calcium channel blockers appear to be equally effective in treating the physiologic effects of Pheo/PGL.
- Several surgical approaches are used to remove Pheo/PGL, and the choice of approach depends on patient and tumor-related factors, as well as surgeon preference.

INTRODUCTION: NATURE OF THE PROBLEM

The terms paraganglioma (PGL) and pheochromocytoma (Pheo) were first mentioned in 1908 and 1912 respectively when pathologists Henri Alezais, Felix Peyron, and Ludwig Pick noted tumors with a positive chromaffin reaction in extra-adrenal and adrenal chromaffin tissue. However, according to Welborne and colleagues[1] it was not until 1922, when Marcel Labbe and colleagues[2] reported a case of symptomatic paroxysmal hypertension in a patient with a Pheo, that the relationship between the tumor and its symptoms was established.

The first successful resection for Pheo was performed by Cesar Roux in February 1926. The patient, Madam S, was 33 years old and had suffered attacks of vertigo

The authors have nothing to disclose.

Division of Surgical Oncology and Endocrine Surgery, Vanderbilt University Medical Center, 597 Preston Research Building, 2220 Pierce Avenue, Nashville, TN 37232, USA

[1] Present address: 597 Preston Research Building, 2220 Pierce Avenue, Nashville, TN 37232, USA.

* Corresponding author. 1161 21st Avenue, CCC-4312 MCN, Nashville, TN 37232.

E-mail address: colleen.m.kiernan@vanderbilt.edu

and nausea for 2 years. At laparotomy, she was found to have a 13-cm adrenal Pheo. Charles Mayo performed the second and perhaps better-known resection for Pheo in October 1926. The patient, Mother Joachim, a nun from Canada, suffered from paroxysmal hypertension, weakness, vomiting, and headaches. At the time, it was felt that her hypertension was mediated through the sympathetic nerves and that sympathectomy may provide relief. She underwent an exploratory laparotomy, and a tumor "the size of a lemon" was found behind the tail of her pancreas. Without preoperative pharmacologic blockade, the entire procedure was completed in 64 minutes and the patient recovered well.[1,3]

By 1934, more than 60 patients had been diagnosed with a Pheo or PGL and by 1940, 20 successful operations had been performed. The operative mortality in these early series was 30% to 45%.[4] These high mortality rates were partly due to a lack of preoperative alpha blockade and modern anesthesia management. Since that time, much has been learned about the management of these rare tumors. Herein we discuss the incidence and prevalence of Pheo/PGL; describe the typical clinical presentation and diagnostic evaluation of these tumors; explore the known genetic associations; and summarize the preoperative, intraoperative, and postoperative management strategies.

EPIDEMIOLOGY

The annual incidence of Pheo and PGL is between 2 and 8 per million and the prevalence in the population is 1:6500 to 1:2500, respectively.[5] Pheo/PGLs are thought to occur in 0.05% to 0.1% of patients with sustained hypertension. However, this accounts for only 50% of people with Pheo/PGL because approximately half of patients will have paroxysmal hypertension or normotension.[5] Pheochromocytomas comprise 4% to 8% of all adrenal incidentalomas.[6–9] The peak age of occurrence is in the third to fifth decade of life. Today, 10% to 49% of Pheo/PGLs are found incidentally during imaging studies obtained for other reasons.[10–14]

In 1951, John Graham[15] analyzed the records of 207 Pheo/PGLs and concluded that Pheo/PGLs follow the "rule of 10s," with 10% occurring in extra-adrenal tissues, 10% bilateral, and 10% malignant. Later, the teaching that 10% of these tumors were familial was added to this rule. Although this teaching persists in many textbooks and medical school lectures, studies have shown that the "rule of 10" no longer applies. Approximately 15% to 25% of Pheo/PGLs originate in extra-adrenal chromaffin tissue,[16,17] 8% of sporadic and 20% to 75% of hereditary Pheo/PGL are bilateral at presentation,[18–20] 5% of adrenal-based and 33% extra-adrenal tumors are malignant,[14] and at least 24% of sporadic Pheo/PGLs have a genetic basis.[18] Today, bilaterality, extra-adrenal location, and prevalence of malignancy depend directly on the underlying genetic mutation.

PATHOPHYSIOLOGY

Pheo/PGLs are neuroendocrine tumors that arise from paraganglia cells derived from the neural crest and are distributed along the paravertebral and para-aortic axis from the base of the skull to the pelvic floor. Adrenal-based Pheos arise in the sympathetic adrenal chromaffin cells. Extra-adrenal sympathetic PGLs most commonly occur around the inferior mesenteric artery or at the aortic bifurcation in the organ of Zuckerkandl, but can occur in any chromaffin tissue in the thorax, abdomen, and pelvis. Almost all adrenal-based Pheos and extra-adrenal sympathetic PGLs produce, store, metabolize, and secrete catecholamines or their metabolites.[5] Extra-adrenal parasympathetic PGLs are most commonly found in the head and neck region and are usually not associated with catecholamine secretion. In this article, head and neck PGLs are not discussed.

The uncontrolled release of catecholamines by Pheo/PGLs leads to several physiologic changes and end-organ effects. Prolonged and repeated norepinephrine release has been associated with long periods of vasoconstriction and contraction of the venous pool, and thus decreased circulating blood volume. The decrease in blood volume can lead to acute hypovolemia on cessation of norepinephrine-induced vasoconstriction when the Pheo/PGL is surgically removed. Tumors that secrete predominantly epinephrine have been associated with tachycardia and tachyarrhythmias in addition to arterial hypertension.[21] Elevated plasma catecholamine levels can result in increased glycogenolysis and inhibition of insulin release by islet cells, resulting in signs and symptoms of diabetes mellitus. Additionally, elevated catecholamines can lead to stress-induced cardiomyopathy (Takotsubo cardiomyopathy) with severe left ventricular dysfunction.[22] Pheochromocytoma crisis is the name given to a constellation of symptoms that can result from uncontrolled release of catecholamines and consists of multisystem organ failure, high fever, encephalopathy, and severe hypertension and/or hypotension. Although rarely seen today, these symptoms can progress to severe metabolic acidosis and death if not recognized and treated.[23]

CLINICAL PRESENTATION AND DIAGNOSIS
Clinical Presentation

The main signs and symptoms of excess circulating catecholamines from Pheo/PGL are headache, palpitations, sweating, pallor, nausea, constipation, flushing, weight loss, fatigue, anxiety, sustained or paroxysmal hypertension, orthostatic hypotension, fever, and hyperglycemia.[5,14] According to the degree of catecholamine excess, patients may present with myocardial infarction, arrhythmia, or stroke. Because similar signs and symptoms are produced by numerous other clinical conditions (**Table 1**), Pheo/PGL is often referred to as the "great mimic."[5] In our experience, patients are often diagnosed with an incidental "asymptomatic" adrenal mass and when a focused history is obtained, the classic symptoms of Pheo/PGL are often elicited in retrospect.

Biochemical Evaluation

Traditional biochemical tests include measurements of urinary and plasma catecholamines, urinary fractionated and plasma-free metanephrines, and urinary vanillylmandelic acid (VMA). When a patient is suspected to have a Pheo/PGL, the recommended initial test is plasma-free metanephrines or 24-hour urinary fractionated metanephrines.[5,14,24] Norepinephrine and epinephrine are metabolized within the tumor by

Table 1	
Differential diagnosis for diagnosis of pheochromocytoma and paraganglioma	
Organ System	**Possible Diagnosis**
Endocrine	Hyperthyroidism, carcinoid syndrome, hypoglycemia, medullary thyroid carcinoma, mastocytosis, menopause
Cardiovascular	Congestive heart failure, arrhythmias, ischemic heart disease, baroreflex failure
Neurologic	Migraine, stroke, meningioma, postural orthostatic tachycardia
Miscellaneous	Porphyria, panic disorder, factitious disorders, monoamine oxidase inhibitor use, clonidine withdrawal, cocaine abuse

catechol-O-methyltransferase to normetanephrine and metanephrine, respectively.[25] The lack of this enzyme in sympathetic nerves means that the O-methylated metabolites are relatively specific markers of chromaffin tumors.[26] These metabolites are produced continuously in the tumor independent of physiologic catecholamine release and therefore have been shown to be both more sensitive and specific diagnostic biomarkers of Pheo/PGL than their parent catecholamine.[5,27,28] There is no consensus that one test is superior.[26] The investigators prefer to start by measuring plasma-free metanephrines because of their high sensitivity and patient convenience. Blood sampling should be performed with the patient in the supine position 15 to 20 minutes after intravenous (IV) catheter insertion. Eight to 12 hours before testing, food, caffeinated beverages, strenuous exercise, and/or smoking should be avoided, to reduce false-positive results from secondary catecholamine release. Providers interpreting tests results should be aware that sympathomimetic agents such as labetalol, sotalol, acetaminophen, buspirone, mesalamine, sulfasalazine, methyldopa, and antidepressants can interfere with the biochemical assays.[25,29] In a multicenter cohort study of 858 patients, Lenders and colleagues[27] found that the use of multiple initial diagnostic tests increases sensitivity at the cost of decreased specificity. A single plasma or urine metanephrine level remains superior to that of a combination of biochemical tests for initial diagnostic workup.

Studies have shown that in comparison with plasma-free metanephrines or urinary fractionated metanephrines, urinary VMA has a lower sensitivity (68%) and therefore it is not used routinely in our practice.[26] Plasma or urinary dopamine and its metabolite (methoxytyramine) may also be elevated in patients with Pheo/PGL. Although they are not used for diagnostic purposes, their elevation has been associated with SDHB and SDHD mutations and therefore may help guide management.[30]

A suggested algorithm for the biochemical evaluation of Pheo/PGL is depicted in **Fig. 1**. If urine and/or plasma metabolites are normal, the diagnosis of Pheo/PGL can be excluded due to the high sensitivity of these tests. If urine and/or plasma metabolite levels are >4 times above the upper limit of normal for any given laboratory, the diagnosis of Pheo/PGL is highly probable.[5,25,31] Patients with slight or moderate elevation (>1 time or less than 3 times above the normal limit) of both or either metabolite should undergo repeat testing once potential causes of false-positive results are removed or addressed. Finally, if repeat testing results in elevation of metabolites, a clonidine suppression test can be considered to confirm the diagnosis. This test is useful in distinguishing between high levels of plasma norepinephrine caused by release from sympathetic nerves and those from Pheo/PGL. It is considered diagnostic if norepinephrine levels remain elevated 3 hours after administration of 0.3 mg of oral clonidine.[25] It is important to note that this test is not useful for tumors that intermittently secrete catecholamines or in patients who have marginally elevated norepinephrine levels. Additionally, diuretics and tricyclic antidepressants can cause false-positive values.[16] When the diagnosis of Pheo/PGL is suspected but not confirmed (lack of >4 times elevation of metabolites) and there is a mass on imaging, our group prefers to forgo the clonidine test and proceed directly to resection, particularly when such patients have indications for surgical intervention, such as a large size and atypical imaging characteristics.[32]

When possible, biochemical testing should always precede imaging, as it is the most cost-effective approach to the diagnosis of Pheo/PGL and if biochemical testing proves negative, the patient is not subject to unnecessary radiation. However, in clinical practice, many patients with Pheo/PGL present with an incidentally discovered mass and are in need of biochemical evaluation after imaging is already complete.[5,26,32]

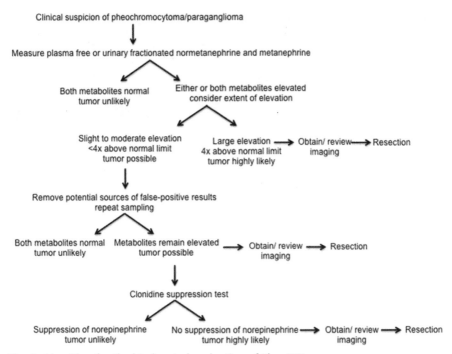

Fig. 1. Algorithm for the biochemical evaluation of Pheo/PGL.

Imaging

The 2 most commonly used imaging modalities in the initial evaluation of Pheo/PGL are computerized tomography scan (CT) with and without IV contrast (adrenal protocol for adrenal lesions) and MRI. Functional imaging, including 123 I-metaiodobenzylguanidine (MIBG), 111-In-Pentetreotide (octreotide scan), and PET combined with CT (PET/CT) using fluorodeoxyglucose (FDG) and other radiolabeled agents are also used for the localization of Pheo/PGL.

Computed tomography

CT provides an excellent initial method for the localization of Pheo/PGL because of its outstanding spatial resolution for the thorax, abdomen, and pelvis. To obtain the best results, CT scans should be performed with and without IV contrast. CT scans are highly sensitive (88%–100%) but lack specificity.[26,33] Pheo/PGL may appear homogeneous or heterogenous, can be necrotic with some calcifications, and may appear solid or cystic (**Fig. 2A**). Pheo/PGLs demonstrate avid contrast enhancement due to their rich capillary network, and most exhibit mean attenuations of more than 10 Hounsfield units on unenhanced CT.[32,34] Some studies suggest that the sensitivity of CT for extra-adrenal or bilateral tumors can be low, and therefore the use of MRI or other functional studies is advised in these populations.[35,36] However, in our practice, CT scan is often the only imaging study necessary to localize lesions and plan for resection of a Pheo/PGL.

MRI

This imaging technique has the same sensitivity and specificity as CT scan in detecting adrenal-based Pheos but has shown superior sensitivity (near 100%) in detecting PGLs and familial adrenal pheochromocytomas.[37] Pheo/PGLs show enhancement on

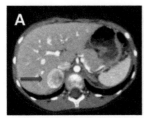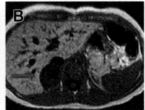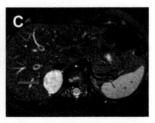

Fig. 2. CT and MRI images of adrenal-based Pheo. (*A*) CT abdomen with IV contrast of right adrenal pheochromocytoma. (*B*) MRI T1-weighted image of right Pheo. (*C*) MRI T2-weighted image of right adrenal Pheo. *Arrows* point to the adrenal based pheochromocytoma.

T2-weighted imaging and may appear heterogenous due to internal hemorrhage and cystic components (**Fig. 2**B, C).[34] MRI is useful in patients with inability to tolerate IV contrast, those with intracorporeal metal or surgical clips, and in patients in whom radiation exposure should be limited; that is, children, pregnant women, patients with germline mutations, or in patients with previous excessive radiation exposure.[26]

Functional imaging
There is debate over the role of functional imaging in the preoperative evaluation of Pheo/PGL. Some groups recommend functional imaging for all Pheo/PGLs except for metanephrine producing a small adrenal-based Pheo (PGLs do not produce epinephrine).[5] Others recommend selective use of functional imaging for patients with a high risk of recurrent, multifocal, or malignant disease and for patients with occult lesions on CT or MRI.[38,39] The field of functional imaging is expanding and some techniques are available only under clinical trials at selected centers.

Metaiodobenzylguanidine with single-photon emission computed tomography
Metaiodobenzylguanidine with single-photon emission CT (MIBG-SPECT) is a guanethidine analog resembling norepinephrine that is taken up and concentrated in sympatho-adrenergic tissue. SPECT data can be fused with CT images to improve spatial resolution and provide anatomic correlation (**Fig. 3**). The 123 I-MIBG is used preferentially over 131 I-MIBG because of its higher sensitivity, shorter half-life, lack of beta emission, lower radiation dose, and better image quality. The 131 I-MIBG can be used to treat MIBG avid metastasis. MIBG displays improved specificity (95%–100%) when compared with CT or MRI. MIBG can be used to identify sites of primary disease, evaluate metastases, and confirm the biochemical diagnosis. However, 123 I-MIBG-SPECT has lower sensitivity (80%–100%, 88%–100%, respectively) when compared with MRI and CT.[26,39–41] Some studies show that the sensitivity of MIBG scans is further reduced in familial PGL syndromes, malignant disease, and extra-adrenal Pheo/PGLs[5,41–45] (**Fig. 4**). Furthermore, up to 50% of normal adrenal

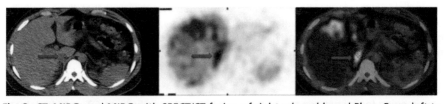

Fig. 3. CT, MIBG, and MIBG with SPECT/CT fusion of right adrenal-based Pheo. From left to right, CT scan, MIBG, MIBG with SPECT/CT fusion. *Arrows* point to the adrenal based pheochromocytoma.

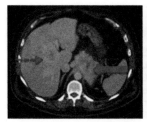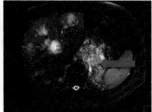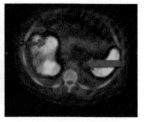

Fig. 4. CT, MRI, and MIBG-SPECT/CT of para-aortic PGL with liver metastases (*solid arrow* points to PGL; *dashed arrow* points to liver metastases.) From left to right: CT scan of abdomen and pelvis, MRI T2-weighted image, MIBG-SPECT/CT.

glands demonstrate physiologic uptake of 123 I-MIBG and thus false-positive results for adrenal-based lesions are a problem.[26,46]

Octreotide scan
The radiolabeled octreotide binds to somatostatin receptors in tumors; however, the extent of the binding is variable and dependent on the presence of such receptors in the Pheo/PGL.

The 123 I-MIBG is more sensitive than octreotide for the site of primary disease; however, octreotide has high sensitivity for metastatic disease and can be positive in tumors that have no MIBG uptake. Therefore, octreotide scans may be useful if MIBG scan is negative and/or metastatic disease is suspected.[34]

PET/computed tomography scan
Depending on the radioactive tracer used, the use of PET/CT scans in Pheo/PGL can have superior sensitivity and specificity when compared with 123 I-MIBG and octreotide scans.

However, because of its limited availability and sometimes high cost, it is not commonly used in the evaluation of Pheo/PGL.[26] There are multiple agents used in PET scanning for Pheo/PGL and include 18F-FDG, 18F-fluorodopamine (18F-FDA), 18-F-fluorodihydroxy-phenylalanine (18F-FDOPA) and 68-gallium 1,4,7,10-teraazacy-clododecane-1,4,5,10-teraacetic acid-octreotate (68-Ga-DOTATATE). The currently known strengths and weaknesses of these imaging agents and the aforementioned imaging modalities are summarized in **Table 2**.

Although some investigators advocate for both positive localization with CT/MRI and 123-MIBG before surgical intervention,[16] most investigators will agree that when there is a high biochemical probability of Pheo/PGL and low likelihood of metastases (small tumor, adrenal location, adrenergic phenotype, non-*SDHB*) that CT or MRI is adequate. If, however, metastatic disease is suspected or when CT or MRI fails to localize the lesion, functional imaging may be warranted.[5,26,47] In our practice, if CT or MRI fails to localize the lesion or a patient is suspected to have a hereditary syndrome or metastatic disease, 123-MIBG, 18F-FDG, or 68-Ga-DOTATATE (on protocol) or a combination may be used.

Genetic Testing
Pheo/PGLs are associated with multiple genetic mutations and familial syndromes (**Table 3**). It is estimated that 20% to 41% of Pheo/PGLs are associated with known genetic mutations.[48–51] Neumann and colleagues[18] studied 298 unrelated patients diagnosed with presumably sporadic Pheo/PGL, and 24% were found to have germline mutations. Hereditary Pheo/PGLs are most commonly associated with Multiple

Table 2
Diagnostic imaging modalities: strengths and weaknesses

	Strengths	Weakness
CT with and without IV contrast	• Localizes Pheo/PGL with 88%–100% sensitivity • Easiest for surgeon to interpret • Often the only imaging modality necessary to localize and plan for resection	• Lacks specificity • Lower sensitivity (64%) for extra-adrenal or bilateral tumors • Requires IV contrast
MRI	• Localizes Pheo/PGL with 88%–100% sensitivity • Localizes extra-adrenal and familial adrenal Pheo/PGL with near 100% sensitivity • Avoids radiation exposure of CT	• Difficult to interpret for surgical planning • Less tolerated by some patients (claustrophobia)
123 I-MIBG-SPECT with or without CT	• Can confirm biochemical diagnosis of Pheo/PGL with 95%–100% specificity	• Lower sensitivity than CT/MRI • 50% of normal adrenal glands demonstrate uptake (false positives) • Sensitivity reduced in familial PGL, malignant disease and extra-adrenal Pheo/PGL
Octreotide scan	• High sensitivity for metastatic disease • Can be positive in tumors that have no MIBG uptake	• Variable uptake in tumors • Less sensitive than 123 I-MIBG for primary disease
18 F-FDG PET/CT	• Superior to 123 I-MIBG, 18 F-FDA in visualization of malignant Pheo/PGL and metastasis; especially in patients with *SDHB* mutations	• Cannot be differentiated between benign and malignant lesions • Expensive
18 F-FDA PET/CT	• Good imaging agent for Pheo/PGL • Superior to 123 or 131 I-MIBG in detection of Pheo/PGL especially for malignant tumors (testing only in VHL)	• Difficult to produce and limited availability • Normal adrenal uptake (false positives) • Expensive
18 F-FDOPA PET/CT	• Superior to 123 I-MIBG in detection of Pheo/PGL • Does not concentrate within normal adrenal tissue	• Low sensitivity for metastatic Pheo/PGL • Limited availability • Expensive
68 Ga-DOTATATE PET/CT	• High sensitivity in patients with high risk of PGL and metastatic disease • Superior to 123-MIBG in detecting lesions in all locations, particularly bone	• Available only in clinical trials • Expensive

Abbreviations: 68-Ga-DOTATATE, 68-gallium 1,4,7,10-teraazacyclododecane-1,4,5,10-teraacetic acid-octreotate; CT, computed tomography; FDA, fluorodopamine; FDG, fluorodeoxyglucose; FDOPA, fluorodihydroxy-phenylalanine; IV, intravenous; MIBG, I-metaiodobenzylguanidine; PGL, paraganglioma; Pheo, pheochromocytoma; SPECT, single-photon emission CT.

Table 3
Genes associated with Pheo/PGL and the associated clinical phenotype and frequency

Gene	Syndrome/Clinical Phenotype	Frequency	Proportion of Malignant Pheo/PGL
FH	Leiomyomas (cutaneous and uterine) and papillary kidney cancer and Pheo/PGL	<1% of all Pheo/PGL patients The % of patients with FH who develop Pheo/PGL is unknown	Unknown
HIF2	Multiple paragangliomas and polycythemia	Unknown—Rare	Unknown
MAX	Pheo/PGL	Unknown—Rare	Unknown
NF1	von Recklinghausen disease: peripheral nervous system tumors, gastrointestinal stromal tumors, malignant gliomas, and juvenile chronic myelogenous leukemia	1% of all Pheo/PGL patients 1%–2% of patients with NF1 develop Pheo/PGL	11% of NF1 Pheo/PGL are malignant
RET	MEN2A: medullary thyroid carcinoma, pheochromocytoma, primary hyperparathyroidism MEN2B: medullary thyroid carcinoma, pheochromocytoma, mucosal neuromas	5% of all Pheo/PGL patients 50% of MEN2a patients develop Pheo/PGL ~ 100% of MEN2b patients develop Pheo/PGL	4% of RET Pheo/PGL are malignant
SDHA	Pheo/PGL	Unknown—Rare	Unknown
SDHB	Pheo/PGL, renal tumors, familial renal cell carcinoma	10%–15% of all patients with Pheo/PGL The % of patients with SDHB who develop Pheo/PGL is unknown	50% of SDHB Pheo/PGL are malignant
SDHC	Head and neck PGL, Pheo/PGL	Unknown—Rare	Unknown
SDHD	Head and neck PGL, Pheo/PGL	5%–10% of all patients with Pheo/PGL The % of patients with SDHD who develop Pheo/PGL is unknown	Unknown
TMEM127	Pheo/PGL	Unknown—Rare	Unknown
VHL	von Hippel-Lindau disease: retinal and cerebellar hemangioblastoma, renal cell carcinoma, Pheo/PGL, pancreatic neuroendocrine tumors, visceral cysts, Pheo/PGL	5%–10% of all patients with Pheo/PGL 20% of VHL patients develop Pheo/PGL	Less frequent than sporadic Pheo/PGL but overall % unknown

Abbreviations: PGL, paraganglioma; Pheo, pheochromocytoma.

Endocrine Neoplasia type 2 syndrome (*RET* proto-oncogene mutation), Von Reckling-hausen disease/neurofibromatosis type 1 (*NF-1* mutation), von Hippel-Lindau disease (*VHL* mutation), and familial Pheo/PGL syndrome due to germline mutations of genes encoding succinate dehydrogenase subunits A, B, C, and D (*SDHA, SDHB, SDHC, SDHD, SDHAF2*). In general, these traits are inherited in an autosomal dominant pattern.[5,52] Less frequently, hereditary Pheo/PGLs are associated with familial Pheo syndrome due to germline mutations in *TMEM127* or *MAX*, polycythemia PGL syndrome due to mutations in the *HIF2* gene, or leiomyomatosis and renal cell cancer due to mutations in the fumarate hydratase gene (*FH*).

Most investigators agree that although it is not cost-effective to obtain genetic testing on every patient with a Pheo/PGL, genetic testing should be considered in all patients with Pheo/PGL.[5,18,26,49] It is our practice to routinely refer Pheo/PGL patients to the Hereditary Cancer Clinic for counseling and consideration of genetic testing. There are several reasons to consider testing in all patients. First, as previously stated, it is estimated that a quarter to a third of all patients with Pheo/PGL have disease-causing germline mutations. Second, mutations in the *SDHB* gene have been associated with metastatic disease in approximately 40% to 50% of affected patients.[53,54] Finally, establishing a hereditary syndrome in the proband may result in earlier diagnosis and treatment of Pheo/PGL and other syndromic manifestations in relatives.[26]

There is no consensus to determine who should be tested and for which genes. However, most agree that there should be an algorithm for genetic testing and that it should include factors such as presence of a clinical syndrome, family history, biochemical profile, and/or metastases at presentation.[26,49,51,52,55] Age at presentation, extra-adrenal tumor location, and patients with multiple tumors also should be considered. In a study of 989 nonsyndromic Pheo cases, age younger than 45 years and extra-adrenal tumor location were independently associated with a fivefold increased likelihood of mutation when compared with patients older than 45 years or those with adrenal-based tumors. Furthermore, the presence of multiple tumors was associated with an eightfold increased likelihood of mutation when compared with patients with a single focus of disease.[56] Based on a review of the literature,[26,49,55,56] a proposed algorithm for genetic testing in patients with Pheo/PGL is depicted in **Table 4**. Recently, a genetic sequencing panel was made commercially available that tests for 10 gene mutations: *MAX, MEN1, NF1, RET, SDHAF2, SDHB, SDHC, SDHD, TMEM127*, and *VHL*. As these panels become more available and cost-effective, they will eliminate the need for a stepwise approach to genetic testing and make genetic testing more accessible to all patients with Pheo/PGL.

PREOPERATIVE MANAGEMENT

It is recommended that all patients with functional Pheo/PGL should receive appropriate preoperative medical management to block the effects of catecholamine release during surgical extirpation.[5] The practice of alpha-blockade was first described in the literature in 1956 when Priestly and colleagues[57] reported on a series of 51 Pheos removed without mortality. The lack of mortality was attributed to routine intraoperative use of alpha-blockade.[58] Due to wide-ranging practices and lack of randomized control trials or large prospective cohort studies, there is no consensus and no specific recommendations regarding the preferred drug to be used for preoperative blockade. However, alpha-blockade, calcium channel blockade, or angiotensin receptor blockade have all been named as options. The main goal of preoperative

Table 4	
Recommended order of genetic testing by clinical presentation, tumor location and biochemical profile	
Clinical Presentation/Biochemical Profile	**Gene(s) to Be Analyzed**
Syndromic presentation/family history	
VHL	*VHL*
MEN2	*RET*
NF1	*NF1*
Metastatic disease	*SDHB if SDHB negative: SDHD, SDHC, VHL, MAX, FH*
Extra-adrenal	
Dopaminergic	*SDHB, SDHD*
Normetanephrine	*VHL, SDHB, SDHC, SDHD*
Adrenal	
Dopaminergic	*SDHB, SDHD*
Normetanephrine	*VHL, SDHD, SDHB*
Metanephrine	*RET, NF1*
Bilateral or age <45	*VHL, RET*

management of Pheo/PGL is to normalize blood pressure, heart rate, and volume status and prevent a patient from surgically induced catecholamine storm and its consequences on the cardiovascular system.[51]

Nonselective Alpha-Blocking Agent

Phenoxybenzamine is the most recognized and widely used alpha-blocking agent for Pheo/PGL resections. It is a nonselective, irreversible, noncompetitive alpha-blocker. It has a long-lasting effect that diminishes only after de novo alpha-receptor synthesis. The typical starting dosage is 10 mg twice daily. This dosage is increased until clinical manifestations are controlled or side effects appear. Typical side effects include postural hypotension, reflex tachycardia, dizziness, syncope, nasal congestion, and headache. In comparison with selective alpha-blocking agents, phenoxybenzamine is expensive, is not readily available in many pharmacies, and has higher side-effect profile.

Selective Alpha-Blocking Agents

Prazosin, terazosin, and doxazosin have been used as an alternative to phenoxybenzamine. These drugs are short-acting alpha-1 antagonists. They offer the advantage of once-daily dosing and are less expensive and more readily available than phenoxybenzamine. We typically start doxazosin at a dosage of 5 mg daily and the dosage is increased until clinical manifestations are controlled. The most common side effect is orthostatic hypotension. Multiple studies have compared the intraoperative and postoperative hemodynamics as well as outcomes of patients treated with nonselective and selective alpha blockade.[59–63] These studies have demonstrated no difference in the incidence of intraoperative or postoperative adverse outcomes when selective alpha blockade is used as an alternative to nonselective phenoxybenzamine. Thus, the choice between phenoxybenzamine versus selective alpha-blocking agents is at the treating physician's discretion. Dosing frequency, side-effect profiles, availability, and cost should be considered when making this decision.

Beta-Blockers

Patients with catecholamine or alpha-blocker–induced tachyarrhythmia can be treated with beta-blocking agents such as atenolol, metoprolol, or propranolol. Beta-blockers should never be knowingly used without a concurrent alpha-blocker because treatment with only beta blockade may result in unopposed alpha vasoconstriction, which can lead to worsening symptoms of hypertension, end-organ malperfusion, and heart failure.[51]

Calcium Channel Blockers

These agents block norepinephrine-mediated calcium influx into vascular smooth muscle, thereby controlling hypertension and tachyarrhythmias. Calcium channel blockers can be used to supplement alpha blockade in patients with inadequate blood pressure control, can replace alpha blockade in patients unable to tolerate the side effects of alpha-blocking agents, can prevent alpha-blocker–induced sustained hypotension in patients with only intermittent hypertension, and may also prevent catecholamine-associated coronary spasm.[51,64] Nicardipine is typically started at 20 mg 3 times daily and can be increased until symptoms are controlled.

Metyrosine

Metyrosine is a less commonly used agent that blocks catecholamine synthesis by inhibiting the enzyme tyrosine hydroxylase. Metyrosine significantly depletes catecholamine stores, exhibiting its maximum effect 3 days after treatment. The typical starting dosage is 250 mg 4 times daily.[51] Although it is not a first-line agent, it can be used to control high blood pressure refractory to more traditional alpha, beta, or calcium channel blocking agents that can result from extensive metastatic disease.

Fluid Management

Increased preoperative fluid intake is recommended because of the depletion of plasma volume that results from chronic vasoconstriction. Experts recommend salt loading and increased fluid intake before surgery. Small retrospective studies report that initiation of high-sodium diet a few days after the start of alpha blockade reverses blood volume contraction, prevents orthostatic hypotension before surgery, and reduces the risk of significant hypotension after surgery.[26,51,65] Historically, patients were admitted preoperatively for IV fluid administration; to our knowledge, there is no evidence to support the use of IV fluid over increased oral intake in combination with a high-sodium diet, and therefore the additional cost of increased length of hospital stay is not warranted.

There is no gold standard for the duration of preoperative therapy or end points to determine adequate preoperative blockade. Most investigators agree that medical management with the chosen blocking agent should begin at least 7 to 14 days before surgical intervention to allow for adequate time to normalize blood pressure and heart rate. The most commonly used end points that demonstrate appropriate blockade are a normal blood pressure, defined as a systolic blood pressure less than 130 mm Hg seated but greater than 90 mm Hg while standing, and heart rate between 60 and 70 beats per minute sitting and 70 to 80 beats per minute while standing.[5,26,51] Some investigators have advocated that in normotensive patients, preoperative alpha blockade is not essential.[66] However, most providers treating patients with Pheo/PGL agree that some form of preoperative medical management is warranted.

SURGICAL TREATMENT OF THE PRIMARY TUMOR

There are several operative approaches available to the experienced surgeon, including laparoscopic (transperitoneal or retroperitoneoscopic), robotic anterior or posterior, open anterior, lateral flank, or posterior. The choice of surgical approach is determined by patient-related and tumor-related factors. For instance, a smaller Pheo can be removed from a retroperitoneoscopic approach, whereas a larger one (>6 cm) may be resected via the transperitoneal laparoscopic, robotic, or open anterior approach. A large tumor or one suspected to be malignant and/or with involvement of other adjacent organs should be removed using the open approach. Morphometric patient factors also play an important role in the choice of video-assisted posterior versus transperitoneal surgical approach. Very obese patients with a large amount of retroperitoneal fat may not be ideal candidates for a retroperitoneoscopic approach. For most adrenal Pheos, laparoscopic adrenalectomy has become the preferred approach. The benefits of laparoscopic adrenalectomy when compared with open adrenalectomy include decreased operative times, blood loss, duration of hospital stay, and complications.[67–72] Although some recommend an open approach for large lesions (>6 cm),[26] several studies have shown that laparoscopic adrenalectomy is safe and effective for larger pheochromocytomas (>6 cm)[73–75]; yet, larger pheochromocytomas pose unique technical challenges during laparoscopic surgery. Larger tumors result in smaller operative space and therefore make mobilization more difficult. In addition, the increased vascularity and friability displayed by these tumors can make the operation quite challenging and should be approached with caution. Because PGLs are more likely to be malignant and are frequently found in areas difficult for laparoscopic resection, they more commonly require open resection, although some investigators have reported the successful use of laparoscopic approaches for PGL.[76] Details of the technical aspects of each operative approach are beyond the scope of this article.

Surgical management of hereditary Pheo/PGL, particularly patients with VHL and MEN2, often necessitates bilateral adrenalectomy. Bilateral Pheo/PGLs have been shown to develop in approximately 50% of patients with MEN2A and 40% to 60% of patients with VHL.[19,77,78] In patients with synchronous presentation of bilateral tumors, there are 3 options for surgical resection: bilateral total adrenalectomy, cortical sparing adrenalectomy of one adrenal and complete resection of the other, or bilateral cortical sparing procedures on both adrenals. The goal of cortical sparing adrenalectomy is to remove all of the adrenal medulla, leaving behind only cortical tissue, which can prevent the need for chronic steroid replacement and adrenal insufficiency. There is, however, an increased risk of recurrence associated with cortical sparing adrenalectomy.[79] In one study of 91 patients with familial Pheo/PGL, 39 patients underwent bilateral cortical sparing adrenalectomy; acute adrenal insufficiency developed in 3% of patients compared with 20% in the bilateral total adrenalectomy group. The risk of recurrence was 7% in the cortical-sparing group compared with 3% in the bilateral total adrenalectomy group.[79]

The surgical management of malignant Pheo/PGL is not covered in this article. A multidisciplinary team should manage such patients. When possible, the medical management should be optimized and the primary and metastatic tumor burden should be surgically debulked. In a recent large database study of 287 patients with malignant Pheo and 221 patients with malignant PGL, the 5-year overall and disease-specific survival rates were 58.1% and 71.1% for patients with malignant Pheo and 80.0% and 86.4% for patients with malignant PGL.[80] Patients with malignant Pheo/PGL should be considered for enrollment in available clinical trials offering novel treatments.

POSTOPERATIVE MANAGEMENT, OUTCOMES, AND FOLLOW-UP

For most patients who undergo resection of a Pheo/PGL, the postoperative course is uncomplicated. In a recent study of 91 patients who underwent resection of adrenal-based Pheo, the average length of hospital stay was 3 days and the overall complication rate was 10%.[63] Other series report complication rates of 8% to 23% and an average length of hospital stay of 3 to 4 days.[13,81,82] In the current era, 30-day postoperative mortality of Pheo/PGL is less than 5%.[81,82] However, postoperative hypotension due to a combination of the abrupt fall in circulating catecholamines after tumor removal, the continued presence of alpha blockade, preoperative volume contraction, and intraoperative blood loss are not uncommon. The initial treatment for hypotension after extirpation of the Pheo/PGL is volume resuscitation.[14] Patients with persistent hypotension in the setting of volume repletion may require short-term vasopressor support. Approximately 11% of patients have hypotension refractory to volume repletion requiring postoperative vasopressors.[63]

Another well-described postoperative complication associated with resection of Pheo/PGL is hypoglycemia. High levels of preoperative catecholamine can cause suppression of alpha and beta cell function[83] and lead to insulin resistance.[84] Removal of the Pheo/PGL can result in excessive rebound secretion of insulin and hypoglycemia.[85] This occurs in 4% to 17% of patients, typically within the first 4 postoperative hours.[85,86] Therefore, patients should undergo regular glucose monitoring and be placed on dextrose-containing fluids until they are tolerating oral intake. Clinicians should have a low threshold for checking the glucose level if a patient demonstrates symptoms of hypoglycemia postoperatively and initiate dextrose infusion if necessary.[86]

Currently there is no method to rule out potential malignancy or recurrence from a Pheo/PGL. Thus, long-term periodic follow-up is recommended for all cases of Pheo/PGL.[5,51] Most Pheo/PGLs do not recur. The incidence of recurrence is 15% to 17%.[14,87] In one retrospective study of 176 patients with Pheo/PGL diagnosed from 1975 to 2003, the 5-year and 10-year probabilities of recurrence were 6% and 16%, respectively.[87] Due to the risk of recurrence, the National Comprehensive Cancer Network recommends that follow-up consists of history and physical, plasma-free, or urinary fractionated metanephrines and consideration of CT, MRI, or FDG-PET scan at 3 to 12 months after resection, every 6 to 12 months for the first 3 years after resection, and annually from years 4 to 10 after resection.[88] In a review of long-term postoperative follow-up in patients with apparently benign Pheo/PGL, Amar and colleagues[87] agree that patients with sporadic Pheo/PGL less than or equal to 5 cm in size should have clinical follow-up with a history and physical focusing on symptoms of catecholamine excess and blood pressure measurements in addition to plasma-free or urinary fractionated metanephrines 1 year after surgery and then every other year for life. However, they recommend that patients with familial/inherited disease (particularly those with SDHB mutations) or with tumors larger than 5 cm should undergo clinical and biochemical follow-up 6 months after surgery and then every year for life because of their increased likelihood of recurrence or malignancy. If a patient is found to have elevated metanephrines he or she should then undergo imaging to localize the recurrent or metastatic disease.[87]

In our practice, patients are seen in clinic at 1 month after resection and undergo measurement of plasma metanephrines. If the patient is asymptomatic and metanephrines are within normal range, the patient is followed in 1 year. Plasma metanephrines are repeated annually with either CT or MRI imaging as first-line modality if abnormalities are noted or suspected. In patients with hereditary Pheo/PGL, the follow-up may be more frequent and tailored to the likelihood of malignancy and recurrence.

SUMMARY

Pheos and PGLs are well-described yet rare neuroendocrine tumors. The classic clinical signs and symptoms of paroxysmal hypertension, headaches, sweating, and palpitations at presentation are becoming less common as more Pheo/PGLs are being diagnosed incidentally on imaging or by genetic testing. When a Pheo/PGL is suspected clinically, plasma-free metanephrines or urinary fractionated metanephrine levels are highly sensitive in confirming the diagnosis. Genetic testing should be considered for all patients with Pheo/PGL. CT or MRI is often the only imaging modality necessary to localize Pheo/PGL and plan for surgical resection. Selective or nonselective alpha-blocking agents and calcium channel blockers appear to be equally effective in treating the physiologic effects of Pheo/PGL and should be used at the discretion of the treating team before surgical resection. There are several surgical approaches used to remove Pheo/PGL and the choice of approach depends on patient-related and tumor-related factors as well as surgeon preference. Overall, resection of Pheo/PGLs in the current era of preoperative and intraoperative management is well tolerated with low morbidity and mortality. After resection, patients with Pheo/PGL should be followed at least annually with plasma or urine metanephrines with CT or MRI if abnormalities are noted or detected.

REFERENCES

1. Welbourn RB. Early surgical history of phaeochromocytoma. Br J Surg 1987; 74(7):594–6.
2. Labbe M, Tinel J, Doumer E. Crises solaires et hypertension paroxystique en rapport avec une tumeur surrenale. Bulletin et memoires de la Societe de Medicine de Paris 1922;46:982–90.
3. Zeiger M, Shen WT, Felger EA. The supreme triumph of the surgeon's art: a narrative history of endocrine surgery. San Francisco (CA): University of California Medical Humanities Press; 2013.
4. Hull CJ. Phaeochromocytoma. Diagnosis, preoperative preparation and anaesthetic management. Br J Anaesth 1986;58(12):1453–68.
5. Chen H, Sippel RS, O'Dorisio MS, et al. The North American Neuroendocrine Tumor Society consensus guideline for the diagnosis and management of neuroendocrine tumors: pheochromocytoma, paraganglioma, and medullary thyroid cancer. Pancreas 2010;39(6):775–83.
6. Mansmann G, Lau J, Balk E, et al. The clinically inapparent adrenal mass: update in diagnosis and management. Endocr Rev 2004;25(2):309–40.
7. Mantero F, Terzolo M, Arnaldi G, et al. A survey on adrenal incidentaloma in Italy. Study group on adrenal tumors of the Italian Society of Endocrinology. J Clin Endocrinol Metab 2000;85(2):637–44.
8. Barzon L, Scaroni C, Sonino N, et al. Risk factors and long-term follow-up of adrenal incidentalomas. J Clin Endocrinol Metab 1999;84(2):520–6.
9. Strosberg JR. Update on the management of unusual neuroendocrine tumors: pheochromocytoma and paraganglioma, medullary thyroid cancer and adrenocortical carcinoma. Semin Oncol 2013;40(1):120–33.
10. Baguet JP, Hammer L, Mazzuco TL, et al. Circumstances of discovery of phaeochromocytoma: a retrospective study of 41 consecutive patients. Eur J Endocrinol 2004;150(5):681–6.

11. Kopetschke R, Slisko M, Kilisli A, et al. Frequent incidental discovery of phaeochromocytoma: data from a German cohort of 201 phaeochromocytoma. Eur J Endocrinol 2009;161(2):355–61.
12. Kudva Y, Young WF Jr, Thompson G, et al. Adrenal incidentaloma: an important component of the clinical presentation spectrum of benign sporadic adrenal pheochromocytoma. Endocrinologist 1999;9(2):77–80.
13. Solorzano CC, Lew JI, Wilhelm SM, et al. Outcomes of pheochromocytoma management in the laparoscopic era. Ann Surg Oncol 2007;14(10):3004–10.
14. Lenders JWM, Eisenhofer G, Mannelli M, et al. Phaeochromocytoma. Lancet 2005;366(9486):665–75.
15. Graham JB. Pheochromocytoma and hypertension; an analysis of 207 cases. Int Abstr Surg 1951;92(2):105–21.
16. Pacak K, Linehan WM, Eisenhofer G, et al. Recent advances in genetics, diagnosis, localization, and treatment of pheochromocytoma. Ann Intern Med 2001; 134(4):315–29.
17. Whalen RK, Althausen AF, Daniels GH. Extra-adrenal pheochromocytoma. J Urol 1992;147(1):1–10.
18. Neumann HP, Berger DP, Sigmund G, et al. Pheochromocytomas, multiple endocrine neoplasia type 2, and von Hippel-Lindau disease. N Engl J Med 1993; 329(21):1531–8.
19. Richard S, Beigelman C, Duclos JM, et al. Pheochromocytoma as the first manifestation of von Hippel-Lindau disease. Surgery 1994;116(6):1076–81.
20. Rodriguez JM, Balsalobre M, Ponce JL, et al. Pheochromocytoma in MEN 2A syndrome. Study of 54 patients. World J Surg 2008;32(11):2520–6.
21. Brunjes S, Johns VJ Jr, Crane MG. Pheochromocytoma: postoperative shock and blood volume. N Engl J Med 1960;262:393–6.
22. Gilsanz FJ, Luengo C, Conejero P, et al. Cardiomyopathy and phaeochromocytoma. Anaesthesia 1983;38(9):888–91.
23. Newell KA, Prinz RA, Pickleman J, et al. Pheochromocytoma multisystem crisis. A surgical emergency. Arch Surg 1988;123(8):956–9.
24. Grossman A, Pacak K, Sawka A, et al. Biochemical diagnosis and localization of pheochromocytoma: can we reach a consensus? Ann N Y Acad Sci 2006;1073: 332–47.
25. Eisenhofer G, Goldstein DS, Walther MM, et al. Biochemical diagnosis of pheochromocytoma: how to distinguish true- from false-positive test results. J Clin Endocrinol Metab 2003;88(6):2656–66.
26. Lenders JW, Duh QY, Eisenhofer G, et al. Pheochromocytoma and paraganglioma: an endocrine society clinical practice guideline. J Clin Endocrinol Metab 2014;99(6):1915–42.
27. Lenders JW, Pacak K, Walther MM, et al. Biochemical diagnosis of pheochromocytoma: which test is best? JAMA 2002;287(11):1427–34.
28. Sawka AM, Jaeschke R, Singh RJ, et al. A comparison of biochemical tests for pheochromocytoma: measurement of fractionated plasma metanephrines compared with the combination of 24-hour urinary metanephrines and catecholamines. J Clin Endocrinol Metab 2003;88(2):553–8.
29. Pappachan JM, Raskauskiene D, Sriraman R, et al. Diagnosis and management of pheochromocytoma: a practical guide to clinicians. Curr Hypertens Rep 2014; 16(7):442.
30. Eisenhofer G, Lenders JW, Timmers H, et al. Measurements of plasma methoxytyramine, normetanephrine, and metanephrine as discriminators of different hereditary forms of pheochromocytoma. Clin Chem 2011;57(3):411–20.

31. van Berkel A, Lenders JW, Timmers HJ. Diagnosis of endocrine disease: biochemical diagnosis of phaeochromocytoma and paraganglioma. Eur J Endocrinol 2014;170(3):R109–19.
32. Zeiger MA, Thompson GB, Duh QY, et al. American Association of Clinical Endocrinologists and American Association of Endocrine Surgeons Medical Guidelines for the Management of Adrenal Incidentalomas: executive summary of recommendations. Endocr Pract 2009;15(5):450–3.
33. Maurea S, Cuocolo A, Reynolds JC, et al. Diagnostic imaging in patients with paragangliomas. Computed tomography, magnetic resonance and MIBG scintigraphy comparison. Q J Nucl Med 1996;40(4):365–71.
34. Baez JC, Jagannathan JP, Krajewski K, et al. Pheochromocytoma and paraganglioma: imaging characteristics. Cancer Imaging 2012;12:153–62.
35. Jalil ND, Pattou FN, Combemale F, et al. Effectiveness and limits of preoperative imaging studies for the localisation of pheochromocytomas and paragangliomas: a review of 282 cases. French Association of Surgery (AFC), and the French Association of Endocrine Surgeons (AFCE). Eur J Surg 1998;164(1):23–8.
36. Sahdev A, Sohaib A, Monson JP, et al. CT and MR imaging of unusual locations of extra-adrenal paragangliomas (pheochromocytomas). Eur Radiol 2005;15(1):85–92.
37. Pacak K, Eisenhofer G, Carrasquillo JA, et al. Diagnostic localization of pheochromocytoma: the coming of age of positron emission tomography. Ann N Y Acad Sci 2002;970:170–6.
38. Greenblatt DY, Shenker Y, Chen H. The utility of metaiodobenzylguanidine (MIBG) scintigraphy in patients with pheochromocytoma. Ann Surg Oncol 2008;15(3):900–5.
39. Meyer-Rochow GY, Schembri GP, Benn DE, et al. The utility of metaiodobenzylguanidine single photon emission computed tomography/computed tomography (MIBG SPECT/CT) for the diagnosis of pheochromocytoma. Ann Surg Oncol 2010;17(2):392–400.
40. Derlin T, Busch JD, Wisotzki C, et al. Intraindividual comparison of 123I-mIBG SPECT/MRI, 123I-mIBG SPECT/CT, and MRI for the detection of adrenal pheochromocytoma in patients with elevated urine or plasma catecholamines. Clin Nucl Med 2013;38(1):e1–6.
41. Lumachi F, Tregnaghi A, Zucchetta P, et al. Sensitivity and positive predictive value of CT, MRI and 123I-MIBG scintigraphy in localizing pheochromocytomas: a prospective study. Nucl Med Commun 2006;27(7):583–7.
42. Bhatia KS, Ismail MM, Sahdev A, et al. 123I-metaiodobenzylguanidine (MIBG) scintigraphy for the detection of adrenal and extra-adrenal phaeochromocytomas: CT and MRI correlation. Clin Endocrinol (Oxf) 2008;69(2):181–8.
43. Brito JP, Asi N, Gionfriddo MR, et al. The incremental benefit of functional imaging in pheochromocytoma/paraganglioma: a systematic review. Endocrine 2015;50:176–86.
44. Mackenzie IS, Gurnell M, Balan KK, et al. The use of 18-fluoro-dihydroxyphenylalanine and 18-fluorodeoxyglucose positron emission tomography scanning in the assessment of metaiodobenzylguanidine-negative phaeochromocytoma. Eur J Endocrinol 2007;157(4):533–7.
45. Van Der Horst-Schrivers AN, Jager PL, Boezen HM, et al. Iodine-123 metaiodobenzylguanidine scintigraphy in localising phaeochromocytomas–experience and meta-analysis. Anticancer Res 2006;26(2b):1599–604.
46. Furuta N, Kiyota H, Yoshigoe F, et al. Diagnosis of pheochromocytoma using [123I]-compared with [131I]-metaiodobenzylguanidine scintigraphy. Int J Urol 1999;6(3):119–24.

47. Timmers HJ, Taieb D, Pacak K. Current and future anatomical and functional imaging approaches to pheochromocytoma and paraganglioma. Horm Metab Res 2012;44(5):367–72.
48. Benn DE, Robinson BG. Genetic basis of phaeochromocytoma and paraganglioma. Best Pract Res Clin Endocrinol Metab 2006;20(3):435–50.
49. Fishbein L, Merrill S, Fraker DL, et al. Inherited mutations in pheochromocytoma and paraganglioma: why all patients should be offered genetic testing. Ann Surg Oncol 2013;20(5):1444–50.
50. Gimenez-Roqueplo AP, Favier J, Rustin P, et al. Mutations in the SDHB gene are associated with extra-adrenal and/or malignant phaeochromocytomas. Cancer Res 2003;63(17):5615–21.
51. Pacak K. Preoperative management of the pheochromocytoma patient. J Clin Endocrinol Metab 2007;92(11):4069–79.
52. Bryant J, Farmer J, Kessler LJ, et al. Pheochromocytoma: the expanding genetic differential diagnosis. J Natl Cancer Inst 2003;95(16):1196–204.
53. Amar L, Baudin E, Burnichon N, et al. Succinate dehydrogenase B gene mutations predict survival in patients with malignant pheochromocytomas or paragangliomas. J Clin Endocrinol Metab 2007;92(10):3822–8.
54. Brouwers FM, Eisenhofer G, Tao JJ, et al. High frequency of SDHB germline -mutations in patients with malignant catecholamine-producing paragangliomas: implications for genetic testing. J Clin Endocrinol Metab 2006;91(11):4505–9.
55. Favier J, Amar L, Gimenez-Roqueplo AP. Paraganglioma and phaeochromocytoma: from genetics to personalized medicine. Nat Rev Endocrinol 2015;11(2):110–1.
56. Erlic Z, Rybicki L, Peczkowska M, et al. Clinical predictors and algorithm for the genetic diagnosis of pheochromocytoma patients. Clin Cancer Res 2009;15(20):6378–85.
57. Kvale WF, Manger WM, Priestley JT, et al. Pheochromocytoma. Circulation 1956;14(4 Part1):622–30.
58. Goldstein RE, O'Neill JA Jr, Holcomb GW 3rd, et al. Clinical experience over 48 years with pheochromocytoma. Ann Surg 1999;229(6):755–64 [discussion: 764–6].
59. Agrawal R, Mishra SK, Bhatia E, et al. Prospective study to compare perioperative hemodynamic alterations following preparation for pheochromocytoma surgery by phenoxybenzamine or prazosin. World J Surg 2014;38(3):716–23.
60. Bruynzeel H, Feelders RA, Groenland TH, et al. Risk factors for hemodynamic instability during surgery for pheochromocytoma. J Clin Endocrinol Metab 2010;95(2):678–85.
61. Prys-Roberts C, Farndon JR. Efficacy and safety of doxazosin for perioperative management of patients with pheochromocytoma. World J Surg 2002;26(8):1037–42.
62. Weingarten TN, Cata JP, O'Hara JF, et al. Comparison of two preoperative medical management strategies for laparoscopic resection of pheochromocytoma. Urology 2010;76(2):508.e6–11.
63. Kiernan CM, Du L, Chen X, et al. Predictors of hemodynamic instability during surgery for pheochromocytoma. Ann Surg Oncol 2014;21(12):3865–71.
64. Siddiqi HK, Yang HY, Laird AM, et al. Utility of oral nicardipine and magnesium sulfate infusion during preparation and resection of pheochromocytomas. Surgery 2012;152(6):1027–36.

65. Lentschener C, Gaujoux S, Tesniere A, et al. Point of controversy: perioperative care of patients undergoing pheochromocytoma removal—time for a reappraisal? Eur J Endocrinol 2011;165(3):365–73.

66. Ulchaker JC, Goldfarb DA, Bravo EL, et al. Successful outcomes in pheochromocytoma surgery in the modern era. J Urol 1999;161(3):764–7.

67. Bittner JGT, Gershuni VM, Matthews BD, et al. Risk factors affecting operative approach, conversion, and morbidity for adrenalectomy: a single-institution series of 402 patients. Surg Endosc 2013;27(7):2342–50.

68. Brunt LM, Doherty GM, Norton JA, et al. Laparoscopic adrenalectomy compared to open adrenalectomy for benign adrenal neoplasms. J Am Coll Surg 1996; 183(1):1–10.

69. Gagner M, Pomp A, Heniford BT, et al. Laparoscopic adrenalectomy: lessons learned from 100 consecutive procedures. Ann Surg 1997;226(3):238–46 [discussion: 46–7].

70. Imai T, Kikumori T, Ohiwa M, et al. A case-controlled study of laparoscopic compared with open lateral adrenalectomy. Am J Surg 1999;178(1):50–3 [discussion: 54].

71. Smith CD, Weber CJ, Amerson JR. Laparoscopic adrenalectomy: new gold standard. World J Surg 1999;23(4):389–96.

72. Kiernan CM, Shinall MC Jr, Mendez W, et al. Influence of adrenal pathology on perioperative outcomes: a multi-institutional analysis. Am J Surg 2014;208(4):619–25.

73. Asari R, Koperek O, Niederle B. Endoscopic adrenalectomy in large adrenal tumors. Surgery 2012;152(1):41–9.

74. Manger WM, Gifford RW. Pheochromocytoma. J Clin Hypertens (Greenwich) 2002;4(1):62–72.

75. Wilhelm SM, Prinz RA, Barbu AM, et al. Analysis of large versus small pheochromocytomas: operative approaches and patient outcomes. Surgery 2006;140(4): 553–9 [discussion: 559–60].

76. Walz MK, Alesina PF, Wenger FA, et al. Laparoscopic and retroperitoneoscopic treatment of pheochromocytomas and retroperitoneal paragangliomas: results of 161 tumors in 126 patients. World J Surg 2006;30(5):899–908.

77. Green JS, Bowmer MI, Johnson GJ. Von Hippel-Lindau disease in a Newfoundland kindred. CMAJ 1986;134(2):133–8, 146.

78. Lairmore TC, Ball DW, Baylin SB, et al. Management of pheochromocytomas in patients with multiple endocrine neoplasia type 2 syndromes. Ann Surg 1993; 217(6):595–601 [discussion: 601–3].

79. Grubbs EG, Rich TA, Ng C, et al. Long-term outcomes of surgical treatment for hereditary pheochromocytoma. J Am Coll Surg 2013;216(2):280–9.

80. Goffredo P, Sosa JA, Roman SA. Malignant pheochromocytoma and paraganglioma: a population level analysis of long-term survival over two decades. J Surg Oncol 2013;107(6):659–64.

81. Shada AL, Stokes JB, Turrentine FE, et al. Adrenalectomy for adrenal-mediated hypertension: national surgical quality improvement program analysis of an institutional experience. Am Surg 2014;80(11):1152–8.

82. Plouin PF, Duclos JM, Soppelsa F, et al. Factors associated with perioperative morbidity and mortality in patients with pheochromocytoma: analysis of 165 operations at a single center. J Clin Endocrinol Metab 2001;86(4):1480–6.

83. Hamaji M. Pancreatic alpha- and beta-cell function in pheochromocytoma. J Clin Endocrinol Metab 1979;49(3):322–5.

84. La Batide-Alanore A, Chatellier G, Plouin PF. Diabetes as a marker of pheochromocytoma in hypertensive patients. J Hypertens 2003;21(9):1703–7.

85. Akiba M, Kodama T, Ito Y, et al. Hypoglycemia induced by excessive rebound secretion of insulin after removal of pheochromocytoma. World J Surg 1990; 14(3):317–24.
86. Chen Y, Hodin RA, Pandolfi C, et al. Hypoglycemia after resection of pheochromocytoma. Surgery 2014;156(6):1404–9.
87. Amar L, Servais A, Gimenez-Roqueplo AP, et al. Year of diagnosis, features at presentation, and risk of recurrence in patients with pheochromocytoma or secreting paraganglioma. J Clin Endocrinol Metab 2005;90(4):2110–6.
88. National Comprehensive Cancer Network. Neuroendocrine Tumors. Available at: http://www.nccn.org/professionals/physician_gls/f_guidelines.asp. Accessed March 1, 2015.

Minimally Invasive Adrenalectomy

Azadeh A. Carr, MD, Tracy S. Wang, MD, MPH*

KEYWORDS

- Minimally invasive • Laparoscopic adrenalectomy • Adrenal incidentaloma
- Posterior retroperitoneoscopic adrenalectomy • Adrenal metastases

KEY POINTS

- Minimally invasive adrenalectomy is the preferred method for benign, accessible adrenal masses.
- Adrenal imaging and biochemical evaluation are essential for characterization of adrenal lesions.
- Patient selection for laparoscopic transabdominal and posterior retroperitoneoscopic adrenalectomy (PRA) should be based on anthropometric parameters and characterization of the adrenal mass.
- Minimally invasive adrenalectomy has been shown to be safe and efficacious for adrenal metastases; however, open adrenalectomy is recommended in suspected or confirmed primary adrenal malignancy for best oncologic outcome.

INTRODUCTION

With the increased use of abdominal imaging, adrenal neoplasms are being identified more frequently.[1,2] Autopsy studies have evaluated the frequency of incidental adrenal masses and found that they are present in up to 6% of patients. There is an increasing prevalence with age, as adrenal masses are present in less than 1% of patients younger than 30 years and up to 7% of patients older than 70 years.[3-8] Minimally invasive adrenalectomy through a laparoscopic transabdominal approach was first introduced in the early 1990s and has transformed the management of adrenal tumors.[9] Since then, minimally invasive adrenalectomy has been shown to have less blood loss, earlier patient mobility, decreased length of stay, and faster return to regular

The authors have nothing to disclose.
Section of Endocrine Surgery, Division of Surgical Oncology, Department of Surgery, Medical College of Wisconsin, 9200 West Wisconsin Avenue, Milwaukee, WI 53226, USA
* Corresponding author.
E-mail address: tswang@mcw.edu

Surg Oncol Clin N Am 25 (2016) 139–152
http://dx.doi.org/10.1016/j.soc.2015.08.007
1055-3207/16/$ – see front matter © 2016 Elsevier Inc. All rights reserved.

activity.[10–12] These advantages have led to increased frequency of surgery and evolution of indications for adrenalectomy.[13–15]

Laparoscopic adrenalectomy has become the gold standard for removal of benign adrenal masses. This article discusses the management of incidentally discovered adrenal masses, indications for surgery, and surgical approaches, with a focus on the transabdominal and retroperitoneal methods.

PATIENT EVALUATION AND INDICATIONS FOR ADRENALECTOMY

The initial presentation of an adrenal mass is frequently an adrenal incidentaloma, defined as the identification of an unsuspected adrenal mass when imaging is performed for other indications. Adrenal incidentalomas have been reported in up to 5% of patients undergoing abdominal computed tomographic (CT) scans for other indications.[16–18] Most adrenal masses are benign, although biochemical evaluation is recommended in all patients with adrenal incidentalomas.[2,19,20] Indications for adrenalectomy include a hormonally active adrenal tumor or a suspected or confirmed malignancy.[2,20,21] Adrenal malignancies may be either a primary adrenocortical carcinoma (ACC) or metastases from another primary cancer.

Imaging of Adrenal Masses

The increased frequency and technological advances in abdominal imaging have led to the increased identification of adrenal masses. Most often the imaging is obtained for other indications and is not optimized for evaluating the adrenal glands.[17] However, some characteristics can be identified to broadly determine the nature of the lesion. Common characteristics attributed to benign adrenal neoplasms are size less than 4 cm, smooth contours with planes between organs intact, and a homogenous density; in contrast, malignant neoplasms are frequently greater than 6 cm in size, have irregular borders without clear planes, and are heterogeneous.[1]

Benign adrenal adenomas contain high amounts of intracytoplasmic fat; approximately 70% of adrenal adenomas are rich in lipids.[22] This high lipid content allows for the use of densitometry, measured as Hounsfield units (HU), to distinguish benign and malignant lesions on unenhanced CT.[1] Initial reports used an HU threshold of less than 0 to indicate a benign lesion, with high specificity (100%) but poor sensitivity (47%).[23] A meta-analysis of 10 studies that evaluated 495 adrenal lesions (272 benign and 223 malignant) by unenhanced CT found that an HU threshold of less than 10 had a sensitivity of 71% and specificity of 98% for the diagnosis of an adrenal adenoma, without further radiologic imaging.[24] This method has become the standard for initial evaluation of incidental adrenal lesions without intravenous contrast.[1]

Approximately 30% of adrenal masses may have an indeterminate HU (between 10 and 30), necessitating contrast-enhanced CT with delayed washouts.[1] Because of neovascularization, malignancies tend to have increased contrast accumulation; as a result, intravenous contrast washes out from adenomas, both lipid rich and lipid poor, more quickly than from adrenal malignancies and pheochromocytomas.[25] Contrast washout can be calculated in 2 ways: absolute percentage washout (APW) requires both noncontrast and contrast scans ([(enhanced HU−delayed HU) ÷ (enhanced HU−noncontrast HU)] × 100), whereas relative percentage washout (RPW) can be calculated based on an initial CT scan with contrast and delayed scans only ([(enhanced HU−delayed HU) ÷ enhanced HU] × 100). In adrenal protocol CT scans, initial noncontrast imaging is followed by contrast imaging; a 15-minute delayed scan is then performed. Adrenal masses with initial noncontrast HU less than 10 do not warrant contrast imaging.[2,26] A 2002 prospective study of 166 adrenal masses imaged using this protocol found that an APW threshold of greater than 60% had a sensitivity of 86% and specificity of 92% for distinguishing lipid-poor adenomas from nonadenomas and an RPW threshold of 40% had a sensitivity of 82% and specificity of 92%.[26,27] Other studies have confirmed these thresholds using 15-minute delayed imaging.[22,25,27–29]

MRI may also be used for the characterization of adrenal lesions. Malignant adrenal lesions tend to contain more water and less fat than benign lesions and therefore have higher signal on T2 images, although pheochromocytomas may also have a similar appearance.[1,20] When gadolinium contrast is used, adenomas appear more homogenous, whereas malignancies are heterogeneous. However, there is significant overlap in the characteristics of benign and malignant lesions; therefore, MRI may not definitively distinguish adenomas from malignant masses.[30]

Adrenal lesions not well characterized by CT or MRI may benefit from radionuclide adrenal imaging with specific radiolabeled compounds that target elements of adrenal function and help characterize lesions.[31,32] These radiotracers may include meta-iodobenzylguanidine (MIBG) for medullary tissue lesions and fludeoxyglucose F 18 (^{18}F FDG) for malignant tumors.[33] MIBG imaging may identify both nonhypersecreting and hypersecreting adrenal medulla lesions with a positive predictive value of 83%.[32] [18]F FDG-PET/CT has a sensitivity 99% to 100% and specificity of 94% to 100% for identifying malignant lesions.[32,34,35]

Biochemical Evaluation of Adrenal Tumors

Initial evaluation of an adrenal mass should be to determine functional status.[5,36] A thorough history and physical examination should be obtained, with specific questions related to eliciting symptoms of excess production of aldosterone, cortisol, or catecholamines (**Table 1**).[2,5] Evaluation should include assessment of other constitutional symptoms, including weight loss, history of cancer, and smoking history, as a primary ACC or adrenal metastases must also be considered in the differential diagnosis.

METASTASES TO THE ADRENAL GLAND

Isolated adrenal metastases are most commonly from a primary lung cancer, but other sites of primary malignancy include breast, melanoma, kidney, colon, stomach, and lymphoma.[37–39] The benefits of surgery for metastatic disease are controversial, but studies have demonstrated improved survival in properly selected patients. Adrenal metastases should be suspected in patients with known history of cancer who are found to have an adrenal mass on initial workup or routine surveillance of the primary malignancy. Evaluation should include comparison to prior imaging and biochemical evaluation for a functional adrenal tumor.[2,40]

According to the American Association of Clinical Endocrinologists (AACE) and American Association of Endocrine Surgeons (AAES) guidelines on the management of adrenal incidentaloma, a thorough evaluation for locoregional recurrence and other metastatic sites is required if an adrenal metastasis is suspected.[2] Adrenalectomy can be considered to improve disease-free survival in appropriately selected patients without significant other sites of disease and good performance status. Given the safety of minimally invasive surgery, it should be considered as a first-line approach for isolated adrenal metastases.

Several studies have examined the outcomes of patients undergoing adrenalectomy for adrenal metastases. A retrospective review from the Mayo clinic matched 166 patients who underwent adrenalectomy for adrenal metastases to Surveillance, Epidemiology, and End Results (SEER) data of similar patients who did not undergo

Table 1
Evaluating for hormonal excess in adrenal tumors

	Signs/Symptoms	Biochemical Evaluation
Cushing's syndrome	• Weight gain • Easy bruising • Acne • Proximal muscle weakness • Striae • Fatigue • Neuropyschological disturbances • Hypertension • Glucose intolerance • Hyperlipidemia • Menstrual abnormalities	• Overnight 1 mg dexamethasone suppression test • 24-h urine free cortisol • Late-night salivary cortisol (at least 2 tests)
Pheochromocytoma	• Severe headache • Weight loss • Anxiety • Sweating • Cardiac arrhythmia • Palpitations • Syncope	• Plasma free metanephrines • 24-h urine fractionated metanephrines and catecholamines
Primary aldosteronism	• Hypertension (often refractory) • Fluid retention • Hypokalemia • Muscle cramps • Polyuria • Palpitations	Plasma aldosterone/renin ratio

Data from Young WF Jr. Clinical practice. The incidentally discovered adrenal mass. N Engl J Med 2007;356(6):601–10; and Zeiger MA, Siegelman SS, Hamrahian AH. Medical and surgical evaluation and treatment of adrenal incidentalomas. J Clin Endocrinol Metab 2011;96(7):2004–15.

adrenalectomy.[41] Patients with primary soft-tissue, kidney, lung, and pancreatic tumors were found to have better overall survival at 3 years: sarcoma (86% vs 30%), kidney (72% vs 27%), lung (52% vs 25%), and pancreas (45% vs 12%). In this study, risk factors for death included shorter interval from primary diagnosis to adrenalectomy, other distant sites of disease, surgery for palliation, and persistent disease. A retrospective European multicenter review identified 317 patients who underwent adrenalectomy for adrenal metastases; the most common primary tumor was non–small cell lung cancer (47%), followed by colorectal (14%) and renal (12%) cancers.[39] Laparoscopic adrenalectomy was performed in 146 (46%) patients. Median overall survival was 29 months, with 3- and 5-year survival of 42% and 35%, respectively. Patients who underwent laparoscopic adrenalectomy had improved survival (hazard ratio, 0.65; 95% confidence interval, 0.47–0.90).

Laparoscopic adrenalectomy has been shown to be safe and oncologically appropriate for adrenal metastases. A retrospective review of 92 patients undergoing adrenalectomy (94 adrenalectomies: 63 open and 31 laparoscopic) for isolated adrenal metastases found a median overall survival of 30 months and 5-year estimated survival of 31%.[42] In comparing laparoscopic with open surgery, there was no difference in local recurrence, margin status, disease-free interval, or overall survival. Laparoscopic adrenalectomy was associated with decreased blood loss (106 vs 749 mL; *P*<.0001), operative time (175 vs 208 minutes; $P = .04$), length of stay (2.8 vs 8.0 days; $P<.0001$), and complication rates (4% vs 34%; $P<.0001$). A more recent study of 90 patients who underwent adrenalectomy for adrenal metastases found that laparoscopic adrenalectomy, performed in 55 (61%) patients, was associated with smaller tumor size and reduced blood loss, operative time, and length of stay.[38] Median overall survival was 2.46 years (range, <1 month to 15 years) and 5-year survival was 38%, with no difference in overall survival between laparoscopic and open adrenalectomy.

PREOPERATIVE PREPARATION

Preoperative preparation depends on the functional status of the mass. For patients with a pheochromocytoma, preoperative α-adrenergic blockade is necessary to decrease risk of perioperative cardiovascular complications.[43] Medication should be started 7 to 14 days before planned surgery for adequate time to correct blood pressure and heart rate. β-Adrenergic blockade should be initiated for reflexive tachycardia only after appropriate α-blockade. Patients should also be encouraged to increase sodium and fluid intake to counteract the catecholamine-induced volume contraction. It is important that preoperative consultation and discussion is arranged with the anesthesia team so they are prepared to manage hemodynamic changes during the procedure. For patients with cortisol production, patients may require perioperative steroids with outpatient follow-up for monitoring and tapering of steroids.

APPROACHES TO SURGERY: LAPAROSCOPIC TRANSABDOMINAL VERSUS POSTERIOR RETROPERITONEOSCOPIC ADRENALECTOMY

The laparoscopic transabdominal and posterior retroperitoneoscopic approaches to adrenalectomy both afford specific advantages and disadvantages (**Table 2**).[44]

Table 2
Advantages and disadvantages of laparoscopic transabdominal and posterior retroperitoneoscopic adrenalectomy

	Advantages	Disadvantages/Contraindications
Retroperitoneoscopic	• Do not have to mobilize other organs • Not affected by prior abdominal surgery • No intraperitoneal insufflation (for patients with potential cardiovascular or respiratory compromise) • Same position for bilateral adrenalectomy	• Not suitable for obese patients • Short distance between 12th rib and iliac crest (<4 cm) • Not suitable for known or highly suspected malignant tumor (ACC or pheochromocytoma); evidence of invasion into adjacent structures
Laparoscopic transabdominal	• Can be combined with other transabdominal procedure • Easier access for conversion to open procedure • More suitable in obese patients	• Need to change position for bilateral adrenalectomy • Need to mobilize abdominal structures • Not suitable for known or highly suspected malignant tumor (ACC or pheochromocytoma); evidence of invasion into adjacent structures

Data from Callender GG, Kennamer DL, Grubbs EG, et al. Posterior retroperitoneoscopic adrenalectomy. Adv Surg 2009;43:147–57.

Proper patient selection is essential, with minimally invasive adrenalectomy not recommended for suspected or known ACC.[45] The transabdominal approach was initially widely adopted as the view is more familiar to most surgeons and allows for combination with other abdominal procedures.[20] This approach requires mobilization of the colon, spleen, and pancreas (left) and liver (right), and intra-abdominal adhesions from prior surgical procedures may be present. Retrospective review of laparoscopic transabdominal adrenalectomy in patients with prior abdominal surgery has shown it to be safe, without significantly increasing operative time, complication rates, conversion to open surgery, or length of stay.[46,47]

PRA provides direct access to the adrenal gland without requiring mobilization and retraction of other organs.[48] A retrospective review suggested a selection algorithm for the 2 procedures by comparing anthropometric parameters between 52 patients who underwent laparoscopic transabdominal adrenalectomy and 30 patients who underwent PRA.[49] They recommended selection for PRA if distance from Gerota's fascia to the skin was less than 5 cm and the 12th rib was at or rostral to the level of the renal hilum. The transabdominal approach was recommended in obese patients with thick perinephric fat, a long distance from Gerota's fascia to skin, and tumors greater than 6 cm, as the limited space in PRA makes this dissection especially challenging. In a retrospective review of 118 PRAs comparing the authors' initial experience with PRA to their more recent experience, the authors noted a decrease in rates of complications (15.9% vs 7.7%, $P = .29$) and conversion to an open procedure (9.5% vs 1.9%, $P = .19$), although neither reached statistical significance.[50] However, the authors did gain increasing comfort with patients with higher body mass index (BMI), successfully performing PRA on 55 patients with BMI 30 or more and 17 patients with BMI 35 or more, despite longer operative times than in patients with BMI less than 30 (106 vs 125 minutes, $P = .01$).

SURGICAL TECHNIQUE: LAPAROSCOPIC TRANSABDOMINAL ADRENALECTOMY
Patient Positioning

Patients should be placed in a supine position on the operating table; a bean bag should be placed below the patient. After the induction of general anesthesia, an orogastric tube and Foley catheter are usually placed, both of which may be removed at the end of the procedure. The patient is turned to a lateral decubitus position with the affected side up. An axillary roll is placed, and the elevated arm is secured on an elevated arm board. Pillows are placed between the legs, with the lower leg flexed and the upper leg straight. The superior iliac spine should be positioned at the break point in the operating table and the bed is flexed to increase working space.

The patient should be prepared and draped down to the midline of the abdomen (**Fig. 1**). Landmarks that should be noted, the costal margin and the midline, are marked. The Veress needle or Hasson technique may be used for access into the abdomen. The initial entry is made at the anterior axillary line, 2 cm below the costal margin. The authors prefer to use the Hasson technique with a balloon-tip adjustable 10- to 12-mm trocar and a 10-mm 30° laparoscope. The abdominal space should be insufflated to 15 mm Hg, and after inspection for intra-abdominal adhesions, additional 5-mm ports are placed medial and lateral to the initial port, making sure that port sites are greater than 5 cm apart to allow for mobility of the laparoscopic instruments.

Right Laparoscopic Transabdominal Adrenalectomy

For a right adrenalectomy, the patient is positioned with the right side up, and after placement of the ports, dissection is begun by incising the right triangular ligament.

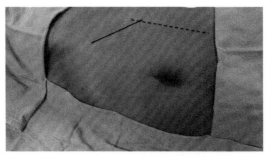

Fig. 1. Positioning for left laparoscopic transabdominal adrenalectomy. Solid line marks the costal margin and dotted line marks the anterior midaxillary line.

Most of the dissection should be performed with an ultrasonic or bipolar device. This incision should be carried up to the level of the diaphragm. A fourth port is often used (placed through the falciform ligament, in the midline of the abdomen), to allow use of a gentle liver retractor. Once the liver is completely mobilized, it should be retracted medially, allowing for visualization of the adrenal gland and the inferior vena cava (IVC). The right adrenal vein empties directly into the IVC and is identified by gentle dissection of the gland on its medial border. The plane between the adrenal gland and IVC should be gently created, using blunt dissection and electrocautery. The adrenal vein should be carefully delineated and be doubly ligated with clips. If the adrenal vein cannot be safely ligated with clips alone, a vascular stapler may be used. After the vein has been secured, the rest of the medial and inferomedial attachments are divided. The gland is then elevated, and the remainder of the avascular posterior and lateral attachments are ligated. The gland is placed in a retrieval bag and removed from the 12-mm port site, which may need to be increased in size to allow for safe removal of larger adrenal glands. The fascia for the 12-mm trocar site should be closed at the end of the procedure.

Throughout the procedure and dissection, it is important to avoid undue pressure, retraction, or grasping of the adrenal gland, as this may cause fracture or tearing of the gland. If surgery is being performed for a pheochromocytoma, constant communication with the anesthesia team is essential, including notifying the team when the adrenal vein is being ligated. The anesthesia and surgical teams must be ready for significant alterations in blood pressure and may need to pause dissection for addressing these needs.

Left Laparoscopic Transabdominal Adrenalectomy

Left adrenalectomy may be performed with 3 ports, although an additional medial port may be used to aid in retraction (**Fig. 2**). The first step is mobilization of the splenic flexure of the colon. This step may need to be performed before the most lateral port can be placed. The splenorenal ligaments are then divided up to the diaphragm to allow the spleen to be retracted medially. Caution must be taken at this point to create a proper plane between the pancreas and the left kidney; Gerota's fascia should not be accessed. With the spleen and tail of the pancreas mobilized medially, an additional medial port may be placed to aid in retraction. The adrenal gland should now be seen adjacent to the superior pole of the kidney. The medial border of the adrenal gland should be dissected free with a combination of blunt dissection and electrocautery, again using the ultrasonic device. On the left, the adrenal vein drains into the renal vein and may be seen inferomedial to the adrenal gland (**Fig. 3**). Once it is

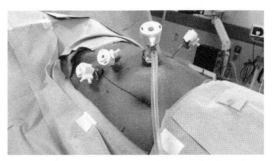

Fig. 2. Port placement for left laparoscopic transabdominal adrenalectomy.

properly dissected free, it should be ligated with a clip applier. The inferior phrenic vein may also enter into the adrenal vein and may require ligation. After the adrenal vein is ligated, the remaining attachments of the gland can be divided. The inferior portion of the gland is elevated to aid in division of the posterior attachments and small arterial branches. Once the gland is completely free, it may be placed into a retrieval bag for removal.

SURGICAL TECHNIQUE: POSTERIOR RETROPERITONEOSCOPIC ADRENALECTOMY

The technique for PRA has been extensively described by Walz and colleagues[51] and is summarized here.[52,53] Patients are intubated in the supine position after placement of sequential compression devices and a Foley catheter. The patient is then turned to the prone, jackknife position on a Cloward table (Surgical Equipment International, Honolulu, HI), which has an open space for the abdomen between the hip support to allow contents to fall forward, being careful to place appropriate padding for the patient's face (**Fig. 4**A). The arms are positioned on arm boards, with elbows bent at 90° angle. The hips and knees are also bent at a 90° angle, ensuring that the knee rest is low enough to limit pressure on knees and prevent the hips from being elevated, which can narrow working space.

The landmarks that should be noted in this position are the 12th rib and iliac crest. The initial incision is made just below the tip of the 12th rib. Using sharp dissection with Metzenbaum scissors, the underlying soft tissue is incised and the retroperitoneum is accessed. The index finger is used to create space, and under direct palpation, a 5-mm port is placed medially, just lateral to the paraspinous musculature. The lateral

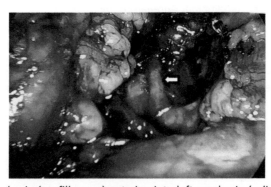

Fig. 3. Left adrenal vein (*no fill arrow*) entering into left renal vein (*solid arrow*).

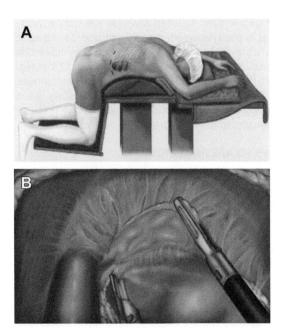

Fig. 4. Right posterior retroperitoneoscopic adrenalectomy. Patient positioning on Cloward table (*A*). After working space is created in the retroperitoneum, dissection begins by separating the lower aspect of the adrenal gland from the superior pole of the kidney (*B*). (*From* Dickson PV, Jimenez C, Chisholm GB, et al. Posterior retroperitoneoscopic adrenalectomy: a contemporary American experience. J Am Coll Surg 2011;212(4):660; [discussion: 665–7]; with permission.)

5-mm port is also placed under direct palpation, 5 cm lateral to the initial incision. A blunt 12-mm trocar with inflatable balloon and adjustable sleeve is then placed through the initial (middle) incision. The retroperitoneal space is then insufflated with high flow to a pressure of 20 to 24 mm Hg. This high insufflation pressure allows the retroperitoneal space to be adequately opened and helps prevent bleeding from smaller veins to aid in dissection. A 10-mm 30° laparoscope is placed in the middle trocar, with the surgeon working through the medial and lateral trocars to ligate the tissues of the retroperitoneum. Once the retroperitoneal space has been developed, a 5-mm 30° laparoscope is used, via the most medial port, and the lateral 2 ports are used by the operating surgeon.

The first landmark to be identified with careful blunt dissection is the superior pole of the kidney. During a right adrenalectomy, the IVC is seen medially, although it may be significantly decompressed because of the high insufflation pressure (see **Fig. 4**B). Mobilization of the adrenal gland should always begin inferiorly; this is done by gently pushing down on the kidney with a laparoscopic peanut and lifting the adrenal superiorly. The tissue along the superior border of the kidney is gently divided using an ultrasonic coagulator or bipolar device. This plane should be created first, as it is easier to accomplish with the other attachments in place with minimal manipulation of the adrenal gland. The adrenal vein should then be identified, medial to the adrenal gland. After it has been carefully dissected free, the vein is grasped on its distal side (closest to the adrenal) with a grasper, clips are doubly placed on the proximal side, and the vein is divided using electrocautery. The rest of the adrenal attachments are then ligated. A retrieval bag is then inserted through the middle port, and the gland is removed. The trocar is then replaced, and the retroperitoneal space is inspected for hemostasis. To visualize any venous bleeding that may have been masked by the high insufflation pressure, the pressure is lowered to 8 to 12 mm Hg. Once hemostasis has been confirmed, the ports are removed, the larger port is closed in layers, and the skin is closed at all sites with absorbable suture. Occasionally, a tear may occur in the peritoneum, which may result in pneumoperitoneum as well. These tears do not have to be closed and usually do not interfere with the procedure.

OTHER APPROACHES TO ADRENALECTOMY

With the continued advances in minimally invasive procedures, there is the drive to identify ways to expand current methods. The first robotic adrenalectomy was reported in 2001.[54] Since then, the robotic approach has been used for both transabdominal adrenalectomy and PRA. Multiple studies have shown no significant difference in rates of conversion to open adrenalectomy, complications, or blood loss between robotic and laparoscopic adrenalectomy, and although operative times may be initially longer, this seems to improve with increasing experience.[55–58] However, use of the robot requires availability of the instrument, specific training, and a learning curve separate from laparoscopy alone. The advantages of robotic adrenalectomy may include improved ability to perform cortical sparing adrenalectomy in patients with familial syndromes who may require bilateral adrenalectomy to avoid steroid dependence and for the posterior approach it may be useful in patients with glands located superior to the 12th rib.[59]

Another area of interest has been single-incision minimally invasive surgery. It has been used for both PRA and for the transabdominal approach. Reported studies have shown overall no significant difference in operative time and complications; however, significant benefits have also not been demonstrated.[60,61] Although this method has been shown to be feasible, further studies are needed to determine risks and benefits.

INDICATIONS FOR OPEN SURGERY

Since the introduction of minimally invasive adrenalectomy, its use for cases of suspected adrenocortical malignancy has been controversial. ACC is a rare malignancy, with an incidence of 1 to 2 per million per year with a high rate of recurrence and poor long-term survival.[62] Proponents of open surgery contend that ACC tends to invade through the tumor capsule with microscopic disease present at the gland surface, which laparoscopy can disrupt and spread.[21] The AACE/AAES recommends that open adrenalectomy be performed for suspected ACC with lymphadenectomy, with a goal to leave the capsule intact to reduce risk of local recurrence.[2,62] However, the European Society of Endocrine Surgeons position statement on malignant adrenal tumors states that laparoscopic resection may be performed for ACC or potentially malignant tumors with preoperative and intraoperative stage I–II ACC and diameter less than 10 cm.[63]

There are inconsistent data on the safety and efficacy of minimally invasive surgery for suspected ACC, which is hindered by the rarity of the disease. Studies have demonstrated increased recurrence rates and decreased disease-free and overall survival in patients undergoing laparoscopic adrenalectomy for ACC.[64–67] Other European studies have found that laparoscopic adrenalectomy may have an outcome similar to open adrenalectomy for ACC, with no significant difference in both local and distant recurrence rates and disease-free or overall survival.[68,69] The differing data and recommendations demonstrate the continued controversy and regional differences.

SUMMARY

Minimally invasive adrenalectomy has become the standard operative approach for adrenal resection in the appropriate clinical setting. Both the laparoscopic transabdominal and posterior retroperitoneoscopic approaches have been shown to be safe and effective for most adrenal pathologies. PRA may be preferred in patients with prior abdominal surgeries or bilateral adrenal disease, whereas laparoscopic transabdominal adrenalectomy is recommended in the obese and morbidly obese. The authors continue to recommend that open adrenalectomy be performed for all patients with known or suspected ACC.

REFERENCES

1. Mazzaglia PJ. Radiographic evaluation of nonfunctioning adrenal neoplasms. Surg Clin North Am 2014;94(3):625–42.
2. Zeiger MA, Thompson GB, Duh QY, et al. The American Association of Clinical Endocrinologists and American Association of Endocrine Surgeons medical guidelines for the management of adrenal incidentalomas. Endocr Pract 2009; 15(Suppl 1):1–20.
3. Young WF Jr. Management approaches to adrenal incidentalomas. A view from Rochester, Minnesota. Endocrinol Metab Clin North Am 2000;29(1):159–85, x.
4. Kloos RT, Gross MD, Francis IR, et al. Incidentally discovered adrenal masses. Endocr Rev 1995;16(4):460–84.
5. Young WF Jr. Clinical practice. The incidentally discovered adrenal mass. N Engl J Med 2007;356(6):601–10.
6. Hedeland H, Ostberg G, Hokfelt B. On the prevalence of adrenocortical adenomas in an autopsy material in relation to hypertension and diabetes. Acta Med Scand 1968;184(3):211–4.
7. Meagher AP, Hugh TB, Casey JH, et al. Primary adrenal tumours – a ten-year experience. Aust N Z J Surg 1988;58(6):457–62.
8. Russi S, Blumenthal HT, Gray SH. Small adenomas of the adrenal cortex in hypertension and diabetes. Arch Intern Med (Chic) 1945;76:284–91.
9. Gagner M, Lacroix A, Bolte E. Laparoscopic adrenalectomy in Cushing's syndrome and pheochromocytoma. N Engl J Med 1992;327(14):1033.
10. Brunt LM, Moley JF, Doherty GM, et al. Outcomes analysis in patients undergoing laparoscopic adrenalectomy for hormonally active adrenal tumors. Surgery 2001; 130(4):629–34 [discussion: 634–5].
11. Guazzoni G, Montorsi F, Bocciardi A, et al. Transperitoneal laparoscopic versus open adrenalectomy for benign hyperfunctioning adrenal tumors: a comparative study. J Urol 1995;153(5):1597–600.
12. Kebebew E, Siperstein AE, Duh QY. Laparoscopic adrenalectomy: the optimal surgical approach. J Laparoendosc Adv Surg Tech A 2001;11(6):409–13.
13. Chavez-Rodriguez J, Pasieka JL. Adrenal lesions assessed in the era of laparoscopic adrenalectomy: a modern day series. Am J Surg 2005;189(5):581–5 [discussion: 585–6].
14. Miccoli P, Raffaelli M, Berti P, et al. Adrenal surgery before and after the introduction of laparoscopic adrenalectomy. Br J Surg 2002;89(6):779–82.

15. Saunders BD, Wainess RM, Dimick JB, et al. Trends in utilization of adrenalectomy in the United States: have indications changed? World J Surg 2004; 28(11):1169–75.
16. Bovio S, Cataldi A, Reimondo G, et al. Prevalence of adrenal incidentaloma in a contemporary computerized tomography series. J Endocrinol Invest 2006;29(4): 298–302.
17. Song JH, Chaudhry FS, Mayo-Smith WW. The incidental adrenal mass on CT: prevalence of adrenal disease in 1,049 consecutive adrenal masses in patients with no known malignancy. AJR Am J Roentgenol 2008;190(5):1163–8.
18. Barzon L, Sonino N, Fallo F, et al. Prevalence and natural history of adrenal incidentalomas. Eur J Endocrinol 2003;149(4):273–85.
19. Brunt LM, Moley JF. Adrenal incidentaloma. World J Surg 2001;25(7):905–13.
20. Mazzaglia PJ, Vezeridis MP. Laparoscopic adrenalectomy: balancing the operative indications with the technical advances. J Surg Oncol 2010;101(8):739–44.
21. Else T, Kim AC, Sabolch A, et al. Adrenocortical carcinoma. Endocr Rev 2014; 35(2):282–326.
22. Taffel M, Haji-Momenian S, Nikolaidis P, et al. Adrenal imaging: a comprehensive review. Radiol Clin North Am 2012;50(2):219–43, v.
23. Lee MJ, Hahn PF, Papanicolaou N, et al. Benign and malignant adrenal masses: CT distinction with attenuation coefficients, size, and observer analysis. Radiology 1991;179(2):415–8.
24. Boland GW, Lee MJ, Gazelle GS, et al. Characterization of adrenal masses using unenhanced CT: an analysis of the CT literature. AJR Am J Roentgenol 1998; 171(1):201–4.
25. Korobkin M, Brodeur FJ, Francis IR, et al. CT time-attenuation washout curves of adrenal adenomas and nonadenomas. AJR Am J Roentgenol 1998;170(3): 747–52.
26. Caoili EM, Korobkin M, Francis IR, et al. Adrenal masses: characterization with combined unenhanced and delayed enhanced CT. Radiology 2002;222(3): 629–33.
27. Park BK, Kim CK, Kim B, et al. Comparison of delayed enhanced CT and chemical shift MR for evaluating hyperattenuating incidental adrenal masses. Radiology 2007;243(3):760–5.
28. Pena CS, Boland GW, Hahn PF, et al. Characterization of indeterminate (lipid-poor) adrenal masses: use of washout characteristics at contrast-enhanced CT. Radiology 2000;217(3):798–802.
29. Sangwaiya MJ, Boland GW, Cronin CG, et al. Incidental adrenal lesions: accuracy of characterization with contrast-enhanced washout multidetector CT–10-minute delayed imaging protocol revisited in a large patient cohort. Radiology 2010;256(2):504–10.
30. Sahdev A, Willatt J, Francis IR, et al. The indeterminate adrenal lesion. Cancer Imaging 2010;10(1):102–13.
31. Lamki LM. Tissue characterization in nuclear oncology: its time has come. J Nucl Med 1995;36(2):207–10.
32. Maurea S, Klain M, Mainolfi C, et al. The diagnostic role of radionuclide imaging in evaluation of patients with nonhypersecreting adrenal masses. J Nucl Med 2001; 42(6):884–92.
33. Gross MD, Gauger PG, Djekidel M, et al. The role of PET in the surgical approach to adrenal disease. Eur J Surg Oncol 2009;35(11):1137–45.
34. Metser U, Miller E, Lerman H, et al. 18F-FDG PET/CT in the evaluation of adrenal masses. J Nucl Med 2006;47(1):32–7.

35. Yun M, Kim W, Alnafisi N, et al. 18F-FDG PET in characterizing adrenal lesions detected on CT or MRI. J Nucl Med 2001;42(12):1795-9.
36. Zeiger MA, Siegelman SS, Hamrahian AH. Medical and surgical evaluation and treatment of adrenal incidentalomas. J Clin Endocrinol Metab 2011;96(7): 2004-15.
37. Creamer J, Matthews BD. Laparoscopic adrenalectomy for cancer. Surg Oncol Clin N Am 2013;22(1):111-24. vi-vii.
38. Romero Arenas MA, Sui D, Grubbs EG, et al. Adrenal metastectomy is safe in selected patients. World J Surg 2014;38(6):1336-42.
39. Moreno P, de la Quintana Basarrate A, Musholt TJ, et al. Adrenalectomy for solid tumor metastases: results of a multicenter European study. Surgery 2013;154(6): 1215-22 [discussion: 1222-3].
40. Sancho JJ, Triponez F, Montet X, et al. Surgical management of adrenal metastases. Langenbecks Arch Surg 2012;397(2):179-94.
41. Vazquez BJ, Richards ML, Lohse CM, et al. Adrenalectomy improves outcomes of selected patients with metastatic carcinoma. World J Surg 2012; 36(6):1400-5.
42. Strong VE, D'Angelica M, Tang L, et al. Laparoscopic adrenalectomy for isolated adrenal metastasis. Ann Surg Oncol 2007;14(12):3392-400.
43. Lenders JW, Duh QY, Eisenhofer G, et al. Pheochromocytoma and paraganglioma: an Endocrine Society clinical practice guideline. J Clin Endocrinol Metab 2014;99(6):1915-42.
44. Callender GG, Kennamer DL, Grubbs EG, et al. Posterior retroperitoneoscopic adrenalectomy. Adv Surg 2009;43:147-57.
45. Shonkwiler RJ, Lee JA. Laparoscopic retroperitoneal adrenalectomy. Surg Laparosc Endosc Percutan Tech 2011;21(4):243-7.
46. Morris L, Ituarte P, Zarnegar R, et al. Laparoscopic adrenalectomy after prior abdominal surgery. World J Surg 2008;32(5):897-903.
47. Mazeh H, Froyshteter AB, Wang TS, et al. Is previous same quadrant surgery a contraindication to laparoscopic adrenalectomy? Surgery 2012;152(6):1211-7.
48. Taskin HE, Siperstein A, Mercan S, et al. Laparoscopic posterior retroperitoneal adrenalectomy. J Surg Oncol 2012;106(5):619-21.
49. Agcaoglu O, Sahin DA, Siperstein A, et al. Selection algorithm for posterior versus lateral approach in laparoscopic adrenalectomy. Surgery 2012;151(5): 731-5.
50. Dickson PV, Jimenez C, Chisholm GB, et al. Posterior retroperitoneoscopic adrenalectomy: a contemporary American experience. J Am Coll Surg 2011;212(4): 659-65 [discussion: 665-7].
51. Walz MK, Alesina PF, Wenger FA, et al. Posterior retroperitoneoscopic adrenalectomy-results of 560 procedures in 520 patients. Surgery 2006;140(6):943-8 [discussion: 948-50].
52. Perrier ND, Kennamer DL, Bao R, et al. Posterior retroperitoneoscopic adrenalectomy: preferred technique for removal of benign tumors and isolated metastases. Ann Surg 2008;248(4):666-74.
53. Cayo A, Wang T. Laparoscopic adrenalectomy: retroperitoneal approach. Curr Surg Rep 2013;1(1):34-9.
54. Horgan S, Vanuno D. Robots in laparoscopic surgery. J Laparoendosc Adv Surg Tech A 2001;11(6):415-9.
55. Brunaud L, Bresler L, Ayav A, et al. Robotic-assisted adrenalectomy: what advantages compared to lateral transperitoneal laparoscopic adrenalectomy? Am J Surg 2008;195(4):433-8.

56. Winter JM, Talamini MA, Stanfield CL, et al. Thirty robotic adrenalectomies: a single institution's experience. Surg Endosc 2006;20(1):119–24.

57. Karabulut K, Agcaoglu O, Aliyev S, et al. Comparison of intraoperative time use and perioperative outcomes for robotic versus laparoscopic adrenalectomy. Surgery 2012;151(4):537–42.

58. Agcaoglu O, Aliyev S, Karabulut K, et al. Robotic vs laparoscopic posterior retroperitoneal adrenalectomy. Arch Surg 2012;147(3):272–5.

59. Morris LF, Perrier ND. Advances in robotic adrenalectomy. Curr Opin Oncol 2012; 24(1):1–6.

60. Hirasawa Y, Miyajima A, Hattori S, et al. Laparoendoscopic single-site adrenalectomy versus conventional laparoscopic adrenalectomy: a comparison of surgical outcomes and an analysis of a single surgeon's learning curve. Surg Endosc 2014;28(10):2911–9.

61. Vidal O, Astudillo E, Valentini M, et al. Single-port laparoscopic left adrenalectomy (SILS): 3 years' experience of a single institution. Surg Laparosc Endosc Percutan Tech 2014;24(5):440–3.

62. Allolio B, Fassnacht M. Clinical review: adrenocortical carcinoma: clinical update. J Clin Endocrinol Metab 2006;91(6):2027–37.

63. Henry JF, Peix JL, Kraimps JL. Positional statement of the European Society of Endocrine Surgeons (ESES) on malignant adrenal tumors. Langenbecks Arch Surg 2012;397(2):145–6.

64. Mir MC, Klink JC, Guillotreau J, et al. Comparative outcomes of laparoscopic and open adrenalectomy for adrenocortical carcinoma: single, high-volume center experience. Ann Surg Oncol 2013;20(5):1456–61.

65. Cooper AB, Habra MA, Grubbs EG, et al. Does laparoscopic adrenalectomy jeopardize oncologic outcomes for patients with adrenocortical carcinoma? Surg Endosc 2013;27(11):4026–32.

66. Leboulleux S, Deandreis D, Al Ghuzlan A, et al. Adrenocortical carcinoma: is the surgical approach a risk factor of peritoneal carcinomatosis? Eur J Endocrinol 2010;162(6):1147–53.

67. Miller BS, Gauger PG, Hammer GD, et al. Resection of adrenocortical carcinoma is less complete and local recurrence occurs sooner and more often after laparoscopic adrenalectomy than after open adrenalectomy. Surgery 2012;152(6): 1150–7.

68. Brix D, Allolio B, Fenske W, et al. Laparoscopic versus open adrenalectomy for adrenocortical carcinoma: surgical and oncologic outcome in 152 patients. Eur Urol 2010;58(4):609–15.

69. Lombardi CP, Raffaelli M, De Crea C, et al. Open versus endoscopic adrenalectomy in the treatment of localized (stage I/II) adrenocortical carcinoma: results of a multiinstitutional Italian survey. Surgery 2012;152(6):1158–64.

Surgical Management of Adrenocortical Carcinoma

An Evidence-Based Approach

Jashodeep Datta, MD, Robert E. Roses, MD*

KEYWORDS

- Adrenocortical carcinoma • Adrenalectomy • Surgery • Multimodality • Localized
- Recurrence • Metastatic • Laparoscopic

KEY POINTS

- Adrenocortical carcinoma is an aggressive malignancy; prognosis is determined by tumor stage at presentation and completeness of surgical resection.
- Complete resection with negative margins is the goal of surgical management and may require multivisceral resection, tumor thrombectomy, or vascular resection with or without reconstruction.
- Extended resection including adjacent organs not obviously involved by tumor is not indicated. Regional lymphadenectomy may provide valuable staging information or be associated with a disease-free or overall survival advantage and is underutilized.
- Minimally invasive approaches have been advocated by select centers with expertise; notwithstanding, likely malignant and locally advanced lesions in particular are most safely managed with an open approach.
- Recurrence is associated with a poor prognosis; however, selected patients with limited or symptomatic disease may benefit from aggressive surgery.

INTRODUCTION

Adrenocortical carcinoma (ACC) is a rare malignancy with an annual incidence of 1 to 2 cases per million individuals.[1] Notwithstanding, frequent presentation with sequelae of steroid precursor overproduction, proclivity for aggressive local growth, early metastasis and recurrence, and the scarcity of effective systemic treatment options contribute to a substantial burden of disease. Women are more affected than men, at a ratio of 1.5:1. Although ACC affects individuals of all ages, cases are clustered

---

The authors have nothing to disclose.

Division of Endocrine and Oncologic Surgery, Department of Surgery, University of Pennsylvania Perelman School of Medicine, 3400 Spruce Street, Philadelphia, PA 19104, USA

* Corresponding author.

E-mail address: robert.roses@uphs.upenn.edu

Surg Oncol Clin N Am 25 (2016) 153–170

http://dx.doi.org/10.1016/j.soc.2015.08.011

1055-3207/16/$ – see front matter © 2016 Elsevier Inc. All rights reserved.

in early childhood or middle age. Most cases are seemingly sporadic; however, ACC may arise in association with hereditary syndromes, including multiple endocrine neoplasia-1 and Li-Fraumeni syndrome.[2] Overall prognosis is poor; estimates of 5-year survival range from 30% to 50%; metastatic disease is associated with a median survival of less than 1 year.[3,4] Surgery is the cornerstone of therapy for localized disease and has a role in selected recurrent cases. Although an association between complete resection with negative margins and survival has been reproduced in numerous series, the frequent presentation with at least locally advanced disease and presence of major vascular invasion or direct invasion of discontiguous structures undermine effective surgical therapy in many cases. Moreover, presence of occult micrometastatic disease at the time of presentation is confirmed by frequent distant failure after apparent negative margin resection.[5] Owing in part to its low incidence, data for many accepted elements of therapy are limited or nonexistent. This review critically considers the existing evidence for elements of the evaluation and treatment of patients with ACC, with a particular focus on surgical management.

WHAT IS THE APPROPRIATE DIAGNOSTIC AND IMAGING WORKUP FOR PATIENTS WITH SUSPECTED ADRENOCORTICAL CARCINOMA?

The presentation of ACC is highly variable. Smaller nonfunctional ACCs are sometimes identified incidentally. Approximately 50% to 60% of ACCs are functional and present with signs or symptoms of hormone excess.[6] As with all tumors of the adrenal gland, directed laboratory testing and high-resolution imaging are critical and allow appropriate management. The former should include serum metanephrines to exclude pheochromocytoma. Glucocorticoid excess may be discerned through measurement of levels of serum cortisol and plasma adrenocorticotropic hormone or 24-hour free urinary cortisol; a more definitive diagnosis may require low-dose dexamethasone suppression. Levels of sex steroids and steroid precursors, including dehydroepiandrosterone sulfate (DHEA-S), 17-OH progesterone, androstenedione, testosterone, and 17-β-estradiol (in men and postmenopausal women), may be elevated in serum. Mineralocorticoid excess may be driven by glucocorticoid-mediated mineralocorticoid receptor activation in the occasional patient with hypercortisolism and is detected through measurement of the plasma aldosterone/renin ratio.[7,8] Urinary steroid metabolomic profiling has emerged as a promising diagnostic tool,[9] but it has yet to be validated in larger prospective multicenter series.

Computed tomography (CT) and MRI are similarly effective at discriminating between benign and malignant adrenal tumors and identifying metastases. The choice of one imaging study over another is largely a question of institutional preference with some caveats: (1) CT is less expensive and (2) MRI is preferable when pheochromocytoma is suspected because of the purported risk of a hypertensive crisis after intravenous infusion of iodinated CT contrast. Hounsfield units less than 10 on unenhanced CT, rapid washout at 15 minutes on delayed contrast-enhanced CT, or signal intensity loss using opposed-phase MRI are consistent with a benign tumor.[10,11] ACCs are typically heterogeneous with irregular margins and irregular enhancement of solid components (**Fig. 1**). With ACC, invasion of adjacent structures or extension into the inferior vena cava (IVC), locoregional lymph node metastases, and distant metastases may be seen. PET with fluorodeoxyglucose F^{18} may have additional sensitivity in identifying metastases.[12] Use of radiolabeled metomidate, highly specific for adrenal cortical cells via targeted binding to both 11β-hydroxylase and aldosterone synthase, for either PET- or single-photon emission CT–based functional imaging is another emerging technique with high sensitivity and specificity for ACC.[13]

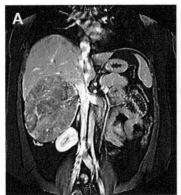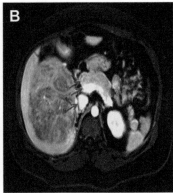

Fig. 1. MRI of a 14 × 12 × 14.1-cm right-sided ACC with sparing of the inferior vena cava (IVC). (*A*) Coronal section with plane between IVC and tumor indicated with arrow, and superior and inferior displacement of the portal vein and right kidney. (*B*) Axial section showing the intimate relationship of tumor with pancreatic head, portal vein, and IVC, indicated by arrows from top to bottom, respectively.

Percutaneous biopsy of a potentially resectable suspected ACC is rarely indicated. It is infrequently helpful owing to poor sensitivity and may result in complications (eg, bleeding and pneumothorax).[14] An increased risk of biopsy site or peritoneal recurrence is often invoked but is largely unproven.[15] In the rare circumstance when biopsy is undertaken (eg, to discriminate a metastasis from a primary adrenal malignancy or in anticipation of neoadjuvant therapy), the diagnosis of pheochromocytoma must first be excluded.

WHAT ARE THE PATHOLOGIC DETERMINANTS OF MALIGNANCY? WHAT FACTORS ARE PROGNOSTIC IN RESECTED ADRENOCORTICAL CARCINOMA?

Histopathologic differentiation between benign and malignant adrenocortical tumors is often challenging. Given that the definitive criteria for malignancy are distant metastasis and local invasion, Weiss proposed a system encompassing 9 morphologic criteria associated with locally recurrent and metastatic adrenocortical tumors (**Box 1**).[16] The subjective identification of 3 of these 9 criteria represents the current standard in establishing adrenocortical malignancy.[17] This classification system, although simple and prognostic,[18] has significant limitations: (1) the criteria do not perform well in the identification of special variants (eg, myxoid, sarcomatoid, pediatric, and oncocytic)[19] and (2) their diagnostic accuracy is lower when by applied by nonexpert pathologists[20]; subjectivity of assessment generates substantial interoperator variability, which limits diagnostic reproducibility.[21] Several immunohistochemical markers have emerged as adjuncts to standard histopathologic analysis and may reduce ambiguity (eg, Ki67 proliferation index, steroidogenic factor-1 [SF-1], tumor protein P53, insulin-like growth factor (IGF) 2, cyclin E, reticulin, E3 ubiquitin-protein ligase [MIB-1]).[20,21] Although promising, these markers have not consistently discriminated ACC from benign adrenal lesions in retrospective studies,[20] and large-scale validation is lacking.

Once malignancy has been established using biochemical, imaging, or pathologic criteria, tumor stage is prognostic of outcome. Although the TNM (tumor, node, metastasis) system from the American Joint Committee on Cancer (AJCC)/Union for

---

Box 1
Weiss criteria

- High nuclear grade (grade 3 or 4)
- Mitosis 6/50 high-powered field or higher
- Atypical mitosis
- Clear cells 25% or less
- Diffuse architecture 33% surface or more
- Confluent necrosis
- Venous invasion
- Sinusoidal invasion
- Capsular infiltration

The identification of 3 of these 9 criteria represents the current standard in establishing adrenocortical malignancy.
From Weiss LM. Comparative histologic study of 43 metastasizing and nonmetastasizing adrenocortical tumors. Am J Surg Pathol 1984;8(3):163–9; with permission.

International Cancer Control (IUCC) was introduced in 2004, the European Network for the Study of Adrenal Tumors (ENSAT) classification has emerged as a more discerning predictor of cancer-specific mortality risk (**Table 1**). Although the two systems classify stage I and II tumors identically (ie, node-negative tumors ≤5 cm or >5 cm, respectively), ENSAT stage III tumors are defined by the presence of positive lymph nodes, infiltration of periadrenal tissue and/or adjacent organs, or venous (ie, IVC or renal vein) tumor thrombus; stage IV ACC includes patients with distant metastasis only. In 492 patients from the German ACC registry, this modification yielded a stage-stratified 5-year disease-specific survival of 82% (stage I), 61% (stage II), 50% (stage III), and 13% (stage IV).[4] The prognostic superiority of the ENSAT, compared with the AJCC/UICC, classification was corroborated in an independent North American cohort of 573 patients.[22] Further improvements to the prognostic value of the ENSAT system, such as addition of tumor grade[23] or molecular markers (eg, SF-1),[24] have been advocated and may be on the horizon.

Beyond ENSAT/AJCC tumor stage, completeness of resection (ie, R0 margin status) is a dominant contributor to disease-free and overall survival in resected ACC.[3,25,26] In a retrospective study of 113 patients, patients undergoing complete primary resection demonstrated significantly improved median (74 vs 12 months) and 5-year actuarial survival (55% vs 5%) compared with those undergoing incomplete resection.[25] In an analysis of 3982 patients with ACC from the National Cancer Data Base (NCDB), R0 resection was associated with a 5-year relative survival rate of 50.4%, compared with rates of 23.2% and 10.8% for R1 and R2 resection, respectively. After adjusting for age, tumor size, grade, nodal involvement, presence of distant metastasis, type of resection, and receipt of multimodality therapy, margin-positive resection remained associated with worse risk-adjusted mortality (hazard ratio [HR], 2.06; 95% confidence interval, 1.74–2.43; P<.0001).[3]

In this and other studies, older age, sex, hormone hypersecretion, poorly differentiated histology, multivisceral resection, and nodal or distant metastasis are also associated with poor prognosis.[3,27] Tumor size, although firmly entrenched in staging classifications, is inconsistently associated with prognosis.[27,28] Conversely, pathologic characteristics such as mitotic rate, atypical mitotic figures, intratumor

Table 1		
TNM classification of adrenocortical carcinoma with comparison of AJCC/UICC/WHO and ENSAT classification systems		
Primary tumor (T)		
TX	Primary tumor cannot be assessed	
T0	No evidence of primary tumor	
T1	Tumor <5 cm in greatest dimension, no extra-adrenal invasion	
T2	Tumor ≥5 cm in greatest dimension, no extra-adrenal invasion	
T3	Tumor of any size with local invasion (periadrenal tissue) but not invading adjacent organs	
T4	Tumor of any size with invasion of adjacent organs (kidney, diaphragm, great vessels, pancreas, spleen, liver)	
Involvement of regional nodes (N)		
NX	Regional lymph nodes cannot be assessed	
N0	No regional lymph node metastasis	
N1	Metastasis in regional lymph nodes	
Distant metastasis (M)		
M0	No distant metastasis	
M1	Distant metastasis	
Stage	**AJCC/UICC/WHO**	**ENSAT**
I	T1, N0, M0	T1, N0, M0
II	T2, N0, M0	T2, N0, M0
III	T3, N0, M0 T1-2, N1, M0	T3-4, N0, M0 T1-4, N1, M0
IV	T3, N1, M0 T4, N0-1, M0 Any M1	Any M1

Abbreviation: WHO, World Health Organization.

hemorrhage, tumor necrosis, and Ki67 index are more reproducibly associated with long-term outcomes.[28,29] Finally, gene expression profiling has identified molecular signatures (eg, *DLG7*, *PINK1*, and *BUB1B*) predictive of malignancy and survival[30]; however, prognostic stratification using such techniques have yet to be widely adopted into clinic practice.

WHAT ARE THE PRINCIPLES OF SURGICAL AND PERIOPERATIVE MANAGEMENT FOR PRIMARY TUMORS? HOW SHOULD PATIENTS WHO HAVE UNDERGONE RESECTION BE SURVEILLED?

Surgical resection remains the cornerstone of treatment and the only curative modality for patients with localized ACC.[18] The surgeon's involvement in the care of these patients should begin in the preoperative setting. In patients with hypercortisolism, perioperative steroid replacement, typically with tapering doses of intravenous hydrocortisone, is recommended to mitigate the risk of adrenal insufficiency following adrenalectomy due to a suppressed contralateral gland.[31,32] The duration of steroid therapy is dictated by time to recovery of the hypothalamic-pituitary axis.[33]

Once the decision to proceed with resection has been made, aggressive local surgical control should be attempted to achieve negative resection margins. Unilateral or bilateral subcostal or J- or L-shaped incisions afford adequate access to sites of potential local invasion and metastatic spread. A thoracoabdominal incision is rarely indicated because of its incident morbidity but may be helpful when concomitant pulmonary metastasectomy is planned (see section "Is there a role for an aggressive surgical approach in locally recurrent or metastatic disease?").[6] En bloc resection of contiguous or discontiguous periadrenal viscera (eg, kidney, colon, spleen, pancreas, stomach) is often required to maintain capsule integrity and prevent tumor spillage.

A unique consideration during surgical resection of ACC is the potential for intracaval extension and/or tumor thrombus (especially for right-sided lesions), observed in up to 25% of cases.[34–36] Although local vascular invasion carries a poor prognosis (ie, approximately 30% 3-year overall survival),[4,35] it is not a contraindication to aggressive surgery per se. Careful preoperative planning is necessary to delineate the location and extent of venous involvement, because the principles of resection vary based on these factors. Tumor thrombectomy in the infrarenal IVC can be achieved by vascular control (via cross-clamping or hepatic vascular exclusion[36]), followed by cavotomy and primary closure or vein resection and reconstruction with or without graft interposition; if tumor extraction is not feasible, the infrarenal IVC can be safely resected with or without replacement.[6] If suprahepatic IVC control is necessary, venovenous bypass is sometimes a useful adjunct. In cases of extension above the diaphragm, or especially into the right atrium, cardiopulmonary bypass may be necessary. Preoperative or intraoperative identification of thrombus in these locations is critical, because clamping of a thrombus-filled IVC can result in tumor thromboembolism, with ensuing hemodynamic instability or tumor dissemination.[6] Management of isolated adrenal vein thrombus (AVT) without caval involvement is laterality specific: (1) for right-sided AVT, resection of a vascular cuff and primary closure of the IVC may be necessary to achieve negative margins; (2) for left-sided AVT, kidney-sparing left renal vein resection may be feasible if the azygous and gonadal venous drainage is intact; if the latter systems are involved, ipsilateral nephrectomy may be necessary (see section "Is there benefit to routine en bloc resection of adjacent organs or aggressive regional lymphadenectomy?").[18,36]

Hormone function should be monitored closely in the postoperative setting. As discussed earlier, postoperative adrenal insufficiency is managed with glucocorticoid and mineralocorticoid replacement as necessary, until recovery of the hypothalamic-pituitary axis. Postoperative hypercortisolism, typically observed after R1/R2 resections for hormonally overactive tumors, may be managed with a variety of agents, including metyrapone, aminoglutethimide, ketoconazole, mitotane (see section "What are the current and emerging options for multimodality management of adrenocortical carcinoma?"), mifepristone (glucocorticoid receptor antagonist), or etomidate.[37] Sex steroid excess can be controlled with androgen receptor inhibitors bicalutamide or finasteride (in virilizing tumors) or antiestrogen therapies, such as tamoxifen or aromatase inhibitors (in estrogen-producing tumors).

Oncologic surveillance of patients who have undergone resection is recommended for up to 10 years and entails cross-sectional imaging with or without biochemical evaluation, depending on the functional status of the primary tumor.[7] Patients with nonfunctional tumors should be under surveillance with periodic CT or MRI because of the risk for early and frequent recurrence (see section "Is there a role for an aggressive surgical approach in locally recurrent or metastatic disease?"). Patients with steroid-producing ACC should be monitored periodically with steroid tumor markers (eg, cortisol, DHEA-S, androstenedione). An increase in hormone levels may indicate recurrence and/or progression before radiographic detection.[6]

IS THERE BENEFIT TO ROUTINE EN BLOC RESECTION OF ADJACENT ORGANS OR AGGRESSIVE REGIONAL LYMPHADENECTOMY?

Although multivisceral resection for margin clearance is clearly indicated, the role for prophylactic organ resection, particularly nephrectomy, is more equivocal. Although early studies advocated for concomitant nephrectomy to improve oncologic outcomes,[38,39] this premise has since been challenged. Bellatone and colleagues[40] reported on 140 patients undergoing radical resection for advanced ACC; 22 (15.7%) underwent ipsilateral nephrectomy. The disease-free interval (16.6 vs 22.3 months) and recurrence rates (36.4% vs 37.3%) did not differ significantly between patients undergoing and not undergoing nephrectomy, respectively. In a preliminarily reported study by Porpiglia and colleagues,[41] 20 of 82 (24.4%) underwent ipsilateral nephrectomy during curative-intent adrenalectomy; at a median follow-up of 60 months, disease-free and overall survival did not differ between nephrectomy and nonnephrectomy cohorts. Based on these limited data, routine ipsilateral nephrectomy is not recommended unless obvious renal infiltration by tumor or associated renal vein tumor thrombus is encountered intraoperatively.

Nodal status is not only an integral component of staging but also an important prognostic feature in resected ACC. Despite this, surgical extirpation of regional lymph nodes is infrequently performed,[3,42] in part owing to lack of consensus regarding the optimal extent of regional lymphadenectomy during primary resection.[36] Based on studies from the German ACC registry and NCDB, nodal metastasis is identified in approximately 25% of patients with resected ACC[3,42]; however, the alarmingly high rates of locoregional failure, up to 85% in some series, despite curative-intent resection[43–45]; substantially greater rates of nodal positivity, as high as 68%, in autopsy studies[46]; and widely variable survival statistics in patients with presumed node-negative stage II resected ACC (ie, indicating overlooked nodal metastasis in worse performers)[18,27,47] suggest that the contribution of surgical understaging to poor long-term outcomes may be underappreciated.

The strongest evidence in support of routine regional lymphadenectomy is derived from a retrospective series of 283 patients who had undergone complete resection from the German ACC registry. In the absence of consensus guidelines defining adequate lymph node dissection (LND), an empiric threshold of 5 or more lymph nodes was chosen to discriminate patients in whom nodes were excised inadvertently from those in whom LND was intended. Using this threshold, only 47 (16.6%) underwent LND during primary resection. Although increased nodal retrieval in these cases may have been self-recommending because of the requirement for more extensive surgery—patients with LND underwent multivisceral resection more frequently and had larger tumors and more locally advanced (ie, ENSAT stage III) disease—removal of at least 5 regional lymph nodes was associated with significant reductions in both risk of recurrence (by 35%) and disease-related mortality (by 46%) despite controlling for age, tumor stage, multivisceral resection, and adjuvant treatment.[42] Despite its methodologic limitations (eg, arbitrary determination of a 5-node LND threshold, lack of knowledge of surgical and/or pathologic quality), the greater than 70% 5-year disease-specific survival in the LND cohort makes a compelling argument for an aggressive surgical approach incorporating regional lymphadenectomy for primary ACC.

The optimal anatomic extent of such nodal dissections remains incompletely understood. Recent efforts to define a systematic approach to regional lymphadenectomy have drawn upon the current anatomic understanding of lymphatic drainage from the adrenal glands, as well as an evolving knowledge of locoregional recurrence patterns following complete resection.[18,36,42] A recent report suggested that first-order drainage pathways from the adrenals encompass renal hilar nodes, nodes associated with the celiac axis, and ipsilateral para-aortic and/or paracaval nodes.[36] These descriptive anatomic pathways correspond closely with actual patterns of postresection locoregional failure, observed most often in the ipsilateral para-aortic/paracaval and renal hilar regions, without contralateral extension.[48] Based on these findings, Gaujoux and Brennan[36] proposed a systematic dissection involving celiac, renal hilum, para-aortic, and/or paracaval lymph nodes ipsilateral to the tumor extending from the aortic hiatus to the renal vein. Reibetanz and colleagues[42] proposed a similar, but laterality-specific, approach: for right-sided ACC, boundaries for lymphadenectomy are the lower edge of liver (upper), border of the IVC (left lateral), and renal pedicle (lower). For left-sided ACC, boundaries are the diaphragmatic crus (upper), border of aorta (right lateral), and renal pedicle (lower).

IS THERE EVIDENCE TO SUPPORT MINIMALLY INVASIVE RESECTION FOR KNOWN OR SUSPECTED MALIGNANCY?

Laparoscopic adrenalectomy (LA) has emerged as the standard of care for management of functioning and nonfunctioning tumors when suspicion for malignancy is low.[49,50] For such indications, LA is associated with reduced postoperative pain, shorter hospital stay, and lower overall costs.[49,51,52] For known or suspected adrenal malignancy, however, open adrenalectomy (OA) has been favored; advocates of this approach purport a decreased risk of capsule breach or tumor fragmentation.[53] The growing expertise with laparoscopy for non-ACC histologies has led to the increased application of minimally invasive approaches in ACC. Early reports, mostly single cases or small series, revealed prohibitive rates of peritoneal and port-site carcinomatosis, local recurrence, R1/R2 resections, tumor fragmentation, and capsule rupture after LA.[54,55]

More recent evidence from high-volume centers, particularly in the United States, recapitulate the dismal outcomes following LA.[53,56–59] In a series of 160 patients (OA, 154; LA, 6) from the MD Anderson Cancer Center, local recurrence and peritoneal carcinomatosis were components of initial failure in 100% and 83% of patients undergoing LA, compared with 35% and 8% undergoing OA, respectively ($P = .0001$).[56] In a contemporary report from the same institution including 302 patients (OA, 256; LA, 46) with ENSAT stage I–III ACC, an increased risk of multifocal peritoneal carcinomatosis was redemonstrated in the LA cohort compared with patients undergoing OA at either the referring or index institution. Moreover, the use of laparoscopy was independently associated with worse recurrence-free and overall survival (both $P<.0001$) on multivariable analysis.[53]

Although these studies have been criticized for including ACCs resected laparoscopically at lower-volume referring hospitals, which may have negatively skewed the observed oncologic results,[60] it seems that outcomes following LA are consistently poor regardless of hospital volume.[57–59] Reporting on their cumulative experience with 156 patients (OA, 110; LA, 46) with ENSAT stage I–III ACC between 2003 and 2008, the high-volume University of Michigan group demonstrated a significantly shorter time to locoregional and peritoneal recurrence ($P = .002$), higher rates of margin-positivity or intraoperative tumor spillage (LA, 30% vs 16%; $P = .04$), and decreased overall survival ($P = .002$) following laparoscopic resection.[58] Mir and colleagues[59] from the Cleveland Clinic reported on 44 patients with ACC (OA, 26; LA, 18); patients selected for LA had smaller tumors and less advanced stage. After controlling for stage by Cox regression, OA was associated with lower risk of recurrence (HR, 0.4; $P = .099$) and improved overall survival (HR, 0.5; P = .122) compared with LA, although these differences did not achieve significance owing to statistical underpowering. Concerns regarding the widespread adoption of LA for ACC are reflected in a position statement from the Society of American Gastrointestinal and Endoscopic Surgeons (SAGES): "For ACC, the best determinant of patient outcomes is an appropriate oncologic resection that includes en bloc resection of any contiguous involved structures and regional lymphadenectomy. Thus, an open approach to resection may be best."[61]

Oncologic outcomes following LA for ACC from select European centers compare favorably with those reported by most US institutions,[50,60,62–64] barring a few exceptions.[65] In a report of 152 (OA, 117; LA, 35) patients with ENSAT stage I–III disease from the German ACC registry, recurrence-free (HR, 0.91; P = .69) and disease-specific (HR, 0.98; P = .92) survival did not differ between OA and LA cohorts in a risk-adjusted model adjusting for stage, tumor size, adjuvant therapy, and presence of glucocorticoid excess.[62] In a multi-institution Italian study of 156 patients (OA, 126; LA, 30) with node-negative (ie, stage I/II) disease, unadjusted 5-year disease-free (P = .12) and overall (P = .2) survival were equivalent between OA and LA cohorts.[64] A French single-institution report examining 34 patients with stage I/II ACC and tumor size less than 10 cm (OA, 21; LA, 13) demonstrated similar unadjusted disease-specific (P = .65) and disease-free (P = .96) survival between the 2 approaches.[60] The latter study emphasized the importance of careful patient selection when considering LA for known/suspected ACC, a position echoed by the European Society of Endocrine Surgeons (ESES): "Laparoscopic resection of ACC...may be performed for pre-and intraoperative stage I–II ACC and tumors with diameter <10 cm."[66]

Given these conflicting data, the oncologic advantages of open resection still seem to outweigh the short-term benefits of a minimally invasive approach for suspected ACC,[53,59] a position that is supported by consensus guidelines from the National Comprehensive Cancer Network.[67] It is possible, however, that experienced laparoscopists may opt for an initial laparoscopic approach in selected patients presenting with smaller well-circumscribed lesions that are diagnostically ambiguous. In such cases, meticulous attention to surgical technique is paramount, and a low threshold should be maintained for open conversion if intraoperative findings are concerning for malignancy.[61]

IS THERE A ROLE FOR AN AGGRESSIVE SURGICAL APPROACH IN LOCALLY RECURRENT OR METASTATIC DISEASE?

Distant metastasis at initial presentation is common in ACC, with 21% to 39% of patients presenting with single-site or multifocal metastatic disease.[3,68,69] Moreover, up to 80% of patients with ACC present with local or distant recurrence following initial radical resection.[70,71] These patients have a similarly poor prognosis; 5-year disease-specific survival is typically less than 15%.[3,18,47,72] Despite these statistics, few data exist on the optimal management of patients with locally recurrent or metastatic disease. The uncertain benefit of salvage chemotherapy and hormonal therapy, poor tolerability of these regimens (particularly mitotane plus etoposide, doxorubicin and cisplatin [EDP-M][73]), short-term efficacy of resection in controlling symptoms of hormone excess, and improvements in perioperative care support an aggressive surgical approach in selected patients.

Outcomes in patients with ENSAT stage IV ACC receiving the best available chemotherapeutic and hormonal agents as sole therapy remain dismal; based on FIRM-ACT (First International Randomized trial in locally advanced and Metastatic Adrenocortical Carcinoma Treatment) trial results, EDP-M treatment yielded response rates of 23%

and median survival around 14 months.[73] Although data regarding the role of aggressive surgery in patients with synchronous metastasis are scarce, it is increasingly applied when complete resection of primary tumor and all metastases is technically feasible.[7,71,74] In a retrospective analysis of 27 patients with synchronous single- or multisite metastasis involving lung, liver, and brain, R0 resection, achieved in 11 (40.7%), was associated with improvements in median (28.6 vs 13.0 months), 1-year (69.9% vs 53.0%), and 2-year (46.9% vs 22.1%, all $P = .02$) overall survival compared with R2 resections. Furthermore, unadjusted analysis demonstrated that receipt of neoadjuvant EDP-M was associated with a trend toward improved survival (5-year, 41.7% vs 8.9%; $P = .1$) compared with surgery alone, although adjuvant mitotane with or without cytotoxic chemotherapy seemed to decrease recurrence in patients selected for a surgery-first approach (see section "What are the current and emerging options for multimodality management of adrenocortical carcinoma?").[74] These data underscore the importance of a multimodality approach, incorporating aggressive surgery with the goal of complete resection. Other studies, although heterogeneous in their design owing to inclusion of both synchronously metastatic patients and those with metachronous metastasis following initial resection, suggest that complete resection may be of benefit in the former group.[25,69,75]

The role of aggressive reoperation for metachronous distant metastasis or local recurrence following initial radical resection is better defined. In a single-institution report of 47 patients undergoing reoperation for distant metastasis (n = 21) or local recurrence (n = 11), completeness of second resection (R0, 74 vs R2, 16 months; $P<.001$) but not pattern of recurrence (distant vs local; $P = .27$) was critically important for long-term survival. Complete repeat resection was more readily accomplished for isolated/oligometastatic distant lesions compared with bulky local recurrences.[25] In a multi-institution Italian cohort of 52 patients with recurrent disease, mean survival (15.9 vs 3.2 months) and 5-year actuarial survival (49.7% vs 8.3%, $P = .00006$) were significantly higher in patients who underwent reoperation (n = 20, 38.5%) compared with patients who did not undergo resection.[40] In a heterogeneous single-institution cohort of 28 patients undergoing hepatectomy for either synchronous (n = 11) or metachronous (n = 17) liver metastasis, all patients had recurrence either locoregionally or in the liver and/or another distant site; of these, recurrence was treated surgically in 11 (39.3%) patients. Surgical treatment of recurrence was an independent prognosticator of overall survival after adjusting for tumor laterality, hormone secretion, and extent of initial hepatectomy.[69] Of 154 patients from the German ACC registry with recurrent disease following initial radical resection, 42 (27%), 57 (37%), and 55 (36%) patients incurred local recurrence alone, metastatic disease alone, and both local recurrence and distant metastasis, respectively; lung and liver were the most common sites of metastasis. In a Cox proportional hazards model adjusting for age, sex, number of affected sites, and receipt of additional therapy, R0 resection (n = 33) was associated with improved progression-free and overall survival.[5]

In the latter study, multivariable analysis also identified time to first recurrence (ie, disease-free interval [DFI]) greater than 12 months as an independent prognosticator of survival; patients (n = 22) with DFI greater than 12 months and R0 resection demonstrated a median progression-free and overall survival of 24 and greater than 60 months, respectively.[5] In parallel with these findings, Datrice and colleagues[75] reported 116 metastasectomies performed in 57 patients at the National Institutes of Health; on univariate analysis, DFI greater than 12 months was associated with longer survival (6.6 vs 1.7 years, $P = .015$) than shorter DFI. In a separate study from the same institution describing 60 pulmonary metastasectomies in 26 patients, median overall survival was significantly longer in patients with time to progression/recurrence greater than 17 months

(P = .015).[76] Based on the available evidence, the authors recommend that, in addition to nuanced clinical judgment regarding the technical feasibility of metastasectomy (ie, ability to perform an R0 resection), aggressive surgery should be restricted to selected patients with DFI of at least 6 months or greater (ie, favorable tumor biology).

Two additional considerations in the surgical management of recurrent/metastatic ACC deserve mention. First, nonresectional ablative modalities (eg, radiofrequency ablation and/or transarterial chemoembolization) may be valuable adjuncts to surgical resection in selected cases.[77,78] Second, in recurrent/metastatic ACC cases in which complete resection is not technically possible, cytoreductive debulking may be considered for symptom palliation when hormone excess is refractory to medical management.[79]

WHAT ARE THE CURRENT AND EMERGING OPTIONS FOR MULTIMODALITY MANAGEMENT OF ADRENOCORTICAL CARCINOMA?

The aggressive behavior of ACC underscore the need for effective adjuvant or neoadjuvant regimens. Probably owing to the low incidence of ACC, level I evidence is lacking. The agent supported by the largest body of available evidence, and the only drug approved by the US Food and Drug Administration for ACC, is mitotane, a potent adrenal corticolytic.[47,80–83] In a multinational retrospective analysis of 177 patients with stage I–III ACC who underwent radical surgery (1985–2005), Terzolo and colleagues[47] compared 47 Italian patients who received adjuvant mitotane with 55 Italian and 75 German patients who did not; receipt of adjuvant mitotane was associated with improved disease-free survival (42 months vs 10 months for Italian control group and vs 25 months for German control group), after adjusting for age, sex, tumor stage, and treatment group in a multivariable analysis. Despite skepticism regarding benefit,[84] poor tolerability, challenging pharmacokinetics (ie, narrow therapeutic window, need to closely monitor drug levels),[85] modest tumor response rates (ie, 10%–30% in most patients),[86] and mixed results with adjuvant use in other uncontrolled studies,[86–88] an international panel recommended that adjuvant mitotane be offered to patients with R1/Rx resection and Ki67 greater than or equal to 10%, but not considered mandatory in groups at presumably low/moderate risk of relapse (eg, stage I–III ACC undergoing R0 resection, Ki67 <10%).[82] The prospective multinational ADIUVO (Efficacy of Adjuvant Mitotane Treatment) trial, which randomizes patients to adjuvant mitotane versus watchful waiting, will assess the benefit of adjuvant mitotane in low- and moderate-risk patients.

Data on cytotoxic chemotherapeutic agents of benefit in ACC are scarce,[89] and regimens demonstrating benefit in the advanced/metastatic setting are typically applied in the adjuvant setting. The FIRM-ACT trial established EDP-M as the first-line treatment in metastatic ACC compared with mitotane and streptozosin; tumor response rates (P<.001) and progression-free survival (P<.001), but not overall survival (P = .07), were significantly improved with EDP-M.[73] Based on the available data, platinum-containing adjuvant regimens, in combination with mitotane, are typically favored in patients at high risk of recurrence who have undergone resection.[8] Cisplatin-mitotane may be a reasonable alternative in patients unfit for EDP-M.[90] Cytotoxic chemotherapy without mitotane is largely ineffective.[91,92] In parallel with developments in other aggressive solid tumors (eg, pancreatic and gastric cancers),[93] there is increasing interest in applying chemotherapy/hormonal therapy in the neoadjuvant setting in ACC, particularly for borderline resectable patients. Preliminary retrospective evidence suggests a potential benefit in select patient subgroups with such an approach.[74,94]

The modest efficacy and poor tolerability of available adjuvant regimens,[8] as well as growing understanding of the molecular underpinnings of adrenal tumorigenesis,[30] have generated interest in directly targeting dysregulated signaling in ACC with molecular-based therapies. The application of tyrosine kinase inhibitors (TKIs) targeting epidermal growth factor receptor–induced downstream signaling (eg, erlotinib, sunitinib) has yielded variable results in advanced ACC.[95,96] Another novel target in ACC is the IGF-1 receptor (IGF1R); anti-IGF1R monoclonal antibodies (ie, figitumumab, cixutumumab) and anti-IGF1R TKI OSI-906 (linsitinib) have been used in chemorefractory metastatic ACC with encouraging results.[97,98] The phase 3 placebo-controlled GALACCTIC trial, evaluating the survival impact of OSI-906 in patients with locally advanced/metastatic ACC, is currently recruiting patients (NCT00924989). It is possible, although unproven, that such targeted therapies may mitigate recurrence if applied in the perioperative or adjuvant settings.

Adjuvant radiotherapy in ACC, previously considered a radioresistant tumor, may be selectively considered in patients with a high risk of local recurrence (ie, R1/Rx resection, ENSAT stage III disease, tumors >8 cm, microvascular invasion, and Ki67 ≥10%),[7,48] although these recommendations are largely based on uncontrolled retrospective data.[99–101] Conversely, the role of radiotherapy in the palliative setting is better defined, particularly for symptomatic bone or cerebral metastasis or in unresectable intra-abdominal recurrences that cause vascular or intestinal obstruction.[48]

PROPOSED APPROACH TO THE MULTIMODAL MANAGEMENT OF LOCALIZED ADRENOCORTICAL CARCINOMA

An algorithm for multimodal management of localized ACC is proposed (**Fig. 2**).

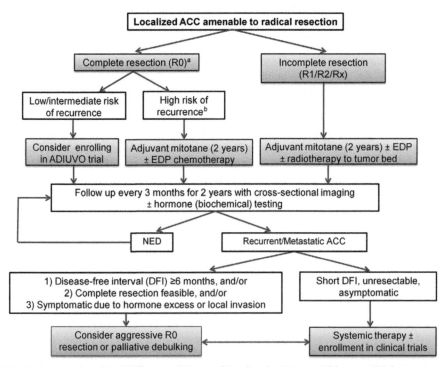

Fig. 2. Proposed multimodal management of localized ACC amenable to radical resection. [a] Consider neoadjuvant combination therapy (mitotane ± EDP chemotherapy) if borderline resectable; [b] high risk: Ki67 index greater than or equal to 10% (EDP, etoposide, doxorubicin, cisplatin; NED: no evidence of disease).

SUMMARY

Preoperative assessment of the patient with suspected ACC should include biochemical workup to characterize functionality and high-resolution imaging to determine extent of disease. Biopsy is rarely indicated. Prognosis is determined by ENSAT/ AJCC tumor stage and completeness of resection. Gene expression profiling is emerging as a powerful predictor of prognosis but is not widely available. Complete resection with negative margins is the goal of surgical management and may require multivisceral resection, tumor thrombectomy, or vascular resection with or without reconstruction. Minimally invasive approaches have been advocated by select centers with expertise and have been extensively applied to the resection of benign or ambiguous lesions; notwithstanding, likely malignant and locally advanced lesions in particular are most safely managed with an open approach. Resection of adjacent organs not obviously involved by tumor is not indicated. Regional lymphadenectomy may provide valuable staging information or be associated with a disease-free or overall survival advantage and is probably underused. Recurrence is associated with poor prognosis; however, selected patients with limited or symptomatic disease may benefit from surgery. Data for specific multimodal approaches are limited; however, a role for adjuvant mitotane after resection of high-risk lesions is widely accepted.

REFERENCES

1. Brennan MF. Adrenocortical carcinoma. CA Cancer J Clin 1987;37(6):348–65.
2. Fassnacht M, Libe R, Kroiss M, et al. Adrenocortical carcinoma: a clinician's update. Nat Rev Endocrinol 2011;7(6):323–35.
3. Bilimoria KY, Shen WT, Elaraj D, et al. Adrenocortical carcinoma in the United States: treatment utilization and prognostic factors. Cancer 2008;113(11): 3130–6.
4. Fassnacht M, Johanssen S, Quinkler M, et al. Limited prognostic value of the 2004 International Union against Cancer staging classification for adrenocortical carcinoma: proposal for a revised TNM classification. Cancer 2009; 115(2):243–50.
5. Erdogan I, Deutschbein T, Jurowich C, et al. The role of surgery in the management of recurrent adrenocortical carcinoma. J Clin Endocrinol Metab 2013; 98(1):181–91.
6. Lafemina J, Brennan MF. Adrenocortical carcinoma: past, present, and future. J Surg Oncol 2012;106(5):586–94.
7. Berruti A, Baudin E, Gelderblom H, et al. Adrenal cancer: ESMO clinical practice guidelines for diagnosis, treatment and follow-up. Ann Oncol 2012;23(Suppl 7): vii131–8.
8. Fassnacht M, Kroiss M, Allolio B. Update in adrenocortical carcinoma. J Clin Endocrinol Metab 2013;98(12):4551–64.
9. Arlt W, Biehl M, Taylor AE, et al. Urine steroid metabolomics as a biomarker tool for detecting malignancy in adrenal tumors. J Clin Endocrinol Metab 2011; 96(12):3775–84.
10. Ilias I, Sahdev A, Reznek RH, et al. The optimal imaging of adrenal tumours: a comparison of different methods. Endocr Relat Cancer 2007;14(3):587–99.
11. Young WF Jr. Conventional imaging in adrenocortical carcinoma: update and perspectives. Horm Cancer 2011;2(6):341–7.
12. Mackie GC, Shulkin BL, Ribeiro RC, et al. Use of [18F]fluorodeoxyglucose positron emission tomography in evaluating locally recurrent and metastatic adrenocortical carcinoma. J Clin Endocrinol Metab 2006;91(7):2665–71.

13. Kreissl MC, Schirbel A, Fassnacht M, et al. [123I]Iodometomidate imaging in adrenocortical carcinoma. J Clin Endocrinol Metab 2013;98(7):2755–64.

14. Williams AR, Hammer GD, Else T. Transcutaneous biopsy of adrenocortical carcinoma is rarely helpful in diagnosis, potentially harmful, but does not affect patient outcome. Eur J Endocrinol 2014;170(6):829–35.

15. Mody MK, Kazerooni EA, Korobkin M. Percutaneous CT-guided biopsy of adrenal masses: immediate and delayed complications. J Comput Assist Tomogr 1995;19(3):434–9.

16. Weiss LM. Comparative histologic study of 43 metastasizing and nonmetastasizing adrenocortical tumors. Am J Surg Pathol 1984;8(3):163–9.

17. Weiss LM, Medeiros LJ, Vickery AL Jr. Pathologic features of prognostic significance in adrenocortical carcinoma. Am J Surg Pathol 1989;13(3):202–6.

18. Chagpar R, Siperstein AE, Berber E. Adrenocortical cancer update. Surg Clin North Am 2014;94(3):669–87.

19. Lin BT, Bonsib SM, Mierau GW, et al. Oncocytic adrenocortical neoplasms: a report of seven cases and review of the literature. Am J Surg Pathol 1998; 22(5):603–14.

20. Papotti M, Libe R, Duregon E, et al. The Weiss score and beyond – histopathology for adrenocortical carcinoma. Horm Cancer 2011;2(6):333–40.

21. Aubert S, Wacrenier A, Leroy X, et al. Weiss system revisited: a clinicopathologic and immunohistochemical study of 49 adrenocortical tumors. Am J Surg Pathol 2002;26(12):1612–9.

22. Lughezzani G, Sun M, Perrotte P, et al. The European Network for the Study of Adrenal Tumors staging system is prognostically superior to the International Union against Cancer-staging system: a North American validation. Eur J Cancer 2010;46(4):713–9.

23. Miller BS, Gauger PG, Hammer GD, et al. Proposal for modification of the ENSAT staging system for adrenocortical carcinoma using tumor grade. Langenbecks Arch Surg 2010;395(7):955–61.

24. Sbiera S, Schmull S, Assie G, et al. High diagnostic and prognostic value of steroidogenic factor-1 expression in adrenal tumors. J Clin Endocrinol Metab 2010; 95(10):E161–71.

25. Schulick RD, Brennan MF. Long-term survival after complete resection and repeat resection in patients with adrenocortical carcinoma. Ann Surg Oncol 1999;6(8):719–26.

26. Icard P, Goudet P, Charpenay C, et al. Adrenocortical carcinomas: surgical trends and results of a 253-patient series from the French Association of Endocrine Surgeons study group. World J Surg 2001;25(7):891–7.

27. Grubbs EG, Callender GG, Xing Y, et al. Recurrence of adrenal cortical carcinoma following resection: surgery alone can achieve results equal to surgery plus mitotane. Ann Surg Oncol 2010;17(1):263–70.

28. Harrison LE, Gaudin PB, Brennan MF. Pathologic features of prognostic significance for adrenocortical carcinoma after curative resection. Arch Surg 1999; 134(2):181–5.

29. Volante M, Bollito E, Sperone P, et al. Clinicopathological study of a series of 92 adrenocortical carcinomas: from a proposal of simplified diagnostic algorithm to prognostic stratification. Histopathology 2009;55(5):535–43.

30. de Reynies A, Assie G, Rickman DS, et al. Gene expression profiling reveals a new classification of adrenocortical tumors and identifies molecular predictors of malignancy and survival. J Clin Oncol 2009;27(7):1108–15.

31. Shen WT, Lee J, Kebebew E, et al. Selective use of steroid replacement after adrenalectomy: lessons from 331 consecutive cases. Arch Surg 2006;141(8): 771–4 [discussion: 774–6].
32. Zeiger MA, Thompson GB, Duh QY, et al. The American Association of Clinical Endocrinologists and American Association of Endocrine Surgeons medical guidelines for the management of adrenal incidentalomas. Endocr Pract 2009; 15(Suppl 1):1–20.
33. Doherty GM, Nieman LK, Cutler GB Jr, et al. Time to recovery of the hypothalamic-pituitary-adrenal axis after curative resection of adrenal tumors in patients with Cushing's syndrome. Surgery 1990;108(6):1085–90.
34. Chiche L, Dousset B, Kieffer E, et al. Adrenocortical carcinoma extending into the inferior vena cava: presentation of a 15-patient series and review of the literature. Surgery 2006;139(1):15–27.
35. Turbendian HK, Strong VE, Hsu M, et al. Adrenocortical carcinoma: the influence of large vessel extension. Surgery 2010;148(6):1057–64 [discussion: 1064].
36. Gaujoux S, Brennan MF. Recommendation for standardized surgical management of primary adrenocortical carcinoma. Surgery 2012;152(1):123–32.
37. Przytulska J, Rogala N, Bednarek-Tupikowska G. Current and emerging therapies for adrenocortical carcinoma - review. Adv Clin Exp Med 2015;24(2):185–93.
38. Icard P, Chapuis Y, Andreassian B, et al. Adrenocortical carcinoma in surgically treated patients: a retrospective study on 156 cases by the French Association of Endocrine Surgery. Surgery 1992;112(6):972–9 [discussion: 979–80].
39. Icard P, Louvel A, Chapuis Y. Survival rates and prognostic factors in adrenocortical carcinoma. World J Surg 1992;16(4):753–8.
40. Bellantone R, Ferrante A, Boscherini M, et al. Role of reoperation in recurrence of adrenal cortical carcinoma: results from 188 cases collected in the Italian National Registry for Adrenal Cortical Carcinoma. Surgery 1997;122(6):1212–8.
41. Porpiglia F, Fiori C, Daffara F, et al. Does nephrectomy during radical adrenalectomy for adrenocortical cancer affect oncologic results? J Urol 2010;183(4, Suppl):e11.
42. Reibetanz J, Jurowich C, Erdogan I, et al. Impact of lymphadenectomy on the oncologic outcome of patients with adrenocortical carcinoma. Ann Surg 2012; 255(2):363–9.
43. Pommier RF, Brennan MF. An eleven-year experience with adrenocortical carcinoma. Surgery 1992;112(6):963–70 [discussion: 970–1].
44. Vassilopoulou-Sellin R, Schultz PN. Adrenocortical carcinoma. Clinical outcome at the end of the 20th century. Cancer 2001;92(5):1113–21.
45. Stojadinovic A, Ghossein RA, Hoos A, et al. Adrenocortical carcinoma: clinical, morphologic, and molecular characterization. J Clin Oncol 2002;20(4):941–50.
46. Didolkar MS, Bescher RA, Elias EG, et al. Natural history of adrenal cortical carcinoma: a clinicopathologic study of 42 patients. Cancer 1981;47(9):2153–61.
47. Terzolo M, Angeli A, Fassnacht M, et al. Adjuvant mitotane treatment for adrenocortical carcinoma. N Engl J Med 2007;356(23):2372–80.
48. Polat B, Fassnacht M, Pfreundner L, et al. Radiotherapy in adrenocortical carcinoma. Cancer 2009;115(13):2816–23.
49. Jacobs JK, Goldstein RE, Geer RJ. Laparoscopic adrenalectomy. A new standard of care. Ann Surg 1997;225(5):495–501 [discussion: 501–2].
50. Sroka G, Slijper N, Shteinberg D, et al. Laparoscopic adrenalectomy for malignant lesions: surgical principles to improve oncologic outcomes. Surg Endosc 2013;27(7):2321–6.

51. Brunt LM, Doherty GM, Norton JA, et al. Laparoscopic adrenalectomy compared to open adrenalectomy for benign adrenal neoplasms. J Am Coll Surg 1996;183(1):1–10.
52. Hazzan D, Shiloni E, Golijanin D, et al. Laparoscopic vs open adrenalectomy for benign adrenal neoplasm. Surg Endosc 2001;15(11):1356–8.
53. Cooper AB, Habra MA, Grubbs EG, et al. Does laparoscopic adrenalectomy jeopardize oncologic outcomes for patients with adrenocortical carcinoma? Surg Endosc 2013;27(11):4026–32.
54. Hamoir E, Meurisse M, Defechereux T. Is laparoscopic resection of a malignant corticoadrenaloma feasible? Case report of early, diffuse and massive peritoneal recurrence after attempted laparoscopic resection. Ann Chir 1998;52(4): 364–8 [in French].
55. Kebebew E, Siperstein AE, Clark OH, et al. Results of laparoscopic adrenalectomy for suspected and unsuspected malignant adrenal neoplasms. Arch Surg 2002;137(8):948–51 [discussion: 952–3].
56. Gonzalez RJ, Shapiro S, Sarlis N, et al. Laparoscopic resection of adrenal cortical carcinoma: a cautionary note. Surgery 2005;138(6):1078–85 [discussion: 1085–6].
57. Miller BS, Ammori JB, Gauger PG, et al. Laparoscopic resection is inappropriate in patients with known or suspected adrenocortical carcinoma. World J Surg 2010;34(6):1380–5.
58. Miller BS, Gauger PG, Hammer GD, et al. Resection of adrenocortical carcinoma is less complete and local recurrence occurs sooner and more often after laparoscopic adrenalectomy than after open adrenalectomy. Surgery 2012; 152(6):1150–7.
59. Mir MC, Klink JC, Guillotreau J, et al. Comparative outcomes of laparoscopic and open adrenalectomy for adrenocortical carcinoma: single, high-volume center experience. Ann Surg Oncol 2013;20(5):1456–61.
60. Donatini G, Caiazzo R, Do Cao C, et al. Long-term survival after adrenalectomy for stage I/II adrenocortical carcinoma (ACC): a retrospective comparative cohort study of laparoscopic versus open approach. Ann Surg Oncol 2014; 21(1):284–91.
61. Stefanidis D, Goldfarb M, Kercher K, et al; Society of American Gastrointestinal and Endoscopic Surgeons. Guidelines for the minimally invasive treatment of adrenal pathology. 2013. Available at: http://www.sages.org/publications/guidelines/guidelines-for-the-minimally-invasive-treatment-of-adrenal-pathology/. Accessed May 26, 2015.
62. Brix D, Allolio B, Fenske W, et al. Laparoscopic versus open adrenalectomy for adrenocortical carcinoma: surgical and oncologic outcome in 152 patients. Eur Urol 2010;58(4):609–15.
63. Porpiglia F, Fiori C, Daffara F, et al. Retrospective evaluation of the outcome of open versus laparoscopic adrenalectomy for stage I and II adrenocortical cancer. Eur Urol 2010;57(5):873–8.
64. Lombardi CP, Raffaelli M, De Crea C, et al. Open versus endoscopic adrenalectomy in the treatment of localized (stage I/II) adrenocortical carcinoma: results of a multiinstitutional Italian survey. Surgery 2012;152(6):1158–64.
65. Leboulleux S, Deandreis D, Al Ghuzlan A, et al. Adrenocortical carcinoma: is the surgical approach a risk factor of peritoneal carcinomatosis? Eur J Endocrinol 2010;162(6):1147–53.
66. Henry JF, Peix JL, Kraimps JL. Positional statement of the European Society of Endocrine Surgeons (ESES) on malignant adrenal tumors. Langenbecks Arch Surg 2012;397(2):145–6.

67. Kulke MH, Benson AB 3rd, Bergsland E, et al. Neuroendocrine tumors. J Natl Compr Canc Netw 2012;10(6):724–64.

68. Kebebew E, Reiff E, Duh QY, et al. Extent of disease at presentation and outcome for adrenocortical carcinoma: have we made progress? World J Surg 2006;30(5):872–8.

69. Gaujoux S, Al-Ahmadie H, Allen PJ, et al. Resection of adrenocortical carcinoma liver metastasis: is it justified? Ann Surg Oncol 2012;19(8):2643–51.

70. Dackiw AP, Lee JE, Gagel RF, et al. Adrenal cortical carcinoma. World J Surg 2001;25(7):914–26.

71. Fay AP, Elfiky A, Telo GH, et al. Adrenocortical carcinoma: the management of metastatic disease. Crit Rev Oncol Hematol 2014;92(2):123–32.

72. Crucitti F, Bellantone R, Ferrante A, et al. The Italian Registry for Adrenal Cortical Carcinoma: analysis of a multiinstitutional series of 129 patients. The ACC Italian Registry Study Group. Surgery 1996;119(2):161–70.

73. Fassnacht M, Terzolo M, Allolio B, et al. Combination chemotherapy in advanced adrenocortical carcinoma. N Engl J Med 2012;366(23):2189–97.

74. Dy BM, Strajina V, Cayo AK, et al. Surgical resection of synchronously metastatic adrenocortical cancer. Ann Surg Oncol 2015;22(1):146–51.

75. Datrice NM, Langan RC, Ripley RT, et al. Operative management for recurrent and metastatic adrenocortical carcinoma. J Surg Oncol 2012;105(7):709–13.

76. Kemp CD, Ripley RT, Mathur A, et al. Pulmonary resection for metastatic adrenocortical carcinoma: the National Cancer Institute experience. Ann Thorac Surg 2011;92(4):1195–200.

77. Wood BJ, Abraham J, Hvizda JL, et al. Radiofrequency ablation of adrenal tumors and adrenocortical carcinoma metastases. Cancer 2003;97(3):554–60.

78. Cazejust J, De Baere T, Auperin A, et al. Transcatheter arterial chemoembolization for liver metastases in patients with adrenocortical carcinoma. J Vasc Interv Radiol 2010;21(10):1527–32.

79. Schteingart DE, Doherty GM, Gauger PG, et al. Management of patients with adrenal cancer: recommendations of an international consensus conference. Endocr Relat Cancer 2005;12(3):667–80.

80. Dickstein G, Shechner C, Arad E, et al. Is there a role for low doses of mitotane (o,p'-DDD) as adjuvant therapy in adrenocortical carcinoma? J Clin Endocrinol Metab 1998;83(9):3100–3.

81. Khorram-Manesh A, Ahlman H, Jansson S, et al. Adrenocortical carcinoma: surgery and mitotane for treatment and steroid profiles for follow-up. World J Surg 1998;22(6):605–11 [discussion: 611–2].

82. Berruti A, Fassnacht M, Baudin E, et al. Adjuvant therapy in patients with adrenocortical carcinoma: a position of an international panel. J Clin Oncol 2010;28(23):e401–2 [author reply: e403].

83. Fassnacht M, Johanssen S, Fenske W, et al. Improved survival in patients with stage II adrenocortical carcinoma followed up prospectively by specialized centers. J Clin Endocrinol Metab 2010;95(11):4925–32.

84. Huang H, Fojo T. Adjuvant mitotane for adrenocortical cancer–a recurring controversy. J Clin Endocrinol Metab 2008;93(10):3730–2.

85. Allolio B, Fassnacht M. Clinical review: adrenocortical carcinoma: clinical update. J Clin Endocrinol Metab 2006;91(6):2027–37.

86. Veytsman I, Nieman L, Fojo T. Management of endocrine manifestations and the use of mitotane as a chemotherapeutic agent for adrenocortical carcinoma. J Clin Oncol 2009;27(27):4619–29.

87. Haak HR, Hermans J, van de Velde CJ, et al. Optimal treatment of adrenocortical carcinoma with mitotane: results in a consecutive series of 96 patients. Br J Cancer 1994;69(5):947–51.
88. Barzon L, Fallo F, Sonino N, et al. Adrenocortical carcinoma: experience in 45 patients. Oncology 1997;54(6):490–6.
89. Khan TS, Imam H, Juhlin C, et al. Streptozocin and o,p'DDD in the treatment of adrenocortical cancer patients: long-term survival in its adjuvant use. Ann Oncol 2000;11(10):1281–7.
90. Bukowski RM, Wolfe M, Levine HS, et al. Phase II trial of mitotane and cisplatin in patients with adrenal carcinoma: a Southwest Oncology Group study. J Clin Oncol 1993;11(1):161–5.
91. Williamson SK, Lew D, Miller GJ, et al. Phase II evaluation of cisplatin and etoposide followed by mitotane at disease progression in patients with locally advanced or metastatic adrenocortical carcinoma: a Southwest Oncology Group study. Cancer 2000;88(5):1159–65.
92. Khan TS, Sundin A, Juhlin C, et al. Vincristine, cisplatin, teniposide, and cyclophosphamide combination in the treatment of recurrent or metastatic adrenocortical cancer. Med Oncol 2004;21(2):167–77.
93. Newton AD, Datta J, Loaiza-Bonilla A, et al. The emerging role for neoadjuvant therapy in gastric cancer: current evidence and future directions. J Gastrointest Oncol 2015. http://dx.doi.org/10.3978/j.issn.2078-6891.2015.047.
94. Bednarski BK, Habra MA, Phan A, et al. Borderline resectable adrenal cortical carcinoma: a potential role for preoperative chemotherapy. World J Surg 2014;38(6):1318–27.
95. Quinkler M, Hahner S, Wortmann S, et al. Treatment of advanced adrenocortical carcinoma with erlotinib plus gemcitabine. J Clin Endocrinol Metab 2008;93(6):2057–62.
96. Kroiss M, Quinkler M, Johanssen S, et al. Sunitinib in refractory adrenocortical carcinoma: a phase II, single-arm, open-label trial. J Clin Endocrinol Metab 2012;97(10):3495–503.
97. Haluska P, Worden F, Olmos D, et al. Safety, tolerability, and pharmacokinetics of the anti-IGF-1R monoclonal antibody figitumumab in patients with refractory adrenocortical carcinoma. Cancer Chemother Pharmacol 2010;65(4):765–73.
98. Naing A, Lorusso P, Fu S, et al. Insulin growth factor receptor (IGF-1R) antibody cixutumumab combined with the mTOR inhibitor temsirolimus in patients with metastatic adrenocortical carcinoma. Br J Cancer 2013;108(4):826–30.
99. Fassnacht M, Hahner S, Polat B, et al. Efficacy of adjuvant radiotherapy of the tumor bed on local recurrence of adrenocortical carcinoma. J Clin Endocrinol Metab 2006;91(11):4501–4.
100. Sabolch A, Feng M, Griffith K, et al. Adjuvant and definitive radiotherapy for adrenocortical carcinoma. Int J Radiat Oncol Biol Phys 2011;80(5):1477–84.
101. Habra MA, Ejaz S, Feng L, et al. A retrospective cohort analysis of the efficacy of adjuvant radiotherapy after primary surgical resection in patients with adrenocortical carcinoma. J Clin Endocrinol Metab 2013;98(1):192–7.

Biochemical Diagnosis and Preoperative Imaging of Gastroenteropancreatic Neuroendocrine Tumors

 CrossMark

Jessica E. Maxwell, MD, MBA[a], Thomas M. O'Dorisio, MD[b],
James R. Howe, MD[a],*

KEYWORDS

- Pancreas neuroendocrine tumors • Carcinoid • OctreoScan • Gut hormones

KEY POINTS

- Many neuroendocrine tumors (NETs) secrete substances that can cause symptoms, but also aid biochemical diagnosis and localization of the primary tumor.
- There are many foods and medications that can interfere with biomarker assays.
- In cases where a pancreas neuroendocrine tumor is suspected, pancreatic polypeptide, chromogranin A (CgA), calcitonin, parathyroid hormone-related peptide, and growth hormone releasing hormone should be drawn during the patient's initial visit.
- When a gastrointestinal NET is suspected, CgA and serotonin levels should be obtained.
- Molecular testing may be used to identify an unknown metastasis as a NET and can be more accurate than traditional histologic procedures in differentiating between primary tumor sites.

INTRODUCTION

There has been a marked increase in the incidence of neuroendocrine tumors (NETs) over the past several decades, from approximately 1 case per 100,000 in 1973 to 5 cases per 100,000 in 2004.[1] The reasons for this increase are unclear and could be

Dr J.E. Maxwell's work is supported by NIH 5T32#CA148062-05. Drs T.M. O'Dorisio and J.R. Howe have nothing to disclose.
^a Department of General Surgery, University of Iowa Hospitals and Clinics, University of Iowa Carver College of Medicine, 200 Hawkins Drive, Iowa City, IA 52242, USA; ^b Department of Internal Medicine, University of Iowa Hospitals and Clinics, University of Iowa Carver College of Medicine, 200 Hawkins Drive, Iowa City, IA 52242, USA
* Corresponding author. University of Iowa Hospitals and Clinics, 200 Hawkins Drive, 4644 JCP, Iowa City, IA 52242.
E-mail address: james-howe@uiowa.edu

Surg Oncol Clin N Am 25 (2016) 171–194
http://dx.doi.org/10.1016/j.soc.2015.08.008
1055-3207/16/$ – see front matter © 2016 Elsevier Inc. All rights reserved.

due to increased environmental exposures, a greater understanding and awareness of these tumors, and the parallel, marked increased use of anatomic imaging studies over this period. Regardless of the cause, these tumors have gone from rare to commonplace, and clinicians need tools to help differentiate NETs from other neoplasms. Furthermore, 30% of patients with small bowel (SBNETs) and 64% of pancreatic NETs (PNETs) present with metastatic disease,[1] and determining the primary NET site of origin is critical for guiding future surgical and medical therapy. This review describes the different modalities commonly used in the diagnosis and follow-up of gastroenteropancreatic (GEP) NETs, including biochemical markers, gene expression tests, and radiologic and nuclear medicine imaging.

BIOCHEMICAL MARKERS FOR GASTROENTEROPANCREATIC NEUROENDOCRINE TUMORS

Approximately 50 years ago, Pearse[2] proposed that all peptide-producing cells of the gut, pancreas, and to a lesser extent, the anterior pituitary gland, belonged to a larger system that shared similar chemical, ultrastructural, and functional characteristics. This system was called the diffuse neuroendocrine cell system, and Pearse held that all of these cells were of neural crest origin. GEP NETs were postulated to derive from a common endocrine progenitor termed amine precursor uptake and decarboxylation cell. Neoplasms arising from this system are defined as epithelial neoplasms with predominant neuroendocrine differentiation.[3] One property shared by these cells and their respective tumors is staining with neuroendocrine immunohistochemical (IHC) markers CgA and synaptophysin.[4] Another property is that approximately 80% of NETs express the somatostatin subtype 2 receptors (SSTR2),[5,6] allowing for the use of synthetic somatostatin (congeners) in the diagnosis and management of these NETs.[5–9] It has been suggested that the long latency period of NETs (up to 9 years for midgut carcinoids)[10] may be related to the inhibitory and antiproliferative action of native somatostatin and its congeners via membrane receptor coupling.[5,7,8,11]

NETs may occur throughout the body, including the lung (bronchial carcinoids), thyroid (medullary thyroid cancer), adrenal gland (pheochromocytoma), gastrointestinal (GI) tract (stomach, duodenum, jejunum, ileum, colon, and rectum), pancreas, and the skin (Merkel cell carcinoma). This occurrence throughout the body is not surprising because the cells of the diffuse neuroendocrine system have come to reside normally in these various organs and tissues. These tumors produce amines and peptides that can be exploited for diagnosis and followed for response to therapy (**Table 1**). These secreted substances may cause symptoms that give clues as to tumor location and are ideal markers to be selected for biochemical testing.[10] This review focuses on NETs of the GEP system, which may be functional (cause symptoms) or nonfunctional. The most frequently encountered GEP NETs are of the small bowel (SBNETs, or carcinoid tumors) and pancreas (PNETs), which account for approximately 70% to 75% of all tumors of the diffuse neuroendocrine system in humans.

Gastrointestinal Neuroendocrine Tumors

The derivation of the term "carcinoid" (carcinoma-like, karzinoide) is credited to Oberndorfer, whose series of 6 cases published in 1907 identified what was thought to be a form of benign neoplasia.[12,13] Carcinoid tumors of the small intestine account for approximately 55% of all adult NETs,[10] and 28% to 44% of all malignant tumors of the small bowel.[14,15] Its incidence has increased 4-fold between 1973 and 2004 (from 2.1 to 9.3 cases per million), and it has transcended adenocarcinoma as the most common cancer type of the small bowel in 2000.[15] The neuroendocrine cell giving

Table 1
Biochemical tests used for gastroenteropancreatic neuroendocrine tumors

(Neuro) Peptide/Amine	Tumor	Value	Interfered with by
Urine 5-HIAA	GI NETs	Elevated in 88% midguts, 30% foreguts, rare in hindguts	Tryptophan-rich foods, caffeine, wine, several medications (see text)
Serotonin	GI NETs Some PNETs	Elevated in 96% midgut, 43% foregut, 20% hindgut	Lithium, MAO inhibitors, morphine, methyldopa, reserpine
CgA	GI NETs PNETs	80%–90% midgut and foregut, most hindgut Useful to follow debulking, recurrence, progression	Somatostatin analogues, PPIs, renal insufficiency, cirrhosis, CHF May also be elevated in HCC and MTC
Pancreastatin	GI NETs PNETs	Elevated in 80% GI NETs Useful to follow debulking, recurrence, progression	Renal insufficiency Medications affecting insulin levels
NKA	GI NETs	Elevated in 21%–70% of midgut carcinoids Indicates poor prognosis if elevated	Medications for hypertension, pain, and GI function
Gastrin	Gastrinoma	Elevated in 98% Should also have hyperchlorhydria, high basal acid output	PPIs; atrophic gastritis/ pernicious anemia, diabetic gastroparesis, gastric outlet obstruction, short bowel syndrome, retained antrum, H pylori infection
Insulin	Insulinoma	Elevated in 98% Hypoglycemia with 72-h fast	Exogenous recombinant insulin
Glucagon	Glucagonoma	Useful when syndrome is present	DM, acute burns and trauma, cirrhosis, renal failure, Cushing syndrome, bacteremia
VIP	VIPoma	Useful when syndrome is present	Recent radioisotope administration
Somatostatin	Somatastatinoma	Useful when syndrome is present	MTC, small cell lung cancer, pheochromocytoma
PP	PPoma	Good marker for nonfunctional PNETs and cosecreted with hormone in many functional PNETs	Other PNETS, nesidioblastosis, PP cell hyperplasia, renal dysfunction

Abbreviations: HCC, hepatocellular carcinoma; MTC, medullary thyroid carcinoma.

rise to small bowel carcinoids of the jejunum and ileum is the Kulchitsky-enterochromaffin (EC) cell,[16] which is a gut epithelial cell that contains secretory granules that store and release serotonin (5-hydroxytryptamine) and other peptides (such as CgA, synaptophysin, and substance P).[4] They are actually derived from enterocyte stem cells, rather than from neural crest cells, as first proposed by Pearse.[17]

Most serotonin in the body (>90%) is produced in the GI tract, which is metabolized by monoamine oxidase (MAO) into its breakdown product 5-hydroxyindole acetic acid (5-HIAA) in the liver and lung, and then excreted into the urine. When SBNETs are metastatic to the liver, serotonin may not be metabolized before its release into the systemic circulation. Sustained serotonin elevation results in the carcinoid syndrome. Serotonin is normally released by EC cells in response to pressure (food), certain nutrients, and bacteria. It acts on the neurons within the gut to stimulate peristalsis.[18] Only 5% to 10% of persons with carcinoid tumors will have carcinoid syndrome, and 76% of these patients will have diarrhea, which may be secretory, hypermotile, malabsorptive, or obstructive.[11] Facial flushing may affect 80% of persons with carcinoid syndrome and is usually episodic. It may be precipitated by catecholamine-driven emotion, excitability, exercise, decongestants, and eating. This symptom is generally mediated by kallikrein, bradykinins, substance P, histamines, and other peptides, rather than serotonin. The episodic spikes of serotonin levels are often associated with hypotension, which worsens the catecholamine-driven serotonin release.[11] Serotonin (and possibly the tachykinin, substance P) is associated with severe bronchial wheezing, which occurs in about 20% of patients with carcinoid syndrome. Cardiac fibrosis with right-sided valvular disease is seen in as many as 50% of patients.[11,19] The primary mediator is thought to be serotonin, but substance P may contribute as well. Some patients may also develop pellagra, due to niacin depletion resulting from tryptophan being shunted to serotonin synthesis rather than nicotinic acid.

LABORATORY TESTS AND BIOMARKERS FOR GASTROINTESTINAL NEUROENDOCRINE TUMORS

In the past, the gold standard for the biochemical diagnosis of carcinoid tumors was the measurement of the serotonin metabolite 5-HIAA in a 24-hour urine collection. This test remains useful, with elevation found in 88% of carcinoid patients,[20] but can be falsely elevated by a variety of tryptophan-rich foods (cheese, bananas, kiwis, walnuts, tomatoes, pineapples, spinach, eggplant, avocados), wine, caffeine, and various medications (acetaminophen, MOA inhibitors, isoniazid, phenothiazines, iodine, 5-fluorouracil). It is less commonly elevated in those with foregut tumors and hindgut tumors.[21] It has a high sensitivity (approaching 100%), but low specificity (35%).[22] Limitations of the test are its inconvenience for the patient and that it may be negative in those with low volume disease (such as a patient with a small bowel primary without nodal or liver metastases). Plasma assays for 5-HIAA are now available and may become another useful tool in the management of these patients.[23]

Most serotonin in the blood is stored within platelets, and measurement of whole blood serotonin has been improved by performing liquid chromatography from platelet-rich plasma.[24] The plasma serotonin assay is now considered very reliable for the diagnosis of carcinoids when performed by Clinical Laboratory Improvement Amendment (CLIA) -licensed and College of American Pathology -approved commercial laboratories in the United States. This test has a positive predictive value of 89% and negative predictive value of 93% in patients with midgut carcinoids, but is less accurate in those with foregut and hindgut carcinoids.[21] It may not correlate as well with the tumor burden as other laboratory assays (eg, chromogranin, pancreastatin) because platelets become saturated at high levels of serotonin. Excess serotonin remains unbound and continues to circulate in the blood.[25] This assay can also be falsely elevated in patients taking lithium, MAO inhibitors, morphine, methyldopa, and reserpine.[26]

CgA is a 457-amino-acid peptide that is widely distributed in endocrine and neuro-endocrine tissues, is present in normal islet cells, and is cosecreted from EC cells with serotonin. Its normal function is to promote formation of secretory granules and it serves as the precursor protein for several negative regulators of neuroendocrine cells (pancreastatin, vasostatin, catestatin). Serum CgA levels are considered one of the most useful markers for diagnosis and surveillance of patients with GI NETs, including hindgut and foregut tumors, where 5-HIAA and serotonin levels are often within normal limits.[27] The sensitivity depends on the specific assay used, but ranges from 67% to 93%, and the specificity from 85% to 96%.[28] Levels of CgA may also be useful for determining prognosis, as patients with CgA greater than 200 U/L have a lower median survival than those less than 200 U/L (2.1 vs 7 years, respectively).[29] CgA is also a useful marker for determining the efficacy of debulking procedures, disease recurrence, and progression.[30,31] Unlike serotonin, CgA levels maintain a good relationship with overall tumor burden, even when circulating levels are high. CgA levels are increased by somatostatin analogues, use of proton pump inhibitors (PPIs; but not H2 blockers), atrophic gastritis/pernicious anemia, and renal insufficiency.[32]

Pancreastatin is a 52-amino-acid derivative of CgA. Its primary function is to decrease cellular glucose uptake.[33] It is a useful marker for diagnosis, the effect of debulking, and tumor progression.[34] It is elevated in as many as 80% of patients with GI NETs.[35] In contrast to the CgA assay, it is not affected by PPI or somatostatin analogue use. The pancreastatin assay does not cross-react with CgA.[36] Pancreastatin is a useful marker for GI NET prognostication[35,37] and more accurately predicted patient outcome in SBNET and PNET patients than did serial measurements of CgA, serotonin, and neurokinin A (NKA) in one recent study.[38] Patients with SBNETs and preoperative elevation of pancreastatin had a median progression-free survival (PFS) of 1.7 years versus 6.5 years when this was normal. If pancreastatin normalized after surgery, PFS improved to 4.2 years (compared with 1.6 years if this remained high postoperatively).

NKA is a tachykinin and bronchoconstrictor that represents an alternatively spliced isoform of substance P. One study examining 73 patients with midgut NETs (80% with metastases) found elevated levels in 70% and that levels seemed to correlate with metastatic tumor burden. Unfortunately, only a minority of patients had both preoperative and postoperative levels drawn.[39] Diebold and colleagues[40] demonstrated that in patients with metastatic midgut NETs (40% with liver metastases), serum NKA levels of less than 50 pg/mL correlated with improved 2-year survival (93% vs 49%) compared with those with more elevated levels. They suggested that when NKA levels normalized after surgery, patient outcomes improved, but survival statistics were not given. Sherman and colleagues[38] did not find a correlation between preoperative NKA levels and PFS or overall survival in 52 midgut patients treated with surgery, and thus, more data are needed to determine the prognostic value of NKA in midgut carcinoid patients.

CURRENT RECOMMENDATIONS FOR BIOCHEMICAL TESTING IN GASTROINTESTINAL NEUROENDOCRINE TUMORS

The National Comprehensive Cancer Network guidelines for GI NETs suggest testing for CgA and collecting a 24-hour urine for 5-HIAA, but do not give specific recommendations for follow-up.[41] The European Neuroendocrine Tumor Society (ENETS) also recommends that the minimal testing performed for GI NETs should include serum CgA and urine 5-HIAA. They also recommend using these assays in follow-up for tumor recurrence and progression. They further suggest that serotonin assays are insensitive and not recommended for either diagnosis or follow-up, but state this biomarker's utility may be improved using the platelet-based assays. They do not comment on pancreastatin and NKA (they suggest that further validation is warranted for newer markers), but do comment that neuron-specific enolase should not be used.[42] The North American Neuroendocrine Tumor Society (NANETS) again only mentions serum CgA and urinary 5-HIAA levels as potentially valuable for measuring response to therapy or progression. They suggest that 5-HIAA may be less useful in foregut (including PNETs) and hindgut NETs, because these tumors tend to not make high levels of serotonin.[43] In patients with midgut and other GI NETs, it is the authors' practice to measure to serum serotonin, CgA, pancreastatin, and less commonly, NKA, preoperatively and at each follow-up visit.[10,34] These biomarkers are readily available and measurable by many CLIA-certified, American College of Pathologists sanctioned laboratories in the United States. Ideally, serial measurements should be from the same laboratory, recognizing that standards and quality control vary.

Pancreatic Neuroendocrine Tumors

PNETs, previously known as islet cell tumors, account for about 1% to 2% of all pancreatic neoplasms and for about 6% of all NETs.[1,44] Their incidence has increased from 1.4 cases per million in 1973 to 3.0 cases per million in 2004.[45] According to the National Cancer Database (NCDB), 85% were classified as nonfunctional, meaning there is no clinical syndrome associated with hormone excess. Because hormone levels are not collected in the database, and tumors classified as pathologically benign (like many insulinomas) are also not included, numbers derived from the NCDB may be overestimated.[46] However, other recent studies suggest that PNETs are nonfunctional in 68% to 90% of cases.[47]

Human adult islet cells produce the hormones insulin, glucagon, somatostatin, vasoactive intestinal peptide (VIP), pancreatic polypeptide (PP), and serotonin; fetal islet cells can produce gastrin. PNETs may secrete any of these hormones, and in addition, rare tumors may secrete adrenocorticotropic hormone, parathyroid hormone-related peptide (PTH-rP), calcitonin, and growth hormone releasing factor (GHRH).[47] About 5% of patients with PNETs have an inherited predisposition, which includes members of multiple endocrine neoplasia type I (MEN1), von Hippel-Lindau, tuberous sclerosis, and neurofibromatosis type I families.[48] Features of each of these more common PNET subtypes and how their biochemical diagnoses are made are covered in the sections that follow.

Gastrinomas

Gastrinomas, which cause Zollinger-Ellison syndrome (ZES), comprise about 15% of all functional PNETs[47] and are the most common PNET associated with MEN1. Approximately 90% of gastrinomas are found in the gastrinoma triangle, an area bordered by the confluence of the cystic and common duct superiorly, the pancreatic neck/body junction medially, and the second and third portions of the duodenum laterally.[49] In patients with sporadic ZES, 50% to 88% of gastrinomas are duodenal in origin versus 70% to 100% of those in MEN1 patients. Approximately 22% to 35% of patients with pancreatic gastrinomas will have liver metastases. The mean size of these tumors is 3.8 cm.[50]

The predominant functional abnormality seen is inappropriately high circulating gastrin causing irreversible hyperchlorhydria (gastric acid overproduction) with subsequent typical or atypical ulcer formation, hemorrhage, and excess acid-induced malabsorptive diarrhea. The hallmarks of a gastrinoma are very elevated gastrin levels as well as gastric acid hypersecretion. More than 98% of gastrinoma patients have elevation of fasting gastrin, but this alone is nondiagnostic. The finding of hyperchlorhydria and basal gastric acid output greater than 15 mEq/h will help to confirm the diagnosis,[50] and a gastric pH of less than 2 is also helpful.[10,51] In the past, secretin infusion resulting in a paradoxic increase of gastrin was a useful way to make the diagnosis of marked hypergastrinemia,[52] but is performed less commonly due to limited availability of this secretogogue.

There are other conditions associated with high levels of gastrin. These conditions include atrophic gastritis/pernicious anemia, gastric outlet syndrome, retained gastric antrum, *Helicobacter pylori* infection, short bowel syndrome, and diabetic gastroparesis.[50] PPIs will also cause significantly elevated gastrin levels through their significant suppression of gastric acid, with subsequent sustained hypergastrinemia and stimulation of CgA from gastric enterochromaffin-like (ECL) cells. Over time, ECL cell nodular hyperplasia can develop with secondary formation of small NETs (usually <1 cm in size). EC cells in the stomach can also be stimulated by high gastrin and result in CgA elevation along with modest levels of serotonin.[10] In MEN1 patients with ZES, hypercalcemia can increase gastrin levels and basal acid secretion. Parathyroidectomy can significantly improve this situation.[53]

Insulinoma

Insulinomas are the most common functional PNET, accounting for approximately 17% of cases.[10,47] Patients are usually symptomatic with episodic hypoglycemia, although some patients can live for years with subclinical disease and have no overt symptoms, or will compensate for hypoglycemia with sugar ingestion. Up to 60% of all insulinomas are found in women, and the average age at diagnosis is 45 years.[11] About 10% are associated with MEN1 and are second to gastrinomas in terms of MEN1-associated PNET frequency. Most are benign adenomas, but malignant insulinomas occur in approximately 10% of patients.

The demonstration of Whipple triad, (1) symptoms of hypoglycemia after fasting, (2) low glucose when symptomatic, and (3) relief of symptoms with ingestion of glucose or food, is strongly suggestive of an insulinoma. Major symptoms may include headache, blurry vision, seizures, confusion, and even coma. Other commonly observed symptoms are due to peripheral catecholamine release and include tremor, diaphoresis, and tachycardia. Approximately 98% of patients with insulinoma will demonstrate inappropriate insulin secretion with symptomatic hypoglycemia within 72 hours, and therefore, a supervised fast within a hospital setting has been recommended as the gold standard for diagnosis.[19,54] Blood sugars should be measured every 4 hours until symptoms occur or blood glucose drops less than 50 mg/dL, and then serum insulin, C-peptide, and glucose levels are drawn. A measurably low blood glucose, symptoms, and inappropriate elevation of insulin (usually >6 uU/ml) or an insulin-to-glucose ratio of 0.3 or greater is highly suspicious for insulinoma. When proinsulin is cleaved by signal peptidase, C-peptide and insulin are formed, which are present in equal amounts in β cells. If a patient has been administered exogenous insulin, C-peptide levels will be low, whereas these levels will be elevated (>200 pmol/L) in insulinoma.[19] Some patients with PNETs and hypoglycemia may have elevated levels of proinsulin rather than insulin.[55] For follow-up of metastatic insulinoma, serial measurement of CgA and pancreastatin can be useful for assessing the extent of metastatic disease.[19]

VIPomas

VIP-secreting PNETs (VIPomas) were independently described by Priest and Alexander,[56] and Verner and Morrison.[57] Initially termed "pancreatic cholera," and later, watery diarrhea, hypokalemia, achlorhydria (most often hypochlorhydria) syndrome, it is now known as watery diarrhea syndrome (WDS). VIP is a neuromodulator (not a hormone in the classical sense), which, in high sustained blood levels, acts as a powerful intestinal secretogogue, resulting in hypokalemia, metabolic acidosis, stool bicarbonate loss, and high-volume alkalotic stool.[11,58,59] VIPoma are an uncommon functional PNET, accounting for 1% to 2% of all functional PNETs.[47,60] They can be seen in MEN1 patients even when other family members may have had gastrinomas or insulinomas.

The diagnosis of VIPoma is suspected in the setting of elevated plasma VIP and severe (often life-threatening) watery diarrhea (usually >1250 cc/d) and profound hypokalemia. Initially, the severe diarrhea may be episodic (tumors may be nonautonomous). Flushing is seen in 20% of patients with WDS, also thought to be a direct action of VIP. Hypochlorhydria, not achlorhydria, is seen in 80% of VIPoma/WDS patients.[60] Both functional and nonfunctional biomarkers from certified commercial laboratories should be measured, to include VIP and PP.[61,62] In the setting of metastasis, CgA and pancreastatin may be helpful to follow for progression and response to therapy. Although most VIPoma in adults arise from the pancreas, there are other nonpancreatic sources of VIP-secreting NETs, including pheochromocytoma, neuroblastoma, ganglioneuroma, bronchogenic carcinoma, and medullary thyroid carcinoma.[10,61]

Glucagonoma

Glucagonoma is a very rare functional tumor, accounting for 1% or less of all PNETs. The clinical manifestations of glucagonoma are very high circulating glucagon levels and a classic necrolytic migratory erythema skin rash, usually on the anterior lower extremity or perianal genital regions. It has come to be known as the "4D syndrome": dementia, diarrhea, deep vein thrombosis (DVT), and depression. Other clinical stigmata include a painful glossitis, weight loss (90%), mild type II diabetes mellitus (DM; 80%), low amino acid concentrations, and DVT (50%). The high circulating glucagon levels do not seem to be the cause of the dermopathy.[10,58,62] Most glucagonomas are large at diagnosis, although they do not often present with classic symptoms. They are more often found in the pancreatic tail and have a very high rate of metastasis at the time of diagnosis. Like many of the functional PNETs, glucagonomas may also be seen in MEN1 patients.

The clinical diagnosis can be made by the finding of a significant elevation of glucagon levels (>500 pg/mL) in the setting of symptoms listed above. Normal fasting levels are generally less than 150 pg/mL, and several conditions may cause mild elevations of glucagon (DM, acute burns and trauma, cirrhosis, renal failure, Cushing syndrome, and bacteremia). PP and insulin levels may also be elevated in association with glucagonoma. As with other metastatic PNETs, serial CgA and pancreastatin levels may be helpful to monitor for progression.[10]

Somatostatinoma

Somatostatinomas are very rare tumors, accounting for less than 1% of PNETs.[47] Although most functional somatostatinomas are of PNET origin (60% of cases), duodenal, ampullary, and less commonly, jejunal somatostatinomas are also recognized. In PNET somatostatinomas, the excess native somatostatin causes hyperglycemia (75% present with DM type II), atony of the gallbladder (59% have gallbladder disease), hypochlorhydria and reduced gastric acid (>80%), steatorrhea and diarrhea (very common, from inhibition of prandial pancreatic enzyme release, bicarbonate, and reduced absorption of fats), and weight loss (possibly due to diarrhea and malabsorption, seen in about 33% of patients). Somatostatinomas are large, which may lead to destruction or loss of islet cells with reduced insulin production. Approximately 80% present with metastatic disease.[10] The diagnosis is commonly made in retrospect by IHC of the tumor, but if there is clinical suspicion, somatostatin levels should be measured. Patients with small cell and bronchogenic carcinomas of the lung have been described with elevated somatostatin levels, as well as up to 25% of patients with pheochromocytoma. PP, CgA, and pancreastatin should also be followed, the latter two for monitoring progression.[10]

Pancreatic polypeptide-secreting tumors and nonfunctional tumors
Pancreatic polypeptide-secreting tumors (PPomas) are a group of nonfunctioning PNETs that comprise about 50% of all PNETs encountered. Although PPomas are not recognized as functional PNETs, diarrhea has been associated with very high levels of PP.[11] One recent report suggested an association of PPomas with DM, because 5 patients with DM and PPoma had improvement or resolution after resection.[63] For the most part, the coassociation of elevated PP in PNETs making other hormones has maintained its value in the diagnosis and follow-up of patients with both functional and nonfunctional PNETs.[19,61,62] Therefore, PP is a good marker to test in all cases of suspected PNETs, in addition to the hormones suggested by a clinical syndrome, if present. Measurement of CgA and pancreastatin is also useful in monitoring the effects of therapy and for progression.

The vast majority of nonfunctional PNETs are diagnosed as a result of nonspecific abdominal pain or symptoms of obstruction of the pancreatic or bile duct. Because of this, nonfunctional PNETs tend to be larger when detected (5.9 cm), and they have a higher rate of metastases (60%) and a poorer prognosis (5-year survival of 33%).[45]

CURRENT RECOMMENDATIONS FOR BIOCHEMICAL TESTING IN PANCREATIC NEUROENDOCRINE TUMORS

The NCNN recommends checking PP, CgA, calcitonin, PTH-rP, and GHRH for generic PNETs. If the patient has a recognizable syndrome, they recommend checking specific hormone levels. When insulinoma is suspected, then insulin, proinsulin, and C-peptide should be checked, and consideration should be given to a 72-hour fast. Serum VIP levels should be checked if one suspects VIPoma, serum glucagon for those with glucagonoma symptoms, and basal or stimulated gastrin for suspected gastrinoma patients.[41] ENETs suggests checking CgA in cases of nonfunctional PNETs, with PP being more uncertain, except in MEN1 patients. Further tests are indicated if the patient demonstrates symptoms.[64] The recommendations from NANETs are similar, although given in more detail for functional tumors. For nonfunctional tumors, they recommend CgA and PP.[53]

BIOMOLECULAR DIAGNOSTICS IN NEUROENDOCRINE TUMORS
WREN Assay

Modlin and colleagues[65] set out to identify a genetic signature for NETs that could be tested from peripheral blood samples that might be useful for diagnosis, assessment of tumor burden, and response to therapy. They retrieved data from tissue-based microarrays from normal tissues, and from 9 primary GEP NETs and 6 GEP NET metastases. They identified a group of genes that showed elevated expression in GEP NETs and then tested these genes in peripheral blood samples as a training set (67 normal samples, 63 GEP NETs). The validation set included 92 normal samples and 143 GEP NETs. They selected 75 genes for further study by quantitative polymerase chain reaction (qPCR; 21 from tissue-based results, 32 from blood-based, and 22 from the literature), which was then further reduced to a 51-gene panel. In PNETs, 79% of samples were accurately identified using the PCR test, as were 88% of GI NETs; the sensitivity was 90% and specificity was 94% for GI NETs, and 80% and 94%, respectively, for PNETs. In comparison with serum CgA levels from 81 GEP NET patients and 95 controls, the PCR-based test outperformed the biomarker (CgA sensitivity 32%, accuracy 60%), even in patients where CgA was low. The investigators concluded that their panel could identify GEP NETs regardless of primary tumor site or metastasis, which could be useful for screening and potential response to therapy. This group is actively recruiting patients to determine how well it might perform under these circumstances.

Biotheranostics Test

A 92-gene molecular assay (CancerTYPE ID, bioTheranostics, Inc, San Diego, CA, USA) was developed for determining the site of unknown primary tumors using qPCR from paraffin-embedded biopsy specimens. In a trial examining 790 tumors comprising 28 different tumor types and 50 subtypes, it was found to have an 87% sensitivity, greater than 98% specificity, and a positive predictive value of 61% to 100%.[66] This test was later applied specifically to 75 NETs (12 GI, 22 pulmonary, 10 pancreas, 10 pheochromocytoma, 11 medullary thyroid carcinoma, and 10 Merkel cell carcinomas), of which 59% were metastases and 41% were primary tumors. This panel correctly classified the tumors as a NET in 74 of 75 cases. The 4 genes that were most important for making this distinction were ELAVL4, CADPS, RGS17, and KCNJ11. Fifteen additional genes were used for further subtyping of NETs, which was accurate in 71 of 75 (95%) cases.[67] One shortcoming of this study is the inability of this test to determine the GI NET subtype—the test does not identify the site of the primary tumor (small bowel vs duodenal vs rectal), only that the tumor is a GI NET. Still, the test performed well overall and shows promise in differentiation of lung, pancreatic, and GI NET primaries from tissue samples of metastases, allowing for more tailored therapy for patients.

Gene Expression Classifiers and Immunohistochemistry to Differentiate Small Bowel Neuroendocrine Tumors from Pancreatic Neuroendocrine Tumors

Sherman and colleagues[68] evaluated the expression of a panel of genes by qPCR in primary tumors and metastases from 61 patients with SBNETs and 25 with PNETs. They were able to refine this panel down to 4 genes in the G-protein-coupled receptor pathway (BRS3, OPRK1, OXTR, and SCTR), and in 136 metastases accurately predicted the origin from SBNETs in 94 of 97 cases (97%) and 34 of 39 PNETs (87%). The algorithm made primary predictions in 122 cases using qPCR of just BRS3 and OPKR1, although when one of the genes had undetectable expression (14 cases), the results for OXTR and/or SCTR were used to come up with a prediction. Maxwell and colleagues[24] compared the results of this gene expression classifier (GEC) to an IHC algorithm that used CDX2, PAX6, and Islet1 in first-tier staining, followed by IHC for PR, PDX1, NESP55, and PrAP if the first-step stains were equivocal. The IHC algorithm was correct in determining the site of origin in 23 of 27 (85%) of SBNET metastases, and 10 of 10 (100%) PNET metastases. Comparison of these results revealed improved performance of the GEC for determining SBNET primaries and of IHC for PNET primaries. Although the overall accuracy was 94% for the GEC and 89% for IHC, they concluded that this IHC algorithm should be used first because of its widespread availability, and that GEC be reserved for cases of indeterminate IHC results. The ability to differentiate SBNET from PNET primaries from a biopsy of a metastatic liver tumor could aid in surgical exploration, and selection of therapy for these patients with metastatic disease, such as Everolimus, Sunitinib, or chemotherapy in patients with PNETs.

IMAGING TESTS FOR DIAGNOSIS AND STAGING OF GASTROENTERICPANCREATIC NEUROENDOCRINE TUMORS

GEP NETs are rare and typically indolent neoplasms that metastasize early. Surgical resection of the primary tumor, regional nodal disease, and distant metastases is the best chance for cure, symptomatic relief, or long-term survival.[69,70] Thus, it is recommended that patients with GEP NETs of any stage be considered for surgery, especially when the primary tumor can be excised and 70% to 90% of their metastatic burden can be debulked.[70–72]

Preoperative imaging is crucial in determining resectability, and the ideal study will identify the primary tumor, define its relationship to surrounding organs and vessels, and detect distant metastases.[73] Conventional imaging modalities, such as computed tomography (CT), MRI, ultrasound (US), or endoscopy, are generally used to define anatomic relationships, whereas somatostatin receptor imaging and PET are used to determine functionality and scan for distant disease. Each of these modalities are reviewed, and their role in the preoperative workup of GEP NETs are discussed.

Computed Tomography

A CT scan is usually the first study ordered in the evaluation of a suspected GEP NET. Whether the primary resides within the pancreas, small bowel, colon, or rectum, a multiphase study should be obtained with intravenous (IV) contrast, as these tumors and their metastases are most often hypervascular and are usually identified in the early arterial phase of a triple-phase scan (**Fig. 1**).[74,75] The later portal venous or delayed phases may detect hypovascular GEP NETs. Diseased mesenteric lymph nodes often develop calcifications, which can help identify them on CT.[76] Oral contrast is also helpful, with conventional radiopaque enteral contrast, or more recently, using negative enteral contrast (methylcellulose for CT enteroclysis, or simply water or polyethylene glycol), which may help to highlight small bowel lesions better.[77]

Primary GEP NETs are detected by CT approximately 73% of the time, although rates vary widely (39%–94%) depending on the study and subset of NETs examined.[78] Study sensitivity is affected by image acquisition protocols, tumor size, location, and contrast with surrounding tissue.[75] SBNETs tend to be small and multifocal and may be missed in approximately 50% of scans.[79] PNETs are more easily detected, with reported rates of approximately 70% for all PNETs and 80% to 100% when the primary is greater than 2 cm in size.[44,80–82] In cases where the location of the primary tumor is unknown, detection rates are much lower (approximately 35%),[51] although inability to detect the primary on imaging should not preclude surgical exploration in most patients, as a recent single-institution study demonstrated that 90% of unknown lesions could be identified intraoperatively.[83] Detection rates for hepatic metastases and soft tissue metastases are approximately 80%.[78,79,84]

MRI

MRI is superior to CT in detailing hepatic metastases and the pancreatic ductal system and is useful in patients with renal failure or an allergy to iodinated contrast (**Fig. 2**).[85–87] It is often unnecessary in the workup of GEP NETs, however, as a CT scan is commonly obtained and sufficient for surgical planning. This study should also be obtained with IV gadolinium contrast, and as with CT, most lesions enhance (are hyperintense) on arterial phases.[82] In a study comparing MRI, CT, and

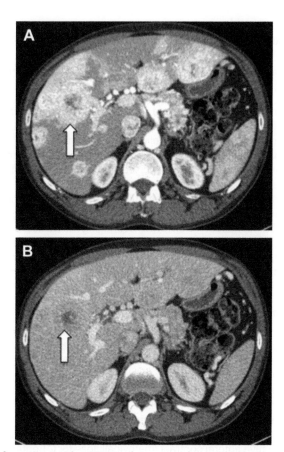

Fig. 1. CT scan of a patient with a PNET and numerous hepatic metastases. (*A*) Early arterial phase demonstrating multiple hypervascular enhancing hepatic metastases. Arrow indicates a large metastasis with a necrotic center. (*B*) Venous phase. In this later phase, contrast has washed out of the hepatic metastases and only the necrotic core of the metastasis indicated by the arrow in (*A*) can be seen as clear evidence of hepatic disease.

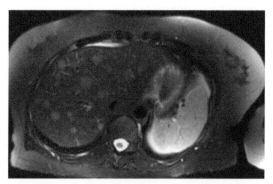

Fig. 2. MRI demonstrating numerous enhancing hepatic metastases on a T2-weighted image.

OctreoScan, MRI detected hepatic metastases with 95.2% sensitivity, compared with sensitivities of 78.5% for CT and 49.3% for OctreoScan.[86] The authors find MRI helpful when planning hepatic debulking, because it generally defines lesions more clearly than CT and also detects hepatic lesions that CT frequently misses. It is not as useful for examining the mesentery and small intestine.

Ultrasound

The primary role of conventional US in the preoperative workup of GEP NETs is for the assessment of hepatic tumor burden. Its sensitivity for detecting primary GEP NETs is only 36%.[84] For hepatic metastases, its sensitivity (88%)[84] is less than contrast-enhanced CT or MRI, although the addition of microbubble contrast agents can improve this to nearly 100%. These small gas bubbles oscillate up to hundreds of meters per second in the blood, perfusing the tumors and enhancing their reflectivity[88]; this is an alternative to standard imaging in patients who cannot tolerate contrast.[89] US is the intraoperative tool of choice to localize hepatic metastases for ablation, or to examine the pancreas for small tumors that were undetectable on CT or MRI.

Endoscopy

Endoscopy is a useful study to localize primary foregut and hindgut GEP NETs and can be used to obtain a tissue diagnosis. In some cases, small (<1 cm) intraluminal tumors that do not invade beyond the mucosa can be treated during this procedure with snare removal.[75,90] It is often combined with US (endoscopic ultrasound, EUS), which may aid in both primary tumor detection and local staging. In PNETs, EUS locates primaries with 93% sensitivity and 95% specificity. For suspected duodenal NETs, it is less sensitive, with detection rates of 45% to 60%.[91] In cases of where the location of the primary is unknown but the small bowel is suspected, either double-balloon enteroscopy (which may need to be done from below and above) or video capsule endoscopy can be used. Unfortunately, double-balloon enteroscopy has a detection rate of only 33% in this context, and capsule endoscopy will uncover only 45% of small bowel primaries.[92,93]

Although it is rarely used as a stand-alone procedure, EUS may add useful information during surgical planning. In a small series of 14 patients with PNETs, EUS was compared with CT to determine whether EUS could be helpful for surgical decision-making. In 36% of cases, EUS altered the surgical plan by identifying either a solitary PNET or additional multifocal PNETs that were missed by CT.[94] EUS has the added benefit of being able to detect tumors less than 2 cm in size, which may be missed by CT or MRI.[91]

18-Fluorodeoxyglucose PET

18-Fluorodeoxyglucose PET (FDG PET) is a functional imaging study that is used to detect a variety of tumor types. It has limited utility for GEP NETs, especially in the preoperative setting, because most of these tumors are of low or intermediate grade and metabolically inactive, and thus do not take up [18]FDG well.[95] High-grade GEP NETs tend to be metabolically active and are most likely to have an uptake on [18]FDG-PET. In this context, uptake identifies lesions likely to have more rapid progression.[96,97] A recent study found shorter overall survival (15 months) in GEP NET patients that had a maximum standardized uptake value (SUV$_{max}$) of 4.5 or greater. Patients with tumors having lower uptake (ie, SUV$_{max}$ <4.5) had an overall survival of 120 months.[98]

Somatostatin Receptor Imaging

Somatostatin is an endogenous peptide that inhibits cellular proliferation and secretion when it binds to 1 of 5 types of somatostatin receptor (SSTR1–SSTR5). These G-protein-coupled receptors are normally expressed by neuroendocrine cells in a wide variety of tissue types, including the brain, pituitary, pancreas, thyroid, spleen, adrenal glands, large and small intestine, kidney, peripheral nervous system, immune cells, and the vasculature.[99–101] SSTR2 is the most highly expressed SSTR subtype on most well-differentiated NETs and is the primary receptor for somatostatin-based imaging and treatment.[99,102]

There are 2 types of somatostatin receptor-based imaging available. Both can be used in the diagnosis and surveillance of GEP NET patients, and also to select candidates for peptide receptor radionuclide therapy.[103] In addition, each uses analogues of endogenous somatostatin to bind to SSTR, because the short half-life of the native peptide precludes its use for this purpose.[102] The most common type of somatostatin-based imaging is a scintigraphic study called the OctreoScan (Mallinckrodt, St. Louis, MO, USA), which uses the radiotracer ^{111}In-DPTA-D-Phe-1-octreotide and binds mainly to SSTR2 but also to SSTR5.[101] Recently, a PET scan has been developed that uses the positron emitter ^{68}Ga to label a variety of somatostatin analogues, which then bind to a variety of SSTR subtypes. The most common of these labeled analogues are ^{68}Ga-DOTATOC, ^{68}Ga-DOTANOC, and ^{68}Ga-DOTATATE. Each has a slightly different affinity for the SSTR subtypes, although this does not translate into variable clinical efficacy.[87,104]

OctreoScan

The OctreoScan is a nuclear medicine study that is available in a large number of centers worldwide and is probably the most commonly used imaging study used in the diagnosis and surveillance of NETs. Patient preparation includes transition to short-acting octreotide 4 to 6 weeks before image acquisition to minimize the drug's interference with the imaging ligand and voiding immediately before the study. In cases of suspected GEP NETs, it may be beneficial to have the patient use an over-the-counter laxative the night before the study to minimize the accumulation of isotope in the lumen of the bowel.[105] The patient is then scanned 4 and 24 hours after IV injection of the analogue.[101]

In its basic form, ligand-receptor binding produces a dark spot on the full-body planar image (**Fig. 3**).[105] Since 1999, however, this scintigraphic image is usually fused with single-photon emission computed tomography (SPECT) and CT to increase its diagnostic accuracy (**Fig. 4**). The addition of SPECT allows for the scintigraphic image to be displayed as tomographic slices, which minimizes the interference physiologic ligand uptake has on NET detection. Fusion with CT increases the anatomic definition of the study.[106–108] A study comparing OctreoScan-SPECT/CT to planar OctreoScan showed that fusing the images positively impacted patient care and altered management decisions in 15% of cases.[109]

Even when fused with SPECT/CT, the anatomic resolution of the OctreoScan is insufficient as the only study used for surgical planning. The primary purpose of this functional imaging is to specifically identify tumors as NETs based on their expression of SSTR2. It is also used as an adjunct to CT or MRI to detect distant metastases and localize primary GEP NETs when the primary tumor site is unknown. The OctreoScan's sensitivity for detection of hepatic metastases ranges from 49% to 91%.[79,84,86,110,111] In comparison to ^{68}Ga-DOTATOC, OctreoScan is more likely to miss small lymph nodes and peritoneal metastases as well as bone metastases.[112] In known primary

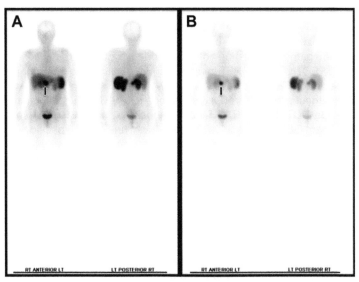

Fig. 3. Planar OctreoScan demonstrating a primary PNET (*arrow*). Physiologic uptake is seen in the liver, spleen, and bladder. (*A*) Image acquired at 4 hours. (*B*) Image acquired at 24 hours.

tumors, OctreoScan has a sensitivity of 80% and specificity of greater than 95%. The study's ability to detect primary tumors seems to be related to tumor size (>2 cm), rather than just SSTR2 expression by the tumor.[113] Its detection rate for unknown primary tumors has been reported to be 24% to 39%.[84,114]

^{68}Ga-PET

Introduction of ^{68}Ga-labeled radioligands to somatostatin receptor-based imaging has enhanced the sensitivity and utility of this type of functional imaging study. The advantages of these radioligands (^{68}Ga-DOTATOC, ^{68}Ga-DOTANOC, and ^{68}Ga-DOTATATE) over the ligand used in the OctreoScan (^{111}In-DPTA-D-Phe-1-octreotide) are the ease and lower cost at which they can be synthesized, enhanced patient convenience (as the image is acquired 1 hour postcontract injection), and ability to quantify lesion uptake of the ligand. This modality better aids preoperative planning

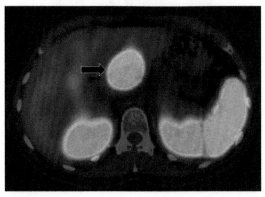

Fig. 4. OctreoScan fused with SPECT/CT. This axial image depicts the same PNET (*arrow*) as is seen in the planar images in **Fig. 3**. Physiologic uptake is seen in the spleen and kidneys.

because it can resolve imaged structures to within millimeters. The more precise spatial resolution is due to the fact that it measures the radiation of 2 photons coincidentally. In comparison, SPECT can only achieve a 1-cm limit of detection and measures the gamma radiation of only one photon directly.[108] Similar to OctreoScan-SPECT/CT, ^{68}Ga-PET images are fused with CT to further improve their anatomic specificity (**Fig. 5**).

One of the largest series (n = 109) comparing ^{68}Ga-PET with conventional imaging found that ^{68}Ga-DOTANOC PET/CT had a sensitivity of 78.3% and specificity of 92.5% for primary GEP-NETs and 97.4% sensitivity and 100% specificity for metastases. In both cases, this was a significant improvement compared with CT, MRI, or US. Furthermore, patient management was altered for 19% of patients on the basis of the ^{68}Ga-DOTANOC PET/CT results. For 5.5% of patients, the primary tumor was detected by ^{68}Ga-DOTANOC PET/CT but missed by other imaging modalities, allowing them to undergo surgical resection. In 6.4% of patients, ^{68}Ga-DOTANOC PET/CT demonstrated new resectable lesions, aiding preoperative planning and potentially improving postoperative outcome. Unnecessary surgery was avoided in 3.6% of patients with evidence of widespread disease on ^{68}Ga-DOTANOC PET/CT.[115]

Despite the excellent image quality and sensitivity of ^{68}Ga-PET/CT, its expense and limited availability make it unlikely to usurp contrast-enhanced CT as the most useful preoperative imaging study. However, it is very helpful in cases where CT or MRI fail to

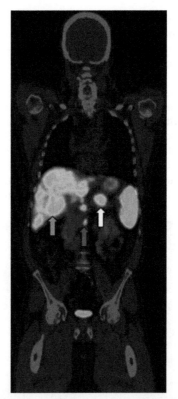

Fig. 5. ^{68}Ga-DOTATOC PET/CT of a patient with innumerable hepatic metastases (*green arrow*), lymph node metastases (*blue arrow*), and a primary PNET (*white arrow*). Physiologic uptake is seen in the spleen.

locate the primary tumor and often uncovers metastases missed by other modalities. In one study, ^{68}Ga-DOTANOC PET/CT found the primary site in 59% of patients with advanced disease but an unknown primary. CT was only able to detect the primary site in 20%.[116] Buchmann and colleagues[117] compared ^{68}Ga-DOTATOC with OctreoScan-SPECT/CT and found that ^{68}Ga-DOTATOC detected more than 279 lesions in their group of 27 patients with histologically proven NETs, whereas OctreoScan-SPECT/CT only detected 157 lesions. When the number of liver metastases detected by each modality was compared, the concordance rate (lesions detected by both modalities) was only 66%. In lymph node metastases, the concordance rate was 40.1%. In both cases, ^{68}Ga-DOTATOC proved to be the superior somatostatin-based imaging study to delineate the extent of patient disease.

Achieving good surgical outcomes requires prudent, meticulous planning. Imaging studies are a crucial part of this process and are required to identify the primary tumor site and the extent of metastatic disease as well as to determine the resectability of the disease. The most practical initial study for GEP NETs is a contrast-enhanced CT scan because it is fast, available at most centers, and excellent in its anatomic detail. For patients that are unable to tolerate iodinated contrast, MRI is a good alternative anatomic study. MRI is also very helpful at defining the extent of hepatic disease in patients selected to undergo hepatic debulking procedures. If extra-abdominal metastases are suspected or require further investigation, ^{68}Ga-PET will likely provide the best supplemental information to the surgeon, although it will take time for this modality to gain US Food and Drug Administration approval and dissemination throughout the United States. Thus, in cases where ^{68}Ga-PET is unavailable, the OctreoScan remains the most helpful NET-specific modality to identify tumors specifically as NETs and to detect metastases. In PNETs and gastric and duodenal NETs, EUS is an excellent adjunct to CT and gives good information regarding primary tumor location, multiplicity, invasion, and likely lymph node involvement. It can also be used to obtain a tissue diagnosis. For GI NETs, endoscopy should be used sparingly, given its moderate sensitivity for locating primary tumors and inability to detect distant disease.

SUMMARY

The increasing incidence of NETs over the past decades, and specifically those of GEP origin, poses several challenges for the clinician. Because a high percentage of patients present with distant disease, one of the difficulties has been in the early identification of these tumors. Increasing recognition of the signs and symptoms characteristic of the specific clinical syndromes associated with functional tumors will promote screening using appropriate NET biochemical markers in the blood, and imaging tests to define the locations of primary tumors. Conversely, the frequent incidental finding of a suspicious lesion on anatomic imaging should lead to appropriate serum testing for functional or nonfunctional NETs, as well as possibly somatostatin-based imaging tests. In metastatic lesions, biopsy samples can now be used to identify the site of unknown primary using qPCR-based tests, which may enhance their discovery and the selection of appropriate surgical or medical therapy.

REFERENCES

1. Yao JC, Hassan M, Phan A, et al. One hundred years after "carcinoid": epidemiology of and prognostic factors for neuroendocrine tumors in 35,825 cases in the United States. J Clin Oncol 2008;26(18):3063–72.

2. Pearse AGE. Common cytochemical properties of cells producing polypeptide hormone, with particular reference to calcitonin and the thyroid C cells. Vet Rec 1966;79:587–90.

3. Klimstra DS, Modlin IR, Coppola D, et al. The pathologic classification of neuroendocrine tumors: a review of nomenclature, grading, and staging systems. Pancreas 2010;39:707–12.

4. Solcia E, Kloppel G, Sobin LH. Histological typing of endocrine tumors. WHO International classification of tumours. 2nd edition. New York: Springer; 2000.

5. Lamberts SW, van der Lely AJ, de Herder WW, et al. Octreotide. N Engl J Med 1996;334(4):246–54.

6. Krenning EP, Kwekkeboom DJ, Oei HY, et al. Somatostatin-receptor scintigraphy in gastroenteropancreatic tumors. An overview of European results. Ann N Y Acad Sci 1994;733:416–24.

7. Rinke A, Muller HH, Schade-Brittinger C, et al. Placebo-controlled, double-blind, prospective, randomized study on the effect of octreotide LAR in the control of tumor growth in patients with metastatic neuroendocrine midgut tumors: a report from the PROMID Study Group. J Clin Oncol 2009;27(28):4656–63.

8. Caplin ME, Pavel M, Cwikla JB, et al. Lanreotide in metastatic enteropancreatic neuroendocrine tumors. N Engl J Med 2014;371(3):224–33.

9. Kwekkeboom DJ, de Herder WW, Kam BL, et al. Treatment with the radiolabeled somatostatin analog [177 Lu-DOTA 0, Tyr3]octreotate: toxicity, efficacy, and survival. J Clin Oncol 2008;26(13):2124–30.

10. Vinik AI, Woltering EA, O'Dorisio TM, et al. Neuroendocrine tumors: a comprehensive guide to diagnosis and management. 5th edition. Inglewood (CA): Inter Science Institute; 2012.

11. O'Dorisio TM, Redfern JS. Somatostatin and somatostatin-like peptides: clinical research and clinical applications. In: Mazzaferri EL, Bar RS, Kreisberg RA, editors. Advances in endocrinology and metabolism, vol. 1. Chicago: Mosby Year Book; 1990. p. 174–230.

12. Oberndorfer S. Karzinoide tumoren des dundarms. Frankf Z Pathol 1907;1: 426–32.

13. Modlin IM, Shapiro MD, Kidd M, et al. Siegfried Oberndorfer and the origins of carcinoid tumors. In: Modlin IM, Oberg K, editors. A century of advances in neuroendocrine tumor biology and treatment. Switzerland: Felsenstein; 2007. p. 22–7.

14. Howe JR, Karnell LH, Menck HR, et al. The American College of Surgeons Commission on Cancer and the American Cancer Society. Adenocarcinoma of the small bowel: review of the National Cancer Data Base, 1985-1995. Cancer 1999;86(12):2693–706.

15. Bilimoria KY, Bentrem DJ, Wayne JD, et al. Small bowel cancer in the United States: changes in epidemiology, treatment, and survival over the last 20 years. Ann Surg 2009;249(1):63–71.

16. Drozdov I, Modlin IM, Kidd M, et al. From Leningrad to London: the saga of Kulchitsky and the legacy of the enterochromaffin cell. Neuroendocrinology 2009; 89(1):1–12.

17. Andrew A. Further evidence that enterochromaffin cells are not derived from the neural crest. J Embryol Exp Morphol 1974;31(3):589–98.

18. Gershon MD. Review article: roles played by 5-hydroxytryptamine in the physiology of the bowel. Aliment Pharmacol Ther 1999;13(Suppl 2):15–30.

19. Vinik AI, Silva MP, Woltering EA, et al. Biochemical testing for neuroendocrine tumors. Pancreas 2009;38(8):876–89.

20. Norheim I, Oberg K, Theodorsson-Norheim E, et al. Malignant carcinoid tumors. An analysis of 103 patients with regard to tumor localization, hormone production, and survival. Ann Surg 1987;206(2):115–25.

21. Meijer WG, Kema IP, Volmer M, et al. Discriminating capacity of indole markers in the diagnosis of carcinoid tumors. Clin Chem 2000;46(10):1588–96.

22. Bajetta E, Ferrari L, Martinetti A, et al. Chromogranin A, neuron specific enolase, carcinoembryonic antigen, and hydroxyindole acetic acid evaluation in patients with neuroendocrine tumors. Cancer 1999;86(5):858–65.

23. Allen KR, Degg TJ, Anthoney DA, et al. Monitoring the treatment of carcinoid disease using blood serotonin and plasma 5-hydroxyindoleacetic acid: three case examples. Ann Clin Biochem 2007;44(Pt 3):300–7.

24. Maxwell JE, Sherman SK, Stashek KM, et al. A practical method to determine the site of unknown primary in metastatic neuroendocrine tumors. Surgery 2014;156(6):1359–65 [discussion: 1365–6].

25. Kema IP, de Vries EG, Slooff MJ, et al. Serotonin, catecholamines, histamine, and their metabolites in urine, platelets, and tumor tissue of patients with carcinoid tumors. Clin Chem 1994;40(1):86–95.

26. Research MFfMEa. Serotonin, Serum. 2015. Available at: http://www.mayomedicallaboratories.com/test-catalog/Clinical+and+Interpretive/84395. Accessed April 30, 2015.

27. Boudreaux JP, Klimstra DS, Hassan MM, et al. The NANETS consensus guideline for the diagnosis and management of neuroendocrine tumors: well-differentiated neuroendocrine tumors of the Jejunum, Ileum, Appendix, and Cecum. Pancreas 2010;39(6):753–66.

28. Stridsberg M, Eriksson B, Oberg K, et al. A comparison between three commercial kits for chromogranin A measurements. J Endocrinol 2003;177(2):337–41.

29. Arnold R, Wilke A, Rinke A, et al. Plasma chromogranin A as marker for survival in patients with metastatic endocrine gastroenteropancreatic tumors. Clin Gastroenterol Hepatol 2008;6(7):820–7.

30. Jensen EH, Kvols L, McLoughlin JM, et al. Biomarkers predict outcomes following cytoreductive surgery for hepatic metastases from functional carcinoid tumors. Ann Surg Oncol 2007;14(2):780–5.

31. Welin S, Stridsberg M, Cunningham J, et al. Elevated plasma chromogranin A is the first indication of recurrence in radically operated midgut carcinoid tumors. Neuroendocrinology 2009;89(3):302–7.

32. Research MFfMEa. Chromogranin A. 2015. Available at: http://www.mayomedicallaboratories.com/test-catalog/Overview/34641. Accessed April 30, 2015.

33. O'Connor DT, Cadman PE, Smiley C, et al. Pancreastatin: multiple actions on human intermediary metabolism in vivo, variation in disease, and naturally occurring functional genetic polymorphism. J Clin Endocrinol Metab 2005;90(9):5414–25.

34. O'Dorisio TM, Krutzik SR, Woltering EA, et al. Development of a highly sensitive and specific carboxy-terminal human pancreastatin assay to monitor neuroendocrine tumor behavior. Pancreas 2010;39(5):611–6.

35. Calhoun K, Toth-Fejel S, Cheek J, et al. Serum peptide profiles in patients with carcinoid tumors. Am J Surg 2003;186(1):28–31.

36. Raines D, Chester M, Diebold AE, et al. A prospective evaluation of the effect of chronic proton pump inhibitor use on plasma biomarker levels in humans. Pancreas 2012;41(4):508–11.

37. Rustagi S, Warner RR, Divino CM. Serum pancreastatin: the next predictive neuroendocrine tumor marker. J Surg Oncol 2013;108(2):126–8.

38. Sherman SK, Maxwell JE, O'Dorisio MS, et al. Pancreastatin predicts survival in neuroendocrine tumors. Ann Surg Oncol 2014;21(9):2971–80.

39. Turner GB, Johnston BT, McCance DR, et al. Circulating markers of prognosis and response to treatment in patients with midgut carcinoid tumours. Gut 2006;55(11):1586–91.

40. Diebold AE, Boudreaux JP, Wang YZ, et al. Neurokinin A levels predict survival in patients with stage IV well differentiated small bowel neuroendocrine neoplasms. Surgery 2012;152(6):1172–6.

41. Kulke MH, Shah MH, Benson AB 3rd, et al. Neuroendocrine tumors, version 1.2015. J Natl Compr Canc Netw 2015;13(1):78–108.

42. Pape UF, Perren A, Niederle B, et al. ENETS Consensus Guidelines for the management of patients with neuroendocrine neoplasms from the jejuno-ileum and the appendix including goblet cell carcinomas. Neuroendocrinology 2012;95(2):135–56.

43. Kunz PL, Reidy-Lagunes D, Anthony LB, et al. Consensus guidelines for the management and treatment of neuroendocrine tumors. Pancreas 2013;42(4):557–77.

44. Kuo JH, Lee JA, Chabot JA. Nonfunctional pancreatic neuroendocrine tumors. Surg Clin North Am 2014;94(3):689–708.

45. Franko J, Feng W, Yip L, et al. Non-functional neuroendocrine carcinoma of the pancreas: incidence, tumor biology, and outcomes in 2,158 patients. J Gastrointest Surg 2010;14(3):541–8.

46. Bilimoria KY, Tomlinson JS, Merkow RP, et al. Clinicopathologic features and treatment trends of pancreatic neuroendocrine tumors: analysis of 9,821 patients. J Gastrointest Surg 2007;11(11):1460–7 [discussion: 1467–9].

47. Ehehalt F, Saeger HD, Schmidt CM, et al. Neuroendocrine tumors of the pancreas. Oncologist 2009;14(5):456–67.

48. Schimmack S, Svejda B, Lawrence B, et al. The diversity and commonalities of gastroenteropancreatic neuroendocrine tumors. Langenbecks Arch Surg 2011;396(3):273–98.

49. Stabile BE, Morrow DJ, Passaro E Jr. The gastrinoma triangle: operative implications. Am J Surg 1984;147(1):25–31.

50. Jensen RT, Niederle B, Mitry E, et al. Gastrinoma (duodenal and pancreatic). Neuroendocrinology 2006;84(3):173–82.

51. Wang SC, Parekh JR, Zuraek MB, et al. Identification of unknown primary tumors in patients with neuroendocrine liver metastases. Arch Surg 2010;145(3):276–80.

52. McGuigan JE, Wolfe MM. Secretin injection test in the diagnosis of gastrinoma. Gastroenterology 1980;79(6):1324–31.

53. Kulke MH, Anthony LB, Bushnell DL, et al. NANETS treatment guidelines: well-differentiated neuroendocrine tumors of the stomach and pancreas. Pancreas 2010;39(6):735–52.

54. Massironi S, Sciola V, Peracchi M, et al. Neuroendocrine tumors of the gastro-entero-pancreatic system. World J Gastroenterol 2008;14(35):5377–84.

55. Piovesan A, Pia A, Visconti G, et al. Proinsulin-secreting neuroendocrine tumor of the pancreas. J Endocrinol Invest 2003;26(8):758–61.

56. Priest WM, Alexander MK. Isletcell tumour of the pancreas with peptic ulceration, diarrhoea, and hypokalaemia. Lancet 1957;273(7006):1145–7.

57. Verner JV, Morrison AB. Islet cell tumor and a syndrome of refractory watery diarrhea and hypokalemia. Am J Med 1958;25:370–80.

58. O'Dorisio TM, O'Dorisio MS. Endocrine tumors of the gastroenteropancreatic (GEP) axis. In: Mazzaferri EL, editor. Endocrinology. New York: Medical Examination Publishing; 1985. p. 76–81.

59. Bloom SR, Polak JM. VIPomas. In: Said SI, editor. Vasoactive intestinal peptide. New York: Raven Press; 1982. p. 457–63.

60. O'Dorisio TM, Mekljian HS. VIPoma syndrome. In: Cohen S, Soloway RD, editors. Contemporary issues in gastroenterology. Edinburgh (United Kingdom): Churchill Livingston; 1984. p. 101–16.

61. O'Dorisio TM, Vinik AI. Pancreatic polypeptides and mixed hormone-producing tumors of the gastrointestinal tract. In: Cohen S, Soloway RD, editors. Contemporary issues in gastroenterology. Endinburgh (United Kingdom): Churchill-Livingston; 1984. p. 117–28.

62. Vinik AI, Strodel WE, O'Dorisio TM. Endocrine tumors of the gastroenteropancreatic axis. In: Santern A, editor. Endocrine related tumors. Amsterdam: Martino Nijolof; 1984. p. 305–45.

63. Maxwell JE, O'Dorisio TM, Bellizzi AM, et al. Elevated pancreatic polypeptide levels in pancreatic neuroendocrine tumors and diabetes mellitus: causation or association? Pancreas 2014;43(4):651–6.

64. Falconi M, Bartsch DK, Eriksson B, et al. ENETS Consensus Guidelines for the management of patients with digestive neuroendocrine neoplasms of the digestive system: well-differentiated pancreatic non-functioning tumors. Neuroendocrinology 2012;95(2):120–34.

65. Modlin IM, Drozdov I, Kidd M. The identification of gut neuroendocrine tumor disease by multiple synchronous transcript analysis in blood. PLoS One 2013; 8(5):e63364.

66. Kerr SE, Schnabel CA, Sullivan PS, et al. Multisite validation study to determine performance characteristics of a 92-gene molecular cancer classifier. Clin Cancer Res 2012;18(14):3952–60.

67. Kerr SE, Schnabel CA, Sullivan PS, et al. A 92-gene cancer classifier predicts the site of origin for neuroendocrine tumors. Mod Pathol 2014;27(1):44–54.

68. Sherman SK, Maxwell JE, Carr JC, et al. Gene expression accurately distinguishes liver metastases of small bowel and pancreas neuroendocrine tumors. Clin Exp Metastasis 2014;31(8):935–44.

69. Givi B, Pommier SJ, Thompson AK, et al. Operative resection of primary carcinoid neoplasms in patients with liver metastases yields significantly better survival. Surgery 2006;140(6):891–7 [discussion: 897–8].

70. Hill JS, McPhee JT, McDade TP, et al. Pancreatic neuroendocrine tumors: the impact of surgical resection on survival. Cancer 2009;115(4):741–51.

71. Mayo SC, de Jong MC, Pulitano C, et al. Surgical management of hepatic neuroendocrine tumor metastasis: results from an international multi-institutional analysis. Ann Surg Oncol 2010;17(12):3129–36.

72. Graff-Baker AN, Sauer DA, Pommier SJ, et al. Expanded criteria for carcinoid liver debulking: maintaining survival and increasing the number of eligible patients. Surgery 2014;156:1369–77.

73. Chambers AJ, Pasieka JL, Dixon E, et al. Role of imaging in the preoperative staging of small bowel neuroendocrine tumors. J Am Coll Surg 2010;211(5):620–7.

74. Bushnell DL, Baum RP. Standard imaging techniques for neuroendocrine tumors. Endocrinol Metab Clin North Am 2011;40:153–62.

75. Sahani DV, Bonaffini PA, Fernandez-Del Castillo C, et al. Gastroenteropancreatic neuroendocrine tumors: role of imaging in diagnosis and management. Radiology 2013;266(1):38–61.

76. Woodbridge LR, Murtagh BM, Yu DFQC, et al. Midgut neuroendocrine tumors: imaging assessment for surgical resection. Radiographics 2014;34:413–26.

77. Sailer J, Zacherl J, Schima W. MDCT of small bowel tumours. Cancer Imaging 2007;7:224–33.

78. Sundin A, Vullierme MP, Kaltsas G, et al. ENETS consensus guidelines for the standards of care in neuroendocrine tumors: radiological examinations. Neuroendocrinology 2009;90(2):167–83.

79. Dahdaleh FS, Lorenzen A, Rajput M, et al. The value of preoperative imaging in small bowel neuroendocrine tumors. Ann Surg Oncol 2013;20(6):1912–7.

80. Khashab MA, Yong E, Lennon AM, et al. EUS is still superior to multidetector computerized tomography for detection of pancreatic neuroendocrine tumors. Gastrointest Endosc 2011;73(4):691–6.

81. Versari A, Camellini L, Carlinfante G, et al. Ga-68 DOTATOC PET, endoscopic ultrasonography, and multidetector CT in the diagnosis of duodenopancreatic neuroendocrine tumors. Clin Nucl Med 2010;35:321–8.

82. Foti G, Boninsegna L, Falconi M, et al. Preoperative assessment of nonfunctioning pancreatic endocrine tumours: role of MDCT and MRI. Radiol Med 2013;118(7):1082–101.

83. Bartlett EK, Roses RE, Gupta M, et al. Surgery for metastatic neuroendocrine tumors with occult primaries. J Surg Res 2013;184(1):221–7.

84. Chiti A, Fanti S, Savelli G, et al. Comparison of somatostatin receptor imaging, computed tomography and ultrasound in the clinical management of neuroendocrine gastro-entero-pancreatic tumours. Eur J Nucl Med 1998;25:1396–403.

85. Manfredi R, Bonatti M, Mantovani W, et al. Non-hyperfunctioning neuroendocrine tumours of the pancreas: MR imaging appearance and correlation with their biological behaviour. Eur Radiol 2013;23(11):3029–39.

86. Dromain C, de Baere T, Lumbroso J, et al. Detection of liver metastases from endocrine tumors: a prospective comparison of somatostatin receptor scintigraphy, computed tomography, and magnetic resonance imaging. J Clin Oncol 2005;23(1):70–8.

87. Sundin A. Radiological and nuclear medicine imaging of gastroenteropancreatic neuroendocrine tumours. Best Pract Res Clin Gastroenterol 2012;26(6):803–18.

88. Ferrara K, Pollard R, Borden M. Ultrasound microbubble contrast agents: fundamentals and application to gene and drug delivery. Annu Rev Biomed Eng 2007;9:415–47.

89. Hoeffel C, Job L, Ladam-Marcus V, et al. Detection of hepatic metastases from carcinoid tumor: prospective evaluation of contrast-enhanced ultrasonography. Dig Dis Sci 2009;54(9):2040–6.

90. Delle Fave G, Kwekkeboom DJ, Van Cutsem E, et al. ENETS Consensus Guidelines for the management of patients with gastroduodenal neoplasms. Neuroendocrinology 2012;95(2):74–87.

91. Anderson MA, Carpenter S, Thompson NW, et al. Endoscopic ultrasound is highly accurate and directs management in patients with neuroendocrine tumors of the pancreas. Am J Gastroenterol 2000;95:2271–7.

92. Bellutti M, Fry LC, Schmitt J, et al. Detection of neuroendocrine tumors of the small bowel by double balloon enteroscopy. Dig Dis Sci 2009;54(5):1050–8.

93. van Tuyl SA, van Noorden JT, Timmer R, et al. Detection of small-bowel neuroendocrine tumors by video capsule endoscopy. Gastrointest Endosc 2006;64(1):66–72.

94. Alsohaibani F, Bigam D, Kneteman N, et al. The impact of preoperative endo-scopic ultrasound on the surgical management of pancreatic neuroendocrine tumors. Can J Gastroenterol 2008;22(10):817–20.

95. Sundin A, Eriksson B, BergstrÖM M, et al. PET in the diagnosis of neuroendo-crine tumors. Ann N Y Acad Sci 2004;1014(1):246–57.

96. Bhate K, Mok WY, Tran K, et al. Functional assessment in the multimodality im-aging of pancreatic neuroendocrine tumours. Minerva Endocrinol 2010;35(1): 17–25.

97. Pasquali C, Rubello D, Sperti C, et al. Neuroendocrine tumor imaging: can 18F-fluorodeoxyglucose positron emission tomography detect tumors with poor prognosis and aggressive behavior? World J Surg 1998;22:588–92.

98. Bahri H, Laurence L, Edeline J, et al. High prognostic value of 18F-FDG PET for metastatic gastroenteropancreatic neuroendocrine tumors: a long-term evalua-tion. J Nucl Med 2014;55(11):1786–90.

99. Reubi JC, Krenning E, Lamberts SWJ. Distribution of somatostatin receptors in normal and tumor tissue. Metab Clin Exp 1990;39(9):78–81.

100. Patel YC. Somatostatin and its receptor family. Front Neuroendocrinol 1999;20: 157–98.

101. Kwekkeboom DJ, Krenning EP, Scheidhauer K, et al. ENETS Consensus Guidelines for the Standards of Care in Neuroendocrine Tumors: somatostatin receptor imaging with (111)In-pentetreotide. Neuroendocrinology 2009;90(2): 184–9.

102. Reubi JC. Somatostatin and other peptide receptors as tools for tumor diagnosis and treatment. Neuroendocrinology 2004;80(Suppl 1):51–6.

103. Lu SJ, Gnanasegaran G, Buscombe J, et al. Single photon emission computed tomography/computed tomography in the evaluation of neuroendocrine tu-mours: a review of the literature. Nucl Med Commun 2013;34(2):98–107.

104. Ambrosini V, Campana D, Tomassetti P, et al. 68Ga-labelled peptides for diag-nosis of gastroenteropancreatic NET. Eur J Nucl Med Mol Imaging 2012;39: s52–60.

105. Theodoropoulou M, Stalla GK. Somatostatin receptors: from signaling to clinical practice. Front Neuroendocrinol 2013;34(3):228–52.

106. Brandon D, Alazraki A, Halkar RK, et al. The role of single-photon emission computed tomography and SPECT/computed tomography in oncologic imag-ing. Semin Oncol 2011;38(1):87–108.

107. Bural GG, Muthukrishnan A, Oborski MJ, et al. Improved benefit of SPECT/CT compared to SPECT alone for the accurate localization of endocrine and neuro-endocrine tumors. Mol Imaging Radionucl Ther 2012;21(3):91–6.

108. Zanzonico P. Principles of nuclear medicine imaging: planar, SPECT, PET, multi-modality, and autoradiography systems. Radiat Res 2012;177(4):349–64.

109. Krausz Y, Keidar Z, Kogan I, et al. SPECT/CT hybrid imaging with 111In-pente-treotide in assessment of neuroendocrine tumours. Clin Endocrinol 2003;59: 565–73.

110. Kumbasar B, Kamel IR, Tekes A, et al. Imaging of neuroendocrine tumors: ac-curacy of helical CT versus SRS. Abdom Imaging 2004;29(6):696–702.

111. Shi W, Johnston CF, Buchanan KD, et al. Localization of neuroendocrine tu-mours with 111In-DTPA-octreotide scintigraphy (Octreoscan): a comparative study with CT and MR imaging. QJM 1998;91:295–301.

112. Gabriel M, Decristoforo C, Kendler D, et al. 68Ga-DOTA-Tyr3-octreotide PET in neuroendocrine tumors: comparison with somatostatin receptor scintigraphy and CT. J Nucl Med 2007;48(4):508–18.

113. Maxwell JE, Sherman SK, Menda Y, et al. Limitations of somatostatin scintigraphy in primary small bowel neuroendocrine tumors. J Surg Res 2014; 190(2):548–53.
114. Savelli G, Lucignani G, Seregni E, et al. Feasibility of somatostatin receptor scintigraphy in the detection of occult primary gastro-entero-pancreatic (GEP) neuroendocrine tumors. Nucl Med Commun 2004;25(5):445–9.
115. Naswa N, Sharma P, Kumar A, et al. Gallium-68-DOTA-NOC PET/CT of patients with gastroenteropancreatic neuroendocrine tumors: a prospective single-center study. AJR Am J Roentgenol 2011;197:1221–8.
116. Prasad V, Ambrosini V, Hommann M, et al. Detection of unknown primary neuroendocrine tumours (CUP-NET) using (68)Ga-DOTA-NOC receptor PET/CT. Eur J Nucl Med Mol Imaging 2010;37(1):67–77.
117. Buchmann I, Henze M, Engelbrecht S, et al. Comparison of 68Ga-DOTATOC PET and 111In-DTPAOC (Octreoscan) SPECT in patients with neuroendocrine tumours. Eur J Nucl Med Mol Imaging 2007;34(10):1617–26.

Minimally Invasive Techniques for Resection of Pancreatic Neuroendocrine Tumors

Gustavo G. Fernandez Ranvier, MD[a], Daniel Shouhed, MD[a],
William B. Inabnet III, MD[b],*

KEYWORDS

- Pancreatic neuroendocrine tumors • Insulinoma • Gastrinoma
- Laparoscopic pancreas resection • Robotic pancreas resection

KEY POINTS

- Surgical resection is the only curative treatment of pancreatic neuroendocrine tumors (PNETs).
- Minimally invasive procedures are a safe modality for the surgical treatment of PNETs.
- Laparoscopy does not compromise oncologic resection, and is associated with decreased postoperative pain, better cosmetic results, a shorter hospital stay, and a shorter postoperative recovery period.
- The overall 5-year and 10-year survival rates for all PNETs are approximately 65% and 45%, respectively.

INTRODUCTION

Pancreatic neuroendocrine tumors (PNETs) are a heterogeneous group of neoplasms that have an incidence of 1 per 100,000 individuals per year, and account for 1% to 2% of all pancreatic neoplasms.[1,2] PNETs can develop at any age, but they are more frequently seen in patients between the fourth and sixth decades of life. Although most tumors are considered sporadic, about 10% to 30% of cases present in patients with familial syndromes such as multiple endocrine neoplasia type 1 (MEN1),von

Disclosures: The authors have nothing to disclose.
[a] Division of Metabolic, Endocrine and Minimally Invasive Surgery, Department of Surgery, Mount Sinai Hospital, Icahn School of Medicine at Mount Sinai, 5 East 98 street, box 1259, New York, NY 10029, USA; [b] Department of Surgery, Mount Sinai Beth Israel, Icahn School of Medicine at Mount Sinai, First Ave at 16th street, Baird Hall, Suite 16BH20, New York, NY 10003, USA
* Corresponding author.
E-mail address: william.inabnet@mountsinai.org

Hippel-Lindau, neurofibromatosis type 1, and tuberous sclerosis, among other more rare syndromes.[3] PNETs can be classified into functional and nonfunctional tumors. Functional tumors are usually detected early because of the symptoms caused by hormonal production. Nonfunctional tumors are more common, but given the absence of hormonal symptoms these tumors are found incidentally or in more advanced stages of the disease, with larger tumors causing mass effect, invading surrounding tissues or presenting with metastatic disease.[4,5]

Surgical resection of the primary tumor remains the treatment of choice for PNETs, because it is associated with increased survival.[4] With the advancement of minimally invasive techniques, an increasing number of laparoscopic surgical resections for pancreatic neuroendocrine tumors are currently performed.[6] Low-risk PNETs in the body and the tail of the pancreas are suitable for minimally invasive surgery, with enough evidence in the literature supporting better outcomes of the laparoscopic approach compared with open surgery.[6,7] However, minimally invasive pancreatic surgery has not yet been widely accepted as the gold standard for all pancreatic resections. Most recently, robotic surgical techniques across different specialties have slowly gained popularity, although the existing experience is only based on reports of small series.[8–12] This article provides an insight into well-established minimally invasive procedures and also those that slowly have gained popularity over the last few years. It also reviews and discusses the different minimally invasive surgical techniques with their benefits and limitations.

DIAGNOSIS
Insulinoma

Insulinomas are the most common functional neuroendocrine tumors of the pancreas as well as the most common cause of hypoglycemia related to endogenous hyperinsulinemia. Most insulinomas are benign, small (<2 cm) tumors with only 10% of cases usually presenting as malignant lesions. They are typically solitary lesions distributed evenly throughout pancreas, except in association with MEN1 syndrome, when they tend to be multifocal. The clinical signs and symptoms of insulinomas are divided into 2 categories. Neuroglycopenic symptoms, which are a direct result of hypoglycemia, may include weakness, confusion, visual disturbances, and in extreme cases seizures and comas. Autonomic symptoms, which are a consequence of catecholamine release from hypoglycemia, include diaphoresis, palpitations, anxiety, and tremor.[13,14]

Establishing a diagnosis of insulinoma has classically relied on satisfying the criteria of the Whipple triad: (1) hypoglycemia (plasma glucose level <50 mg/dL), (2) neuroglycopenic symptoms, and (3) prompt resolution of symptoms following administration of glucose.[15] At present, biochemical measurement of plasma glucose, insulin, C peptide, and proinsulin levels during a 72-hour fast can detect up to 99% of insulinomas and has become the gold standard of diagnosis.[16] However, in more than 97% of cases, biochemical testing in conjunction with a supervised 48-hour fast is sufficient to diagnose an insulinoma.[17] Other conditions, such as the factitious use of insulin or oral hypoglycemic agents, can be ruled out through the measurements of plasma proinsulin, C peptide, and sulfonylurea.

Gastrinoma

Gastrinomas, along with insulinomas, account for most functional PNETs. Most of these tumors are found sporadically, although 20% to 30% are found in conjunction with MEN1. They are the most common pancreatic tumor found in patients with MEN1.[18] Gastrinoma syndrome, also known as Zollinger-Ellison syndrome, has a slight male preponderance and is most commonly diagnosed in the fifth decade of life.[19] Patients most often present with peptic ulcer disease, particularly multiple ulcers and ulcers that are resistant to medical treatment. Up to 75% of patients present with diarrhea, and occasionally this is the chief complaint. Most (up to 60%–90%) of these lesions are malignant, with up to 20% to 30% presenting with liver metastasis at the time of diagnosis. Ninety percent of gastrinomas are found within the gastrinoma triangle, which is formed by the borders of the second and third portions of the duodenum inferiorly, the junction of the cystic and common bile duct superiorly, and the junction between the neck and body of the pancreas medially.[20]

The biochemical diagnosis of gastrinomas can be difficult because many conditions can cause hypersecretion of gastrin, such as the use of proton pump inhibitors, renal failure, and gastric outlet obstruction.[21] Nonetheless, initial testing should be targeted at measuring serum gastrin levels. Increased fasting serum gastrin levels (>500 pg/mL) should prompt further testing, whereas levels greater than 1000 pg/mL are highly suspicious for gastrinoma. A finding of normal gastrin levels is often sufficient to rule out the syndrome. A high fasting serum gastrin level should prompt provocative testing to confirm the diagnosis, most commonly using secretin or calcium gluconate infusion. Secretin does not stimulate the secretion of gastrin from G cells of the stomach; however, it does lead to hypersecretion of gastrin from gastrinomas. An increase in fasting serum gastrin levels to more than 200 pg/mL is assumed to be diagnostic.[22]

Glucagonoma

Glucagonomas, the alpha-cell counterparts of insulinomas, are rare tumors of the pancreas. Unlike insulinomas, these tumors are typically bulky, large malignant lesions, often localized to the body and tail of the pancreas. The most common presenting symptoms include mild glucose intolerance manifesting as diabetes mellitus, weight loss, normocytic anemia, and a distinct skin rash, referred to as necrolytic migratory erythema.[23] Biochemical diagnosis is established through the serum measurement of glucagon, with levels greater than 500 pg/mL characteristic of glucagonomas.

Vasoactive Intestinal Peptideoma

Vasoactive intestinal peptideomas (VIPomas) are exceedingly rare tumors, with an estimated incidence of only 1 in 10 million per year.[24] Approximately 70% of patients present with malignant tumors, as shown by hepatic, distant, or lymph node metastasis.[25] Most tumors are at least 3 cm, with a mean of about 5 cm at initial presentation. Most tumors are found primarily in the body and tail of the pancreas; however, tumors can be identified in the head as well as outside the pancreas. Nearly all patients present with watery diarrhea, with most patients also presenting with hypokalemia and achlorhydria, hence the designation of WDHA syndrome. The diagnosis is established through the measurement of increased fasting serum vasoactive intestinal peptide levels (75–150 pg/mL) in the setting of secretory diarrhea.[26]

Somatostatinoma

Neuroendocrine tumors of the pancreas secreting somatostatin are the rarest of the PNETs, with an incidence of only 1 in 40 million people per year.[1] Most tumors are located in the head of the pancreas; however, it is common to find a lesion within the tail or outside the pancreas. At initial presentation, tumors are large (>5 cm) and nearly half are malignant. Somatostatinomas may lead to diarrhea and/or steatorrhea, cholelithiasis, and diabetes mellitus. However, most commonly patients typically present with signs or symptoms directly related to the tumor, such as abdominal pain, weight loss, or intestinal obstruction.[27] The diagnosis is established through measurement of fasting plasma somatostatin levels, with a level greater than 160 pg/mL strongly suggestive of a somatostatinoma, particularly in the presence of a mass seen on imaging.[27]

PREOPERATIVE EVALUATION
Localization

Management of PNETs depends heavily on a thorough preoperative evaluation. Various imaging studies, including MRI, computed tomography (CT), PET, endoscopic ultrasonography (EUS), and octreotide scans play an important role in localizing the primary tumor and identifying potential sites of metastases. Imaging is also important to assess response to treatment and as a screening tool for recurrence. The utility of each imaging modality differs based on the tumor type.

CT scanning is the most widely accepted and used imaging modality for localizing and staging PNETs. Compared with nonfunctional PNETs, functional PNETs are typically small at the time of diagnosis, creating more of a challenge for proper identification. These smaller tumors seldom alter the contour of the pancreas; therefore obtaining thinly sliced images enhances the ability to detect smaller tumors and should be used routinely. Fidler and colleagues[28] showed that multiphasic imaging with early and late arterial phases as well as portal venous–phase CT had a higher sensitivity for detecting islet cell tumors. The classic CT findings of islet cell tumors are an isodense lesion during the precontrast phase and a hyperattenuating mass in both the arterial and portal venous phases (**Fig. 1**). Depending on the biology and characteristics of the tumor, they may be more apparent during either phase.[29]

Insulinomas are typically small on presentation and particularly difficult to diagnose. Up to 10% to 20% of these lesions are not identifiable during surgical exploration, which emphasizes the importance of preoperative localization of these tumors. With the use of more advanced helical, thinly sliced, multidimensional CT scanning, insulinomas are diagnosed with a sensitivity of 94%; combined with EUS, the sensitivity of identifying insulinomas in one study was 100%.[30] Gastrinomas, like insulinomas, tend to be small at presentation and are more difficult to find when they are present in extrapancreatic locations. They often do not alter the contour of the pancreas. As described earlier, 90% of gastrinomas are found within the gastrinoma triangle and careful attention should be given to this area during imaging review.[29] Other functioning tumors, namely VIPomas, somatostatinomas, and glucagonomas, as well as nonfunctioning neuroendocrine tumors of the pancreas, are often easier to identify because they

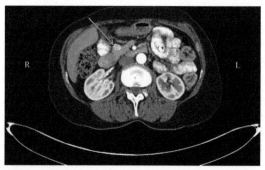

Fig. 1. CT of the abdomen showing a 1-cm arterially enhancing lesion in the head of the pancreas consistent with a PNET (*green arrow*).

commonly present as large, malignant lesions. They tend to show central necrosis, discrete nodular calcifications, and cystic areas.[31] Unlike pancreatic adenocarcinomas, PNETs are hypervascular tumors and rarely cause ductal obstruction.[32]

MRI can play a complimentary role to CT imaging, particularly for small tumors. Relative to the pancreas, PNETS frequently present as low-intensity lesions on T1-weighted sequences and high-intensity lesions on T2-weighted sequences (**Fig. 2**). MRI has been effective at identifying PNETs with a sensitivity of about 93% (range, 85%–100%) and a specificity of about 88% (range, 75%–100%) among 7 studies.[33] Magnetic resonance cholangiopancreatography can be included for the local assessment of PNETs to evaluate the relation of the tumor to the pancreatic and main bile duct.[34]

EUS should be performed in every patient in whom minimally invasive surgery is recommended. EUS provides useful anatomic information that may influence the operative plan, especially pertaining to the pancreatic ductal and vascular anatomy. Fine-needle aspiration can be readily performed if indicated to assist with PNET diagnosis; this is especially helpful in the setting of multifocal disease. Similar to MRI, one of the benefits of EUS is the lack of patient exposure to radiation. Ultrasonography can now be performed with intravenous contrast enhancement using microbubbles, which can be highly effective in depicting smaller tumors, and provides a method to perform needle biopsies for diagnosis, if needed.[35] The first study to report the efficacy of EUS in localizing PNETs was done in 1992 by Rösch and colleagues,[36] showing a sensitivity and specificity of 82% and 92%, respectively, among 50 patients. EUS is particularly useful for identification of small pancreatic tumors as small as 2 to 5 mm, particularly insulinomas and gastrinomas.[36] Despite the various benefits of EUS, it is a more invasive form of imaging study than the other modalities already listed and is highly operator sensitive.

PET imaging has been gaining popularity but may be difficult to obtain because most third party payers do not reimburse for PET scanning. Although the use of PET imaging is controversial, there is emerging evidence that increased intensity, and therefore glucose metabolism, in PNETs indicates a higher likelihood of tumor invasion and metastasis, and poorer prognosis.[34] One study showed that most patients with PET-positive lesions also had early progressive disease.[34] Although not yet conclusive, PET imaging may play an important role in the future in predicting outcomes and management of PNETs.

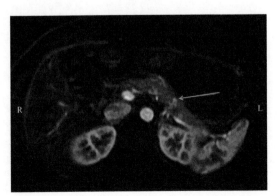

Fig. 2. Gadolinium-enhanced T2-weighted MRI showing a 3.2-cm subtle hypervascular lesion with focal area of enhancement in the body of the pancreas consistent with an insulinoma (*green arrow*).

Patient Selection and Choice of Procedure

Surgical resection is the only curative treatment of patients with PNETs. Surgery may also alleviate symptoms from hormonal production of functioning tumors or symptoms caused by the mass effect frequently seen with nonfunctioning tumors. The planned surgical procedure is mainly mandated by the preoperative localization studies, but it may change according to intraoperative findings. No consensus has been established regarding the indications of minimally invasive surgery for the treatment of PNETs; however, the presence of a malignant PNET could represent a relative contraindication for a minimally invasive approach.[37] Laparoscopic surgery for small and solitary PNETs is feasible and safe.[38] Laparoscopic enucleation is generally recommended in well-circumscribed lesions smaller than 3 cm, with noninvasive features and a peripheral location without involvement of the main pancreatic duct.[38,39] If the tumor is in close proximity to the main pancreatic duct, enucleation is not recommended in light of its high incidence of pancreatic fistula.[40]

Solitary insulinomas are particularly amenable to laparoscopic enucleation because of their small size and benign nature. Intraoperative laparoscopic ultrasonography is routinely performed to confirm tumor location and its relationship to the pancreatic duct and peripancreatic vessels, in order to plan the margin of resection before enucleation[37] (Fig. 3). If enucleation is not possible, a formal pancreatic resection is recommended.[6] In tumors involving the head of the pancreas, pancreaticoduodenectomy is indicated. Pancreaticoduodenectomy has proved to be among the most complex procedures in general surgery, with high rates of morbidity and mortality.[41] However, many studies have shown the effectiveness and safety of this procedure when performed through minimally invasive techniques in high-volume institutions by experienced surgeons.[42–45]

In tumors that are located in the body or tail of the pancreas, which are not amenable for enucleation, laparoscopic distal pancreatectomy (LDP) is the procedure of choice. There are 3 variations of the distal pancreatectomy: spleen-preserving distal pancreatectomy with splenic vessel preservation, spleen-preserving distal pancreatectomy

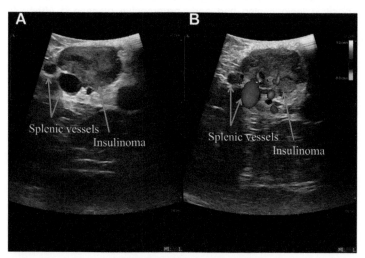

Fig. 3. Intraoperative sonographic appearance of a 3-cm insulinoma involving the pancreatic body and its anatomic relationship to the splenic vessels (*A*) without Doppler effect, (*B*) with Doppler effect.

without splenic vessel preservation, and distal pancreatectomy with splenectomy.[46,47] The anatomic relationship between the tumor within the pancreatic body or tail and the splenic vessels and hilum are factors that determine the appropriate procedure to perform. In addition, the presence or suspicion of a malignant tumor favors a more aggressive approach.

SURGICAL TECHNIQUE
Enucleation (Head)

Once the laparoscopic ports have been placed, exposure of the pancreas is accomplished by opening the gastrocolic ligament, thereby gaining access to the lesser sac. Subsequently, intraoperative laparoscopic ultrasonography is performed to help accurately localize the tumor, rule out the presence of additional lesions, and to identify the exact location of the tumor and its relation to the pancreatic duct and major vessels. Special care is taken to avoid injury to the pancreatic duct and the mesenteric/splenic vessels during the dissection. The use of a combination of blunt dissection, electrocautery, and high-energy cautery devices are recommended to perform the enucleation. Bleeding is common during enucleation (**Fig. 4**). A drain is almost routinely left in the surgical bed.

Enucleation (Body and Tail)

Laparoscopic ports are placed and laparoscopic ultrasonography is performed for tumor localization and its relationship with surrounding structures. The spleen is mobilized superiorly and laterally while the splenic flexure is taken down inferiorly. When the tumor is located anteriorly, an opening is created in the anterior visceral peritoneum of the pancreas and careful dissection is performed between the tumor and the normal pancreatic parenchyma until successful enucleation of the mass is accomplished. For tumors located in the posterior aspect of the pancreatic body or the tail, the inferior margin of the pancreas is dissected and the pancreas is mobilized and lifted up, allowing exposure of the posterior pancreatic surface (**Fig. 5**). After enucleation, the tumor bed must be examined for any evidence of pancreatic duct injury. Tumors located in the distal portion of the tail of the pancreas are in close proximity to the pancreatic duct. Therefore, if in doubt about potential ductal injury, a distal pancreatectomy should be performed.

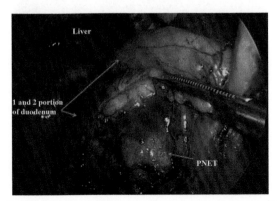

Fig. 4. Intraoperative complication of bleeding during laparoscopic enucleation of a PNET in the head of the pancreas.

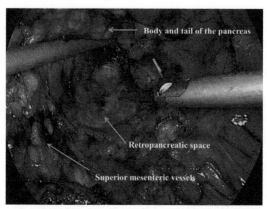

Fig. 5. Laparoscopic exposure of the retropancreatic space with visualization of the tail of the pancreas and the anatomic location of the superior mesenteric vessels.

Laparoscopic Distal Pancreatectomy (Spleen-preserving with Splenic Vessel Preservation)

When possible, spleen-preserving distal pancreatectomy with splenic vessel preservation is performed for distal tumors; however, this procedure requires more advanced technical expertise, with separation of the splenic vessels from the pancreatic parenchyma (see **Fig. 5**), and division of the branching vessels supplying the pancreas. As a result, this procedure is associated with a longer operating time.[48,49] The pancreatic tail is exposed as described earlier. Special care is taken to preserve the short gastric and the left gastroepiploic vessels. After mobilizing the inferior margin of the pancreas, the pancreas is mobilized and lifted up, allowing exposure of the posterior pancreatic surface (see **Fig. 5**).

At this time, the superior mesenteric vein (SMV) and the splenic vein can be identified forming the portal vein (**Fig. 6**). Blunt dissection around the splenic vein is performed, with ligation of the small tributaries coming from the pancreas. After identification and preservation of the splenic artery, the pancreas is divided to the

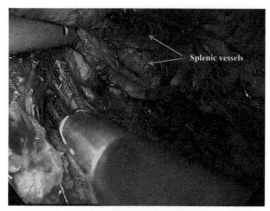

Fig. 6. Laparoscopic exposure of the retropancreatic space. The body and tail of the pancreas has been lifted, allowing exposure and visualization of the splenic vessels.

left of the SMV using an endoscopic stapler device. The body/tail of the pancreas is then anteriorly retracted, allowing separation of remaining small bridging vessels between the pancreas and the splenic vessels. The resection is completed after reaching the splenic hilum. A surgical drain is left in the surgical bed in proximity to the pancreatic stump.

Laparoscopic Distal Pancreatectomy (Spleen-preserving Distal Pancreatectomy Without Splenic Vessel Preservation)

This procedure follows the same course mentioned earlier until obtaining visualization of the posterior aspect of the pancreas and the confluence of the splenic vein and SMV.

At this time, the splenic vein and artery are clipped and ligated. The pancreas is then divided with an endoscopic stapler. The pancreatic body and tail are retracted upwards (along with the attached splenic artery and vein), and the vessels between the pancreatic tail and the splenic hilum are clipped and divided. Blood supply to the spleen depends on the short gastric and left gastroepiploic vessels; therefore, special care is taken to preserve these vessels; this is crucial for the success of this procedure.

Laparoscopic Distal Pancreatectomy with Splenectomy

This procedure is similar to the previous technique (spleen-preserving distal pancreatectomy without splenic vessel preservation) with a few exceptions. Unlike in spleen-preserving procedures, the short gastric and left gastroepiploic vessels can be ligated. In addition to mobilizing the splenic flexure, the lateral attachments of the spleen are divided up to the left crus of the diaphragm, allowing medialization of the spleen. The splenic vessels can be divided separately if an easy plane of dissection is encountered or along with the pancreas if separation of the vessels is difficult. The specimens are removed en bloc from the abdominal cavity in an endoscopic specimen bag. A surgical drain is left in the surgical bed in proximity to the pancreatic stump.

Laparoscopic Central Pancreatectomy

The initial dissection is performed laparoscopically through 5 trocars. Once the anterior surface of the gland is cleared from the head distal to the lesion, a tunnel over the portal vein is created. The lesion is resected with an endoscopic stapler on the proximal margin and cautery on the distal margin with care to avoid thermal injury to the duct. The reconstruction is then performed via a pancreaticogastrostomy or with Roux-en-Y pancreaticojejunostomy reconstruction.

Laparoscopic Pancreaticoduodenectomy

One of the largest series of laparoscopic pylorus-preserving pancreaticoduodenectomy comes from 100 consecutive cases performed in Korea.[42] In their first 10 cases, reconstruction was partially performed extracorporeally, whereas the last 90 cases were performed completely intracorporeally. The patient was positioned supine with the surgeon on the patient's right and the assistant and scrub technician on the left. The operator ports were placed in the right flank area and 1 near the umbilicus with a camera placed in between in the right lower quadrant. Assistant ports were placed in the left flank area.

After evaluation of the abdomen, the gastrocolic omentum was dissected to allow entry into the lesser sac. The hepatic flexure was mobilized and the duodenum was kocherized. The pancreatic dissection began at the inferior border and was continued over the retropancreatic portal vein. The duodenum was mobilized to the ligament of

Treitz and the duodenum was transected 2 cm distal to the pylorus. Next, the common bile duct was isolated within the hepatoduodenal ligament. A cholecystectomy was performed separately. The common bile duct was divided and the common hepatic artery was dissected from the pancreas. The gastroduodenal and right gastric arteries were transected with 2 titanium clips and the pancreas was divided at the neck with an endoscopic linear stapler or Harmonic scalpel. With retraction of the pancreatic head toward the right side of the patient, the intrapancreatic portal vein was dissected. The jejunum was divided 10 to 15 cm distal to the ligament of Treitz with another load of the endoscopic stapler. An endoscopic linear stapler or ultrasonic shears was used to divide the soft tissue and arterial branches between the superior mesenteric artery and the uncinate process to complete the resection.

For totally intracorporeal laparoscopic pancreaticoduodenectomy (LPD), a pancreaticojejunostomy was performed using the double-layered, end-to-side dunking method in normal-sized ducts or using the duct-to-mucosa method in dilated pancreatic ducts. An intracorporeal laparoscopic choledochojejunostomy was performed using interrupted absorbable sutures and an extracorporeal knot pusher in the initial cases and continuous suturing for later cases, except for very small ducts. An internal stent was used if the diameter of the common bile duct was too small. Duodenojejunostomies and jejunojejunostomies were performed intracorporeally or extracorporeally using the specimen extraction site from the umbilical port site. Closed suction drains were placed near the pancreaticojejunostomy and choledochojejunostomy sites.

Robotic Surgery

Robotic systems were first introduced in the late 1990s, and since then the popularity and number of robotic procedures has increased exponentially.[10,11] Since its first reported application in 2003, the appeal of robotic pancreatic surgery has increased.[9] The most popular robotic-assisted minimally invasive surgical platform (da Vinci system, Intuitive Surgical, Sunnyvale, CA) offers multiple advantages, such as, a three-dimensional high-definition view with significant magnification of the surgical field; elimination of tremor with improved dexterity, particularly with the use of articulating instruments that provide 540° range of motion; stereotactic binocular visualization; and improved surgeon comfort.[50]

Most series reporting their experience of robotic surgery describe similar techniques to those listed earlier through the laparoscopic technique. Zeh and colleagues[51] reported their series of 51 robotic-assisted pancreaticoduodenectomies performed at the University of Pittsburgh, 9 of which were performed for neuroendocrine tumors. They emphasized the importance of teamwork in obtaining a successful outcome. They also admitted to several limitations of robotic surgery compared with standard laparoscopic surgery, including the difficulty of working in multiple abdominal quadrants with the robot; frequent collisions between the arms of the robot caused by their large size and suboptimal positioning; the inability to change the position of the table once the robot is docked, preventing gravity from being used as a retractor of viscera; and the lack of tactile feedback. Future generations will potentially address some of these issues, thus improving the flow of robotic-assisted surgery.

Radiofrequency Ablation for Pancreatic Neuroendocrine Tumors

With the goal of developing less invasive techniques, the use of radiofrequency ablation (RFA) has been proposed for the treatment of PNETs, because it has been applied for the treatment of adenocarcinomas of the pancreas.[52–56] More specifically, the use of RFA has been proposed in those patients with PNETs who are ineligible for surgical resection.[57] Radiofrequency ablation can be performed percutaneously under ultrasonography guidance or intraoperatively. The available experience on this procedure is limited and the evidence has been documented in a recent study.[57] The use of RFA is associated with known adverse effects, which include thermal-induced pancreatitis as well as potential injuries to surrounding tumor structures such as the duodenum, pancreatic duct, and major blood vessels.

In the only prospective pilot study currently available, the use of RFA in selective PNETs has shown encouraging results.[57] The study included 10 patients (7 women and 3 men) aged 38 to 75 years old, with 3 functioning PNETs (1 gastrinoma and 2 insulinomas) and 7 nonfunctioning PNETs. Tumor size ranged from 0.9 to 2.9 cm in diameter. Selective criteria to receive treatment with RFA included patients with pathologically confirmed PNETs, those patients ineligible for or who refused surgery, single tumors less than or equal to 3 cm in diameter, and tumor location greater than 1 cm from the wall of the stomach, intestine, or bile ducts. The ultrasonography-guided RFA was performed percutaneously in 7 cases, endoscopically in 1, and intraoperatively in 2 patients.

Endoscopic Ultrasonography-directed Alcohol Ablation

Ethanol ablation has also been used as a treatment modality for PNETs. Ethanol has gained interest as an ablative agent because it is inexpensive and readily available. Alcohol ablation works by causing coagulation necrosis of the tumor as a result of cellular dehydration, protein denaturation, and vascular occlusion.[58,59] Major limitations of alcohol ablation include the possibility of late recurrence, incomplete ablation, and risk of progression during follow-up. As with RFA, ethanol ablation has the potential to cause acute pancreatitis. In a pilot study performed on 11 patients with 14 tumors by a group in Korea, 3 patients developed postoperative pancreatitis. Seven (54%) of the 13 tumors responded to treatment, with the remainder showing residual viable enhancing tissue at 3-month radiologic imaging follow-up.[60]

OUTCOMES
Laparoscopic Pancreatic Resections

Minimally invasive surgery continues to gain popularity as surgeons become more comfortable with and realize the benefits of such techniques. Laparoscopic and robotic surgeries for pancreatic resections are among the slowest to evolve given the complexity of these procedures and fear of suboptimal oncologic resection. Although surgeons continue to extend the limits of what is possible, only a limited number of reported series exist within the literature for minimally invasive pancreatic surgery, particularly for neuroendocrine tumors. Clinicians have yet to reach a consensus on the efficacy and safety of minimally invasive techniques for PNETs; however, several studies describing the outcomes of these operations currently exist and are discussed here.

LDP was first performed in 1994 by Cuschieri[61] in a case of benign disease. Gagner and colleagues[62] subsequently reported on their experience with LDP for the specific treatment of islet cell tumors. Since these initial studies, several series have been reported, with only a few involving more than 30 patients and even a smaller number of malignant cases described.[63–65] The first LPD was reported in 1994 by Gagner and Pomp.[66] Since then, more than 285 cases have been reported in the literature, including hand-assisted and robotic-assisted cases.[67]

LDP seems to be more popular than LPD, perhaps because of the lack of anastomoses and the ability to more easily control major sources of intraoperative hemorrhage, if encountered. Published data, although limited, show that the LDP might be performed with superior results to the open approach in patients with benign disease, resulting in shorter hospital stays, reduced blood loss, and equivalent rates of complications.[68–70] At present, almost all surgical resections for PNETs of the body or tail of the pancreas are performed laparoscopically or through other minimally invasive techniques.[38,40,71,72]

An early report on 17 cases of laparoscopically treated PNETs showed a perioperative complication rate of 23%, and a postoperative pancreatic fistula (POPF) rate of 15.3%. No mortality or recurrence was seen, although this series did not include patients with malignant neuroendocrine tumors.[46] In the same study the investigators reviewed the literature and reported the outcomes on an additional 93 reported cases of laparoscopically managed PNETs, showing an overall perioperative complication rate of 28% and a POPF rate of 17.9%. Following enucleation, the fistula rate was higher than that following distal pancreatectomy (30.7% vs 5.1%, respectively). No mortality was observed in this study.[46]

A group from the University of Barcelona reported their series in 2008. Among 49 patients undergoing laparoscopic surgery for PNETs, a higher perioperative complication rate was seen in patients undergoing laparoscopic enucleation compared with those who underwent LDP (42.8% vs 22%, respectively; $P<.001$).[72] The main complication was POPF, which also occurred more frequently in the enucleation group (38% vs 8.7%; $P<.001$). However, all fistulas following enucleation were successfully managed conservatively. No perioperative mortality was shown.

DiNorcia and colleagues[7] reported on a total 85 open and 45 laparoscopic procedures for PNETs performed at the same institution. This study showed no statistically significant difference in overall morbidity, mortality, or survival rate between the two groups. However, complications were more prevalent in the open surgery group (11.1% vs 28.2%; $P = .03$). No perioperative mortality was seen in the laparoscopic group, whereas in patients who underwent open surgery, the perioperative mortality was 3.5% ($P = .55$). Length of hospital stay was shorter in the laparoscopic group (6 days vs 9 days; $P = .01$). Within the 25.4-month follow-up period, a 4.4% (2 patients) recurrence rate was seen in the laparoscopic group, compared with a 15.3% (13 patients) recurrence rate after a median follow-up of 42.7 months in the open surgery group. Nonetheless, a statistically significant difference was observed with regard to pathologic characteristics of the tumors, with the laparoscopically operated group having smaller, lower-grade tumors, with less local and lymph node invasion.

In a recently published series, 75 laparoscopic procedures for PNETs were documented, of which 65 pancreatic resections or enucleations were performed.[38] The most common operation performed was distal pancreatectomy with splenectomy (n = 28), followed by distal pancreatectomy without splenectomy (n = 23). Enucleation of a PNET of the head was performed in 7 cases, and of the body or tail in another 7 patients. The most common surgical complication was POPF, occurring in 21% of patients. This complication was more common in patients undergoing enucleation (7 of 14 [50%]), with a reported incidence of 13% to 50% following enucleation.[38,40,71] Other nonfistula surgical complications had an incidence of 21%, but no perioperative mortality was shown. In this study, the 5-year disease-specific survival was 90%.

Laparoscopic central pancreatectomy has not been studied extensively, probably because of 2 main factors: first, dual pancreatic transected surfaces could be at an increased risk of leak if handled laparoscopically; and second, lesions of the pancreatic neck that do not require distal pancreatectomy are rare. However, the potential benefits of decreasing or avoiding the incidence of surgically induced diabetes and exocrine insufficiency attributable to loss of pancreatic parenchyma added to the possible benefits of laparoscopy have led to a small number of reports on the subject.[73] Sa Cunha and colleagues[74] and Rotellar and colleagues[75] reported on the 2 largest series of 6 and 9 patients, respectively.[74,75] Experience was fairly similar between the two groups, with median blood loss of 125 mL and less than 100 mL respectively. The median operating times were 225 minutes and 435 minutes; this large discrepancy is probably related to the difference in pancreatic anastomoses, because the first group performed a pancreaticogastrostomy, whereas the second performed a Roux-en-Y reconstruction with a sutured pancreaticojejunostomy and stapled jejuno-jejunostomy. Median hospital length of stay (LOS) was 13 and 18 days, and the fistula rates were 33% and 22%, respectively.[74,75]

Robotic Pancreaticoduodenectomy

The first reported case of a robotic-assisted pancreatic resection of a PNET was described in 2003 by Melvin and colleagues.[9] One the earliest series included 8 patients who underwent robotic pancreaticoduodenectomy (RAPD),[76] and outcomes were compared with open operations at the same institution. The robotic operations took considerably more time (mean, 718 minutes vs 420 min minutes) but the blood loss was less, with a mean of 153 mL versus 210 mL. The R0 resection was 100% in their small series. Fistulas occurred in 2 patients and there were no perioperative deaths. LOS was higher than average at 16 days. No short-term or long-term survival data were described.

Buchs and Giulianotti and colleagues[77–80] evaluated important facets of pancreatic surgery, including robotic versus open outcomes, surgery in the elderly, and the feasibility of the robotic approach in cases of vascular involvement. Buchs and colleagues[77] performed 44 RAPDs and compared these patients with a group who underwent open surgery (n = 39). Patients within the robotic group were older, had higher body mass indices (BMIs), and higher American Society of Anesthesiologists (ASA) scores than patients in the open group. The robotic group had a significantly shorter operative time (444 minutes vs 559 minutes), less blood loss (387 mL vs 827 mL), and a higher number of lymph nodes harvested (16.8 vs 11) than the open group. No difference was found between the 2 groups in terms of complications, perioperative mortality, or LOS.

In the series by Giulianotti and colleagues,[80] the rate of conversion of robotic to open surgery was 7.7% to 18.3%. The overall fistula rate was 36.5%. Mean LOS was 21.8 days in the Italian group and ranged from 9.3 days to 14.3 days in the US cohorts. The mortality at 90 days was 4.5%. Oncologic outcomes were similar to those of large open studies: R0 resection of 90% to 92% with 14 to 21 lymph nodes harvested. In patients with adenocarcinoma of the pancreatic head (n = 27), 2 patients died in the perioperative period, 8 were lost to follow-up, 5 died within 2 years, 3 were alive with recurrences at 1 year, and 9 patients were disease free at a mean follow-up of 16.8 months. Fifteen patients with ampullary carcinoma were followed up for a mean of 50 months. Three patients died within 3 years, but only 1 as a result of disease recurrence. The other 10 patients were disease free at follow-up. These follow-up data preclude meaningful conclusions on long-term outcomes after RAPD because of the small numbers of patients. The group also compared RAPD performed in patients greater than 70 years of age (n = 15) with RAPD performed in younger patients (n = 26). Perioperative complications, morbidity, and mortality were equivalent, suggesting that elderly patients can safely undergo complex robotic procedures.[77]

The University of Pittsburg has also published its experience on robotic pancreatectomies.[51,81–83] In a series of 50 RAPDs for periampullary lesions, the patients included had a mean age of 68 years, an average BMI of 27% and 56%, and a mean ASA score of 3. The operating time was higher than in the Giulianotti experience,[80] with a median operative duration of 568 minutes. Median blood loss was 350 mL. Of the RAPDs, 16% were converted to an open procedure. The fistula rate was 22% with a preponderance of soft glands (73%), and a median pancreatic duct diameter of 3 mm. LOS was 10 days and 90-day mortality was 2% (1 patient). The series showed an 87% R0 resection rate with a median of 18 lymph nodes resected, compared with the Johns Hopkins R0 resection rate of 58%. Of 15 patients who qualified for adjuvant chemotherapy, 11 (73%) received this treatment within 11 weeks of surgery. Long-term outcomes are pending.

In conclusion, both of the large RAPD series discussed earlier compare well with reported laparoscopic and open data. RAPD does not seem to result in increased morbidity or mortality, or compromise short-term oncologic outcomes of margin-negative resection and lymph node harvest. However, these data awaits long-term survival follow-up. It is important to highlight that reported fistula rates for laparoscopic and robotic resections seem to be considerably higher than the rates reported by the group from Johns Hopkins. This finding might reflect heightened awareness by surgeons in detecting leaks (via consistent assessment of drain output and amylase levels) with these new platforms. Moreover, it was only in 2005 that a consensus was reached on stringent guidelines for defining and detecting postoperative fistulas. Even with these criteria some studies only report clinically important fistulas.[84] It is also noteworthy that there is probably a selection bias within the fistula data presented. For example, there were a disproportionate number of soft glands with smaller duct size reported within their series. Furthermore, this leak rate might represent the learning curve for robotic-assisted pancreatic anastomoses. The long operative times will probably improve with newer generations of the robotic platform, providing a reticulating ligation energy device and reticulating stapler, which will enable reduced dissection times.

Robotic Distal Pancreatectomies

The data for robotic distal pancreatectomy (RDP) are also limited.[79,80,85–88] Waters and colleagues[88] evaluated their series of 77 distal pancreatectomies between 2008 and 2009 for both outcome and cost, comparing open distal pancreatectomy (ODP; n = 32) with LDP (n = 28) and RADP (n = 17). The operative times were longer in the RADP group, with a mean of 298 minutes versus 245 minutes in the ODP cohort and 222 minutes in the LDP cohort. Blood loss was less in the RADP group, with a mean of 279 mL versus 681 mL and 661 mL in the ODP and LDP groups, respectively, although this value was not statistically significant. The spleen was preserved in 65% of RADP procedures versus only 29% in the LDP group and 12% in the ODP group. No fistulas were found in the patients who underwent RADP versus 11% in the LDP group and 18% in the ODP cohort. LOS was significantly less in the RADP group, with an average hospital stay of 4 days versus 8 days and 6 days in the LDP and ODP groups, respectively. Oncologic outcomes were similar, with R0 resection in 100%, 82%, and 100% of patients in the RADP, LDP, and ODP groups, respectively. Note that the differences in mean lymph node harvest approached statistical significance, with fewer harvested in the robotic cohort than in the LDP or ODP groups (5 vs 14 and 11). The potential major confounder in this study was that the RADP group had much smaller lesions and no invasive cancers compared with patients treated with the other techniques; patients who underwent LDP resection similarly had smaller lesions than those who underwent ODP (3 cm vs 5 cm and 2 cm for LDP, ODP, and RADP, respectively).

Giulianotti and colleagues[80] published a series of 46 patients undergoing RADP. Their results showed that 6.3% of operations were converted to an open procedure and fistulas occurred in 20% of patients. Thirty nine percent of patients underwent RADP for malignancy, with 6 of these for adenocarcinoma. Other, smaller case reports have shown similar results to the series mentioned earlier regarding duration of operation, blood loss, and short-term oncologic outcomes (R0 resection and lymph node harvest) with longer operative duration seen in malignant cases.[9]

In a retrospective review of 45 patients who underwent laparoscopic or robotic-assisted surgery at Yonsei University, Seoul, South Korea, from 2006 to 2010, Kang and colleagues[87] identified 20 patients who underwent RADP and 25 who underwent LDP.[86] Mean operation length was greater in the RADP group than in the LDP group (258 minutes vs 348 min), which was statistically significant. Mean blood loss was greater in the LDP group than in the RADP group (420 mL vs 372 mL) but did not reach significance, and LOS was the same. Neither fistula rate nor details of the complications were given, and the cumulative mortality was zero in both groups. The investigators did note a superior splenic conservation rate of 95% (19 of 20) in the robotic cohort compared with 64% (16 of 25) in the laparoscopic group ($P = .027$). Operative time was longer for RADP than for LDP, and the LOS reported by Kang and colleagues[87] was longer than that reported by Waters and colleagues.[88]

Investigators from the University of Pittsburgh compared their experience in the first 30 cases of RADP (performed between 2008 and 2011) with a historical control group of 94 laparoscopic cases (2004–2007).[85] The length of hospital stay after surgery and rates of pancreatic fistula, blood transfusion, and readmission were not significantly different. The mean time to complete RADP (including time to dock the robot) was significantly shorter than for LDP (293 minutes vs 371 minutes; $P<.01$). No conversions to open surgery occurred in the RADP group compared with 16% in the LDP group ($P<.05$). More pancreatic ductal adenocarcinomas were approached robotically than laparoscopically (43% vs 15%; $P<.05$). Oncologic outcomes were superior for the RADP group compared with the LDP group, with higher rates of margin-negative resection and improved lymph node yield for both benign and malignant lesions ($P<.01$). RADP was equivalent to LDP in nearly all measures of outcome and safety but significantly reduced the risk of conversion to open resection despite a statistically greater probability of malignancy in the robotic cohort.

In conclusion, RADP seems to have similar results to LDP in the short term. The robotic approach seems to have lower blood loss and higher splenic preservation, although the operative time is higher. Similar to RAPD, limited data are available on long-term follow-up.

Robotic Central Pancreatectomies

Very limited data are available to date on robotic central pancreatectomy (RCP) for PNETs. Giulianotti and colleagues[89] presented their experience in 3 cases. The mean operating time was 320 minutes with 233 mL of blood loss. One patient developed a fistula. Mean LOS was 15 days with no perioperative mortalities. R0 resection was obtained in all 3 patients. The patients showed neither endocrine nor exocrine deficiencies during a mean follow-up of 44 months. In the largest published series, which included 5 patients, Kang and colleagues[90] report a mean operating time of 480 minutes with blood loss of 200 mL. One patient developed a fistula. Mean LOS was 12 days. No patients reported endocrine dysfunction during the follow-up period of almost 2 years. The investigators compared this experience with 10 open central pancreatectomies that were performed at their institution. Within this small series comparison, tumors were significantly larger and blood loss significantly greater in the open cohort; however, operating times were significantly longer in the robotic group.

Overall Prognosis

The 5-year and 10-year survival rates for all PNETs are about 65% and 45%, respectively.[91,92] The 5-year survival rate for functioning PNETs is about 80%, whereas the 5-year and 10-year survival rates for nonfunctioning PNETs are about 60% and 30%, respectively.[92,93] Curative surgical resection of the primary tumor, absence of liver metastases, metachronous liver metastases, and aggressive treatment of the liver metastases are all favorable effect factors of long-term survival in patients with PNETs.[94]

SUMMARY

Minimally invasive procedures are a safe modality for the surgical treatment of PNETs. Multiple studies have shown a lower overall complication rate among benign, small tumors (<2 cm) undergoing minimally invasive surgery compared with the open technique. In malignant PNETs, laparoscopy, although requiring advanced surgical skills, is not associated with a compromise in terms of oncologic resection, and provides the benefits of decreased postoperative pain, better cosmetic results, shorter hospital stay, and a shorter postoperative recovery period. Further prospective, multicenter, randomized trials are required for the analysis of these minimally invasive surgical techniques for the treatment of PNETs and their comparison with traditional open pancreatic surgery.

REFERENCES

1. Milan SA, Yeo CJ. Neuroendocrine tumors of the pancreas. Curr Opin Oncol 2012;24(1):46–55.
2. Yao JC, Hassan M, Phan A, et al. One hundred years after "carcinoid": epidemiology of and prognostic factors for neuroendocrine tumors in 35,825 cases in the United States. J Clin Oncol 2008;26(18):3063–72.
3. Panzuto F, Nasoni S, Falconi M, et al. Prognostic factors and survival in endocrine tumor patients: comparison between gastrointestinal and pancreatic localization. Endocr Relat Cancer 2005;12(4):1083–92.
4. Hill JS, McPhee JT, McDade TP, et al. Pancreatic neuroendocrine tumors: the impact of surgical resection on survival. Cancer 2009;115(4):741–51.
5. D'Haese JG, Tosolini C, Ceyhan GO, et al. Update on surgical treatment of pancreatic neuroendocrine neoplasms. World J Gastroenterol 2014;20(38): 13893–8.
6. Drymousis P, Raptis DA, Spalding D, et al. Laparoscopic versus open pancreas resection for pancreatic neuroendocrine tumours: a systematic review and meta-analysis. HPB 2014;16(5):397–406.
7. DiNorcia J, Lee MK, Reavey PL, et al. One hundred thirty resections for pancreatic neuroendocrine tumor: evaluating the impact of minimally invasive and parenchyma-sparing techniques. J Gastrointest Surg 2010;14(10):1536–46.
8. Giulianotti PC, Coratti A, Angelini M, et al. Robotics in general surgery: personal experience in a large community hospital. Arch Surg Chicago, IL 1960 2003; 138(7):777–84.

9. Melvin WS, Needleman BJ, Krause KR, et al. Robotic resection of pancreatic neuroendocrine tumor. J Laparoendosc Adv Surg Tech A 2003;13(1):33–6.
10. Wayne M, Steele J, Iskandar M, et al. Robotic pancreatic surgery is no substitute for experience and clinical judgment: an initial experience and literature review. World J Surg Oncol 2013;11:160.
11. Winer J, Can MF, Bartlett DL, et al. The current state of robotic-assisted pancreatic surgery. Nat Rev Gastroenterol Hepatol 2012;9(8):468–76.
12. Abood GJ, Can MF, Daouadi M, et al. Robotic-assisted minimally invasive central pancreatectomy: technique and outcomes. J Gastrointest Surg 2013;17(5): 1002–8.
13. Dizon AM, Kowalyk S, Hoogwerf BJ. Neuroglycopenic and other symptoms in patients with insulinomas. Am J Med 1999;106(3):307–10.
14. Service FJ, McMahon MM, O'Brien PC, et al. Functioning insulinoma–incidence, recurrence, and long-term survival of patients: a 60-year study. Mayo Clin Proc 1991;66(7):711–9.
15. Rostambeigi N, Thompson GB. What should be done in an operating room when an insulinoma cannot be found? Clin Endocrinol (Oxf) 2009;70(4):512–5.
16. Service FJ, Natt N. The prolonged fast. J Clin Endocrinol Metab 2000;85(11): 3973–4.
17. Hirshberg B, Livi A, Bartlett DL, et al. Forty-eight-hour fast: the diagnostic test for insulinoma. J Clin Endocrinol Metab 2000;85(9):3222–6.
18. Gibril F, Jensen RT. Zollinger-Ellison syndrome revisited: diagnosis, biologic markers, associated inherited disorders, and acid hypersecretion. Curr Gastroenterol Rep 2004;6(6):454–63.
19. Cameron AJ, Hoffman HN. Zollinger-Ellison syndrome. Clinical features and long-term follow-up. Mayo Clin Proc 1974;49(1):44–51.
20. Norton JA, Jensen RT. Current surgical management of Zollinger-Ellison syndrome (ZES) in patients without multiple endocrine neoplasia-type 1 (MEN1). Surg Oncol 2003;12(2):145–51.
21. Berna MJ, Hoffmann KM, Serrano J, et al. Serum gastrin in Zollinger-Ellison syndrome: I. Prospective study of fasting serum gastrin in 309 patients from the National Institutes of Health and comparison with 2229 cases from the literature. Medicine (Baltimore) 2006;85(6):295–330.
22. Berna MJ, Hoffmann KM, Long SH, et al. Serum gastrin in Zollinger-Ellison syndrome: II. Prospective study of gastrin provocative testing in 293 patients from the National Institutes of Health and comparison with 537 cases from the literature. Evaluation of diagnostic criteria, proposal of new criteria, and correlations with clinical and tumoral features. Medicine (Baltimore) 2006;85(6):331–64.
23. Wermers RA, Fatourechi V, Wynne AG, et al. The glucagonoma syndrome. Clinical and pathologic features in 21 patients. Medicine (Baltimore) 1996;75(2): 53–63.
24. Friesen SR. Update on the diagnosis and treatment of rare neuroendocrine tumors. Surg Clin North Am 1987;67(2):379–93.
25. Mekhjian HS, O'Dorisio TM. VIPoma syndrome. Semin Oncol 1987;14(3):282–91.
26. Adam N, Lim SS, Ananda V, et al. VIPoma syndrome: challenges in management. Singapore Med J 2010;51(7):e129–32.
27. House MG, Yeo CJ, Schulick RD. Periampullary pancreatic somatostatinoma. Ann Surg Oncol 2002;9(9):869–74.
28. Fidler JL, Fletcher JG, Reading CC, et al. Preoperative detection of pancreatic insulinomas on multiphasic helical CT. AJR Am J Roentgenol 2003;181(3): 775–80.

29. Sheth S, Hruban RK, Fishman EK. Helical CT of islet cell tumors of the pancreas: typical and atypical manifestations. AJR Am J Roentgenol 2002;179(3):725–30.
30. Gouya H, Vignaux O, Augui J, et al. CT, endoscopic sonography, and a combined protocol for preoperative evaluation of pancreatic insulinomas. AJR Am J Roentgenol 2003;181(4):987–92.
31. Buetow PC, Parrino TV, Buck JL, et al. Islet cell tumors of the pancreas: pathologic-imaging correlation among size, necrosis and cysts, calcification, malignant behavior, and functional status. AJR Am J Roentgenol 1995;165(5): 1175–9.
32. Stark DD, Moss AA, Goldberg HI, et al. CT of pancreatic islet cell tumors. Radiology 1984;150(2):491–4.
33. Sundin A, Vullierme M-P, Kaltsas G, et al. Mallorca Consensus Conference participants, European Neuroendocrine Tumor Society. ENETS consensus guidelines for the standards of care in neuroendocrine tumors: radiological examinations. Neuroendocrinology 2009;90(2):167–83.
34. Lopez Hänninen E, Amthauer H, Hosten N, et al. Prospective evaluation of pancreatic tumors: accuracy of MR imaging with MR cholangiopancreatography and MR angiography. Radiology 2002;224(1):34–41.
35. Kim MK. Endoscopic ultrasound in gastroenteropancreatic neuroendocrine tumors. Gut Liver 2012;6(4):405–10.
36. Rösch T, Lightdale CJ, Botet JF, et al. Localization of pancreatic endocrine tumors by endoscopic ultrasonography. N Engl J Med 1992;326(26):1721–6.
37. Patterson EJ, Gagner M, Salky B, et al. Laparoscopic pancreatic resection: single-institution experience of 19 patients. J Am Coll Surg 2001;193(3):281–7.
38. Haugvik S-P, Marangos IP, Røsok BI, et al. Long-term outcome of laparoscopic surgery for pancreatic neuroendocrine tumors. World J Surg 2013;37(3):582–90.
39. Al-Kurd A, Chapchay K, Grozinsky-Glasberg S, et al. Laparoscopic resection of pancreatic neuroendocrine tumors. World J Gastroenterol 2014;20(17):4908–16.
40. Crippa S, Bassi C, Salvia R, et al. Enucleation of pancreatic neoplasms. Br J Surg 2007;94(10):1254–9.
41. Whipple AO, Parsons WB, Mullins CR. Treatment of carcinoma of the ampulla of Vater. Ann Surg 1935;102(4):763–79.
42. Kim SC, Song KB, Jung YS, et al. Short-term clinical outcomes for 100 consecutive cases of laparoscopic pylorus-preserving pancreatoduodenectomy: improvement with surgical experience. Surg Endosc 2013;27(1):95–103.
43. Keck T, Wellner U, Küsters S, et al. Laparoscopic resection of the pancreatic head. Feasibility and perioperative results. Chirurg 2011;82(8):691–7 [in German].
44. Jacobs MJ, Kamyab A. Total laparoscopic pancreaticoduodenectomy. JSLS 2013;17:188–93.
45. Lai ECH, Yang GPC, Tang CN. Robot-assisted laparoscopic pancreaticoduodenectomy versus open pancreaticoduodenectomy–a comparative study. Int J Surg 2012;10(9):475–9.
46. Assalia A, Gagner M. Laparoscopic pancreatic surgery for islet cell tumors of the pancreas. World J Surg 2004;28(12):1239–47.
47. Fernández-Cruz L. Distal pancreatic resection: technical differences between open and laparoscopic approaches. HPB 2006;8(1):49–56.
48. Fernández-Cruz L, Sáenz A, Astudillo E, et al. Outcome of laparoscopic pancreatic surgery: endocrine and nonendocrine tumors. World J Surg 2002;26(8): 1057–65.
49. Tagaya N, Kasama K, Suzuki N, et al. Laparoscopic resection of the pancreas and review of the literature. Surg Endosc 2003;17(2):201–6.

50. Hanly EJ, Talamini MA. Robotic abdominal surgery. Am J Surg 2004;188(4A Suppl):19S–26S.
51. Zeh HJ, Bartlett DL, Moser AJ. Robotic-assisted major pancreatic resection. Adv Surg 2011;45:323–40.
52. Bown SG, Rogowska AZ, Whitelaw DE, et al. Photodynamic therapy for cancer of the pancreas. Gut 2002;50(4):549–57.
53. Wu Y, Tang Z, Fang H, et al. High operative risk of cool-tip radiofrequency ablation for unresectable pancreatic head cancer. J Surg Oncol 2006;94(5): 392–5.
54. Varshney S, Sewkani A, Sharma S, et al. Radiofrequency ablation of unresectable pancreatic carcinoma: feasibility, efficacy and safety. JOP 2006;7(1):74–8.
55. Spiliotis JD, Datsis AC, Michalopoulos NV, et al. Radiofrequency ablation combined with palliative surgery may prolong survival of patients with advanced cancer of the pancreas. Langenbecks Arch Surg 2007;392(1):55–60.
56. Girelli R, Frigerio I, Salvia R, et al. Feasibility and safety of radiofrequency ablation for locally advanced pancreatic cancer. Br J Surg 2010;97(2):220–5.
57. Rossi S, Viera FT, Ghittoni G, et al. Radiofrequency ablation of pancreatic neuroendocrine tumors: a pilot study of feasibility, efficacy, and safety. Pancreas 2014; 43(6):938–45.
58. Zhang W-Y, Li Z-S, Jin Z-D. Endoscopic ultrasound-guided ethanol ablation therapy for tumors. World J Gastroenterol 2013;19(22):3397–403.
59. Gelczer RK, Charboneau JW, Hussain S, et al. Complications of percutaneous ethanol ablation. J Ultrasound Med 1998;17(8):531–3.
60. Park DH, Choi J-H, Oh D, et al. Endoscopic ultrasonography-guided ethanol ablation for small pancreatic neuroendocrine tumors: results of a pilot study. Clin Endosc 2015;48(2):158–64.
61. Cuschieri A. Laparoscopic surgery of the pancreas. J R Coll Surg Edinb 1994; 39(3):178–84.
62. Gagner M, Pomp A, Herrera MF. Early experience with laparoscopic resections of islet cell tumors. Surgery 1996;120(6):1051–4.
63. Fernández-Cruz L, Cosa R, Blanco L, et al. Curative laparoscopic resection for pancreatic neoplasms: a critical analysis from a single institution. J Gastrointest Surg 2007;11(12):1607–21 [discussion: 1621–2].
64. Kooby DA, Hawkins WG, Schmidt CM, et al. A multicenter analysis of distal pancreatectomy for adenocarcinoma: is laparoscopic resection appropriate? J Am Coll Surg 2010;210(5):779–85, 786–7.
65. Jayaraman S, Gonen M, Brennan MF, et al. Laparoscopic distal pancreatectomy: evolution of a technique at a single institution. J Am Coll Surg 2010;211(4):503–9.
66. Gagner M, Pomp A. Laparoscopic pylorus-preserving pancreatoduodenectomy. Surg Endosc 1994;8(5):408–10.
67. Gumbs AA, Rodriguez Rivera AM, Milone L, et al. Laparoscopic pancreatoduodenectomy: a review of 285 published cases. Ann Surg Oncol 2011;18(5): 1335–41.
68. Kim SC, Park KT, Hwang JW, et al. Comparative analysis of clinical outcomes for laparoscopic distal pancreatic resection and open distal pancreatic resection at a single institution. Surg Endosc 2008;22(10):2261–8.
69. Borja-Cacho D, Al-Refaie WB, Vickers SM, et al. Laparoscopic distal pancreatectomy. J Am Coll Surg 2009;209(6):758–65 [quiz: 800].
70. Nigri GR, Rosman AS, Petrucciani N, et al. Metaanalysis of trials comparing minimally invasive and open distal pancreatectomies. Surg Endosc 2011;25(5): 1642–51.

71. Dedieu A, Rault A, Collet D, et al. Laparoscopic enucleation of pancreatic neoplasm. Surg Endosc 2011;25(2):572–6.
72. Fernández-Cruz L, Blanco L, Cosa R, et al. Is laparoscopic resection adequate in patients with neuroendocrine pancreatic tumors? World J Surg 2008;32(5): 904–17.
73. Speicher JE, Traverso LW. Pancreatic exocrine function is preserved after distal pancreatectomy. J Gastrointest Surg 2010;14(6):1006–11.
74. Sa Cunha A, Rault A, Beau C, et al. Laparoscopic central pancreatectomy: single institution experience of 6 patients. Surgery 2007;142(3):405–9.
75. Rotellar F, Pardo F, Montiel C, et al. Totally laparoscopic Roux-en-Y duct-to-mucosa pancreaticojejunostomy after middle pancreatectomy: a consecutive nine-case series at a single institution. Ann Surg 2008;247(6):938–44.
76. Zhou N, Chen J, Liu Q, et al. Outcomes of pancreatoduodenectomy with robotic surgery versus open surgery. Int J Med Robot 2011;7(2):131–7.
77. Buchs NC, Addeo P, Bianco FM, et al. Outcomes of robot-assisted pancreaticoduodenectomy in patients older than 70 years: a comparative study. World J Surg 2010;34(9):2109–14.
78. Buchs NC, Addeo P, Bianco FM, et al. Robotic versus open pancreaticoduodenectomy: a comparative study at a single institution. World J Surg 2011;35(12): 2739–46.
79. Giulianotti PC, Addeo P, Buchs NC, et al. Robotic extended pancreatectomy with vascular resection for locally advanced pancreatic tumors. Pancreas 2011;40(8): 1264–70.
80. Giulianotti PC, Sbrana F, Bianco FM, et al. Robot-assisted laparoscopic pancreatic surgery: single-surgeon experience. Surg Endosc 2010;24(7):1646–57.
81. Zureikat AH, Nguyen KT, Bartlett DL, et al. Robotic-assisted major pancreatic resection and reconstruction. Arch Surg Chicago, IL. 1960 2011;146(3):256–61.
82. Zeh HJ, Zureikat AH, Secrest A, et al. Outcomes after robot-assisted pancreaticoduodenectomy for periampullary lesions. Ann Surg Oncol 2012;19(3): 864–70.
83. Nguyen KT, Zureikat AH, Chalikonda S, et al. Technical aspects of robotic-assisted pancreaticoduodenectomy (RAPD). J Gastrointest Surg 2011;15(5): 870–5.
84. Bassi C, Dervenis C, Butturini G, et al. Postoperative pancreatic fistula: an international study group (ISGPF) definition. Surgery 2005;138(1):8–13.
85. Daouadi M, Zureikat AH, Zenati MS, et al. Robot-assisted minimally invasive distal pancreatectomy is superior to the laparoscopic technique. Ann Surg 2013;257(1):128–32.
86. Kim DH, Kang CM, Lee WJ, et al. The first experience of robot assisted spleen-preserving laparoscopic distal pancreatectomy in Korea. Yonsei Med J 2011; 52(3):539–42.
87. Kang CM, Kim DH, Lee WJ, et al. Conventional laparoscopic and robot-assisted spleen-preserving pancreatectomy: does da Vinci have clinical advantages? Surg Endosc 2011;25(6):2004–9.
88. Waters JA, Canal DF, Wiebke EA, et al. Robotic distal pancreatectomy: cost effective? Surgery 2010;148(4):814–23.
89. Giulianotti PC, Sbrana F, Bianco FM, et al. Robot-assisted laparoscopic middle pancreatectomy. J Laparoendosc Adv Surg Tech A 2010;20(2):135–9.
90. Kang CM, Kim DH, Lee WJ, et al. Initial experiences using robot-assisted central pancreatectomy with pancreaticogastrostomy: a potential way to advanced laparoscopic pancreatectomy. Surg Endosc 2011;25(4):1101–6.

91. Ekeblad S, Skogseid B, Dunder K, et al. Prognostic factors and survival in 324 patients with pancreatic endocrine tumor treated at a single institution. Clin Cancer Res 2008;14(23):7798–803.
92. Phan GQ, Yeo CJ, Hruban RH, et al. Surgical experience with pancreatic and peripancreatic neuroendocrine tumors: review of 125 patients. J Gastrointest Surg 1998;2(5):473–82.
93. Liang H, Wang P, Wang X-N, et al. Management of nonfunctioning islet cell tumors. World J Gastroenterol 2004;10(12):1806–9.
94. Chu QD, Hill HC, Douglass HO, et al. Predictive factors associated with long-term survival in patients with neuroendocrine tumors of the pancreas. Ann Surg Oncol 2002;9(9):855–62.

Treatment of Neuroendocrine Liver Metastases

Heather A. Farley, MD, Rodney F. Pommier, MD*

KEYWORDS

- Neuroendocrine • Liver • Metastasis • Resection • Ablation • Embolization

KEY POINTS

- Traditional hepatic surgical resection guidelines are not applicable to resection of neuroendocrine tumors, and all patients with metastases should have a surgical consultation.
- Patients with neuroendocrine liver metastases benefit from an aggressive surgical approach even if they do not receive a complete resection and have extrahepatic disease.
- Radiofrequency ablation is an important adjunct to resection and can be used in patients that are not surgical candidates.
- Patients with function tumors and who have R0 and R1 resection derive the most benefit from surgical resection.

INTRODUCTION: NATURE OF THE PROBLEM

Neuroendocrine tumors are rare and slow-growing tumors that arise from neuroendocrine cells, with approximately 70% arising in the gastrointestinal tract. They have a high propensity to spread to the liver. They are also capable of producing hormones that when released from the liver cause hormonal syndromes that reduce quality of life. The vast majority of patients who die of disease will die of liver failure. Therefore, a thorough understanding of treatment options for patients with neuroendocrine liver metastases is essential to achieving the best possible outcomes for symptom control and survival.

TREATMENT OPTIONS: LIVER RESECTION AND DEBULKING

Because neuroendocrine liver metastases are usually numerous and bilobar, it has often been estimated only 20% of patients are eligible for liver resection. Even if this

Disclosures: Dr Pommier is a consultant for Novartis Oncology Pharmaceuticals. Dr Farley has nothing to disclose.
Division of Surgical Oncology, Oregon Health & Science University, 3181 Southwest Sam Jackson Park Road, Mail Code L 619, Portland, OR 97329, USA
* Corresponding author.
E-mail address: pommierr@ohsu.edu

percentage is correct, hepatic resection is still being vastly underused. Patients are often not even referred for surgical consultation. A lack of understanding of major differences in eligibility criteria between patients with neuroendocrine tumors and other types of cancers may be responsible for much of the discrepancy.

With other types of cancer, the eligibility criteria for liver resection are fairly strict. Primary tumors must be resected or potentially resectable. Patients with extrahepatic disease are considered ineligible. Even if patients have no extrahepatic disease on preoperative staging scans, if it is discovered at operation, they become ineligible. All liver disease must be completely resectable. Generally, disease should be limited to one portion of the liver, so it can be completely resected via wedge resection, lobectomy, trisegmentectomy, or combinations thereof, leaving an adequate hepatic remnant free of disease. Wide margins of resection are also required because primary liver tumors and colorectal metastases are infiltrative, with microscopic extensions continuing a considerable distance beyond the grossly visible tumor. Positive margins of resection lead to rapid recurrence and poor outcomes.

However, as seen from the following review of the literature, these principles are hardly applicable to neuroendocrine liver metastases. In some patients, the primary tumor may never be found. They have still been considered eligible for liver surgery and included in the published major series. Negative margins are not required. Neuroendocrine liver metastases are not infiltrative, but expansive. They push the surrounding liver parenchyma aside rather than invade it, making it possible to separate many tumor masses from the surrounding liver tissue and essentially enucleating them (**Fig. 1**). This is borne out by the fact that the published series generally show no difference in survival outcomes between R0 and R1 resections. Complete resection of all liver disease is not required. Several series have shown that the results of surgically debulking most of the liver metastases yields survival results equivalent to those obtained with complete resection. Even the presence of extrahepatic disease is not a contraindication to liver resection. The vast majority of patients with metastatic neuroendocrine tumors die of liver failure and not from the extrahepatic disease, and many series show no difference in survival between those with and those without extrahepatic disease.

LIVER RESECTION AND DEBULKING: REVIEW OF THE LITERATURE

Prospective randomized data on the outcomes of surgical treatment of neuroendocrine liver metastases are lacking. Surgical treatment recommendations were initially

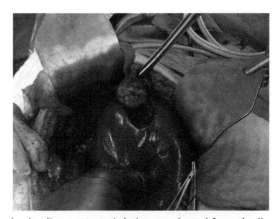

Fig. 1. A neuroendocrine liver metastasis being enucleated from the liver.

based on single-institution experiences compared with historical controls. Published series between 1990 and 2001 had small numbers of patients, ranging from 4 to 34, with a mean of 19, and patients usually had complete resections of all liver disease.[1–3] Reported rates of symptomatic relief were high (88%–100%) and survival rates at 3 to 5 years were encouraging.

Because complete resection of all disease was often not possible, McEntee and colleagues[4] were among the first, in 1990, to advocate surgical debulking when at least 90% of the grossly visible tumor could be resected. Relief of hormonal symptoms in patients with functional tumors was considered the chief justification for proceeding with less than complete resection.

In 2003, Sarmiento and colleagues[5] published a landmark retrospective series of 170 patients who underwent surgical resection with a debulking threshold of 90% of the grossly visible disease. The investigators pointed out that it was difficult to justify incomplete surgical resection solely on the basis of symptom management, particularly for patients with nonfunctional tumors, and endeavored to see if a survival advantage could also be demonstrated. They further endeavored to determine if the operations could be done with acceptable morbidity and mortality.

Their series included patients with liver metastases from carcinoid and pancreatic neuroendocrine primaries and both functional and nonfunctional tumors. The series also included patients with unknown primary tumors and patients with extrahepatic disease. Seventy-six percent had bilobar liver metastases, and 54% underwent some form of major hepatic resection. Forty-four percent of patients had complete resection of all known disease and, among the remainder, 96% had residual disease in the liver, either alone or in combination with other sites. Median blood transfusion was 0 units, ranging up to 17 units. The major and minor complication rates were 17% and 4%, respectively, and the mortality was 1.2%.

Ninety-six percent of patients had improvement or complete relief of their hormonal symptoms. These responses were durable with a median time to recurrence of 45.5 months and a recurrence rate of 59% at 5 years. In carcinoid patients, the improvement in symptoms correlated strongly with a marked reduction in preoperative versus postoperative urinary 5'-hydroxy-indole acetic acid (5'-HIAA) levels from a mean of 585 to a mean of 21 mg per 24 hours. Symptom recurrence rates were lower in patients with compete resection.

Tumor progression and recurrence rates, based on imaging or recurrence of symptoms, were high at 84% at 5 years and 95% at 10 years. There were no differences in recurrence rates between carcinoid and pancreatic neuroendocrine tumor patients.

The 5-year and 10-year overall survival rates were 61% and 35%, respectively, and the median survival was 81 months. No significant differences in survival rates were noted between patients with pancreatic neuroendocrine tumors and carcinoid tumors or between patients who had functional and nonfunctional tumors. The investigators compared their results to historical data from patients with untreated neuroendocrine liver metastases showing 5-year survival rates of 30% to 40% and median survival times of 24 to 48 months. The investigators concluded their data provided evidence that surgical debulking doubles the survival of patients with neuroendocrine liver metastases, with acceptable morbidity and mortality rates, and is therefore justified.

A similar series was published by Glazer and colleagues[6] in 2010. The series included 182 patients with carcinoid and pancreatic neuroendocrine liver metastases, 140 of whom who underwent some type of hepatic resection. Some patients had radiofrequency ablation (RFA) of some lesions. Forty-nine percent had bilobar disease. No patients had extrahepatic disease. The complication rate was 24%, and there were no perioperative deaths. Forty-seven percent had recurrence of their disease. The 5-year and 10-year survival rates were 77% and 50%, respectively, and the median survival was 9.6 years.

The investigators noted that positive margins (R1 or R2) were not associated with significantly worse recurrence-free or overall survival. Thus, the investigators concluded that patients with neuroendocrine liver metastases benefit from an aggressive surgical approach, even if they do not receive a complete resection.

Also in 2010, Mayo and colleagues[7] published a review of surgical treatment of neuroendocrine liver metastases by compiling the databases of 8 international major hepatobiliary centers. This large cohort included 339 patients, of whom 40% had pancreatic primaries and 25% had small bowel primaries. Seventy-eight percent of patients had hepatic resection; 3% had ablation, and 19% had hepatic resection combined with ablation. Forty-five percent of hepatic resections were major resections. Sixty percent of patients had bilobar disease. The debulking threshold was not defined, but patients were divided into groups based on whether they had R0, R1, or R2 resections; 19% had R2 resections.

Ninety-four percent of patients had recurrence at 5 years. The 5-year and 10-year overall survival rates were 74% and 51%, respectively, and the median survival was 125 months. This median survival time was therefore more than 3 times that of the historical median survival times in patients with untreated neuroendocrine liver metastases to which Sarmiento and colleagues[5] compared their results. Patients with functional tumors and R0 or R1 resections derived the most benefit from surgery. On multivariate analysis, synchronous liver metastases, nonfunctional tumors, and extrahepatic disease were significantly associated with decreased survival. However, survival rates for those groups were still very good. Median survival time for patients with extrahepatic disease was 85 months. The median survival time for patients with nonfunctional tumors and R2 resections, a combination of 2 adverse factors, was in excess of 84 months.

In an effort to expand the pool of patients with neuroendocrine liver metastases eligible for liver debulking, the authors' institution published a series of 52 carcinoid patients in whom the eligibility criteria were expanded to include a debulking threshold of 70%, allowing positive margins and extrahepatic disease.[8] Ninety percent of patients had bilobar disease. Sixty-five percent had extrahepatic disease, and 35% still had extrahepatic disease after operation. The mean number of tumors resected per patient was 22 and ranged from 1 to 131. More than 200 resected metastases were histologically graded and 33% of patients had at least one intermediate grade metastasis despite all reviewed primary tumors being low grade.

The median time to liver progression was 71.6 months. Progression did not correlate with the number or size of tumors resected, grade of metastases, type of hepatic resection, percentage of disease debulked, or the presence of extrahepatic disease. The only factor that correlated with time to liver progression was age. Patients less than 50 years of age had a median time to liver progression of 39 months, whereas the median time to liver progression in patients age 50 and older has not yet been reached.

The 5-year disease-specific survival rate was 90%. All disease-specific deaths were due to liver failure; no patient died of extrahepatic disease. Again, none of the clinical or pathologic factors correlated with survival, except age. Patients less than 50 years of age had a 5-year survival rate of 73%, similar to the overall 5-year survival rates reported in many of the series above. However, the 5-year survival rate for patients age 50 and older was a remarkable 97%.

The complication rates for hepatic resection have generally been reported to be 16% to 24%. The most commonly reported complications are hemorrhage, bile leak, intra-abdominal abscess, pleural effusion, cardiac arrhythmia, and urinary tract infection.

TREATMENT OPTIONS: RADIOFREQUENCY ABLATION

RFA is another technique used to treat neuroendocrine metastases of the liver, but it has limitations. One can ablate a limited number of lesions (generally up to 5), of limited size (generally <5 cm in diameter), provided they are not in close proximity to major hepatic veins and portal radicals. Usually, lesions that fit those criteria can be surgically resected, so it is not preferred over surgery unless the patient is not a good surgical candidate. In such cases, the procedure can be done by an interventional radiologist. In circumstances where major resection of the liver would be required to remove the disease, but the patient lacks adequate hepatic reserves, the procedure can be done open, or even laparoscopically, by a surgeon.[9,10]

Data on treating neuroendocrine liver metastases by RFA alone indicate it is well tolerated with a 4% to 5% morbidity. Complications include bleeding, wound infections, pneumonias, urinary tract infections, and liver abscess. Mean hospital stay for RFA is 1.1 days.[10] Some degree of subjective relief of symptoms is reported in up to 95% of patients,[9] with significant symptom relief occurring in 70% to 80% of patients.[9,10] Sixty-five percent to 75% of patients show reduction in their tumor markers, such as 24-hour urinary 5′-HIAA or serum chromogranin A levels.[11] Survival data for patients with neuroendocrine tumors treated primarily by RFA are scant, but the Cleveland Clinic group reports a median survival time of 3.9 years from the time of first ablation among 63 patients undergoing 80 ablation procedures.[10]

The real utility of RFA in the treatment of neuroendocrine liver metastases for surgeons is as an adjunct to surgical resection. As seen in the surgical series reviewed above, it is sometimes combined with surgical resection. The highest usefulness of the technique comes in cases in which substantial liver debulking will require a major hepatic resection; nevertheless, there is a lesion or lesions deep in the future hepatic remnant that would also require a major hepatic resection. RFA offers a reasonable way to still achieve the debulking goal and not compromise the hepatic remnant.

SURGICAL TECHNIQUE

The authors recommend operations for liver debulking surgery begin with exploratory laparoscopy, if possible. Patients with neuroendocrine liver metastases usually have more tumors detected at operation than are appreciated on preoperative imaging. Laparoscopy assists the surgeon in determining if the debulking threshold can still be met. If the liver passes visual inspection, then laparoscopic intraoperative ultrasonography should be performed to assess the number and location of deeper lesions not visible on the surface and continue to assess if the debulking threshold can be met through some combination of tumor enucleations, wedge resections, and major hepatic resections and ablations. The operation is then converted to an open procedure. Visual detection of miliary liver metastases is the most frequent reason for not being able to proceed (**Fig. 2**).

Because neuroendocrine liver metastases are often numerous and bilobar, full mobilization of the liver should be performed. Full mobilization permits a more thorough inspection of all surfaces of the liver by inspection, palpation, and open intraoperative ultrasonography to complete the assessment of the location and volume of liver metastases. Any new findings should be used to modify the plan for achieving the bebulking threshold, as necessary. Deeper lesions can often be simply excised by hepatotomy, in which the capsule overlying the lesion is incised, the hepatic parenchyma between the capsule and the surface of the lesion is divided in linear fashion, and then dissection is carried out around the periphery of the lesion until it can be enucleated (**Fig. 3**).

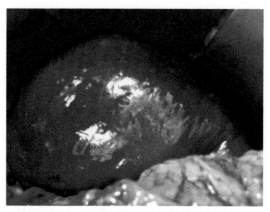

Fig. 2. Miliary liver metastases precluding surgical resection.

TREATMENT OPTIONS: INTRA-ARTERIAL THERAPIES

Intra-arterial therapies are liver-directed therapies delivered by interventional radiologists. They include embolization of the hepatic arteries in which the arteries are occluded (bland embolization), chemoembolization in which the embolic material is also laced with chemotherapeutic agents, and radioembolization in which microspheres with radioisotopes are delivered into the tumors via the arterial route. Treatment can be given to improve symptoms from hormonal syndromes and to improve survival. The major questions are whether one form of intra-arterial treatment is superior to the others in terms of toxicities and outcomes and how the results compare with surgical treatment. Generally, intra-arterial therapy should be reserved for patients who are not surgical candidates.

Gupta and colleagues[12] reported treatment of 123 patients with carcinoid and pancreatic neuroendocrine tumors with bland embolization or chemoembolization. Patients with carcinoid tumors had a significantly higher response rate of 67%, compared with 35% for pancreatic tumors. Median survival for carcinoid patients was significantly higher at 33.8 months compared with 23.2 months for pancreatic patients. Response

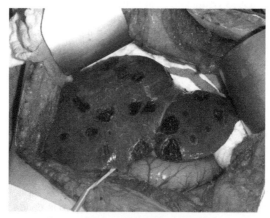

Fig. 3. Forty-two neuroendocrine liver metastases resected via wedge resection, enucleations, and hepatotomies.

rates for chemoembolization were not higher than for bland embolization. Also, survival times were not significantly better for chemoembolization than bland embolization.

Ruutiainen and colleagues[13] also compared bland embolization to chemoembolization in a series of 67 neuroendocrine patients undergoing 219 embolization procedures not only in terms of response rate and survival but also in terms of toxicity. Grade 3 or higher toxicity occurred in 25% of patients after chemoembolization compared with 22% after bland embolization, but the difference was not significant. Mean length of stay was 1.5 days in both groups. There were no significant differences in response rates, response durations, symptom relief, or survival rates. The investigators concluded that chemoembolization is not more toxic than bland embolization, but also does not produce significantly better outcomes.

A newer type of intra-arterial therapy is radioembolization, where microscopic glass or resin beads embedded with the radioisotope yttrium-90 are injected via the hepatic arteries. The beads preferentially flow into the tumors, passing through smaller and smaller arterioles until they reach the capillary level, where they are too large to pass and become lodged. The yttrium-90 decays, with a half-life of 64 hours, by emitting a high-energy electron that travels a very short distance. Unlike bland embolization and chemoembolization, it is not occlusive to the hepatic arteries and therefore may be more repeatable than standard bland embolizations or chemoembolizations. It also does not preclude subsequent bland embolization or chemoembolization, whereas the opposite may not be true. A preliminary multicenter report also suggests that radioembolization may be better tolerated than bland embolization or chemoembolization with only 14% of patients experiencing grade 3 or higher toxicity.[14,15] Ninety-two percent to 94% of patients were reported have an objective response or stabilization of disease. Median survival times were 22 to 28 months.

After collecting data on surgical outcomes from 8 international major hepatobiliary centers for the article on surgery, reviewed above, Mayo and colleagues[15] went on to collect data on intra-arterial therapy from 9 such centers in order to make comparisons between patients and outcomes. They found major differences in characteristics between patients treated with surgery and patients with intra-arterial therapy. Twenty-eight percent of patients treated with surgery had functional tumors, compared with 48% for patients treated with intra-arterial therapy. Fifty-two percent of patients treated with surgery had greater than 25% liver involvement compared with 72% for patients treated with intra-arterial therapies. The 5-year survival rate for patients treated with surgery was 73% and the median survival time was 123 months compared with 30% and 34 months for intra-arterial therapies, but most of this difference is attributed to the differences in patient characteristics. They used quartiles of propensity scores to find a patient cohort in which 11 relevant clinical factors, such as tumor type, bilobar disease, liver tumor involvement, extrahepatic disease, and clinical symptoms, were matched between patients treated with surgery and intra-arterial therapy. Within this cohort, they found symptomatic patients with greater than 25% liver involvement benefited more from surgery than intra-arterial therapy, with median survival times of 81 months compared with 51 months, respectively. However, asymptomatic patients with greater than 25% liver involvement did not derive a comparative benefit from surgery compared with arterial therapy, with median survival times of 16.7 months and 18.5 months, respectively.

SUMMARY

Many physicians may not be aware of the differences in eligibility criteria and technical aspects for liver resection in patients with neuroendocrine metastasis versus other cancers. Patients with extensive bilobar disease and extrahepatic disease are not automatically excluded. Improved symptoms and survival can be achieved with incomplete resection. Enucleation of liver lesions can spare liver parenchyma and reduce blood loss compared with major hepatic resections with wide margins required for other tumors. RFA is a useful adjunct to surgical resection to achieve the debulking threshold without compromising the hepatic remnant. Unfortunately, in many patients, liver metastasis and extrahepatic disease are inappropriately deemed unresectable. Failure to consult a surgeon familiar with these principles could result in denial of appropriate treatment.[16] Application of these principles could greatly expand the pool of eligible patients for liver debulking surgery.

Intra-arterial therapy should be considered for patients that are no longer surgical candidates. Therefore, one must be cautious about using intra-arterial therapy without surgical consultation because it could preclude surgical resection. Intra-arterial therapies can relieve symptoms and delay the progression of disease. However, in the case of high-volume nonfunctional disease that is surgically debulkable, intra-arterial therapy yields result equivalent to surgery.

It is hoped that a better understanding of the principles outlined in this article will lead to appropriate treatment of patients with neuroendocrine liver tumors, which will result in improved quality of life and increased survival.

REFERENCES

1. Chen H, Hardacre JM, Uzar A, et al. Isolated liver metastases from neuroendocrine tumors: does resection prolong survival? J Am Coll Surg 1998;187: 88–93.
2. Chamberlain RS, Canes D, Brown KT, et al. Hepatic neuroendocrine metastases: does intervention alter outcomes? J Am Coll Surg 2000;190:432–45.
3. Yao KA, Talamonti MS, Nemcek A, et al. Indications and results of liver resection and hepatic chemoembolization for metastatic gastrointestinal neuroendocrine tumors. Surgery 2001;130:677–85.
4. McEntee GP, Nagorney DM, Brown KT, et al. Cytoreductive hepatic surgery for neuroendocrine tumors. Surgery 1990;108:1091–6.
5. Sarmiento JM, Heywood G, Rubin J, et al. Surgical treatment of neuroendocrine metastases to the liver: a plea for resection to increase survival. J Am Coll Surg 2003;197:29–37.
6. Glazer ES, Tseng JF, Al-Refaie W, et al. Long-term survival after surgical management of neuroendocrine hepatic metastases. HPB (Oxford) 2010;12:427–33.
7. Mayo SC, de Jong MC, Pulitano C, et al. Surgical management of hepatic neuroendocrine tumor metastasis: results from an international multi-institutional analysis. Ann Surg Oncol 2010;17:3129–36.
8. Graff-Baker AN, Sauer DA, Pommier SJ, et al. Expanded criteria for carcinoid liver debulking: maintaining survival and increasing the number of eligible patients. Surgery 2014;156:1369–77.
9. Berber E, Flesher N, Siperstein AE. Laparoscopic radiofrequency ablation of neuroendocrine liver metastases. World J Surg 2002;26(8):985–90.
10. Mazzaglina PJ, Berber E, Milas M, et al. Laparoscopic radiofrequency ablation of neuroendocrine liver metastases: a 10-year experience evaluation predictors of survival. Surgery 2007;142(1):10–9.
11. Eriksson J, Stålberg P, Nilsson A, et al. Surgery and radiofrequency ablation for treatment of liver metastases from midgut and foregut carcinoids and endocrine pancreatic tumors. World J Surg 2008;32(5):930–8.

12. Gupta S, Johnson MM, Murthy R, et al. Hepatic arterial embolization and chemo-embolization for the treatment of patients with metastatic neuroendocrine tumors: variables affecting response rates and survival. Cancer 2005;104(8):1590–602.
13. Ruutiainen AT, Soulen MC, Tuite CM, et al. Chemoembolization and bland embo-lization of neuroendocrine tumor metastases to the liver. J Vasc Interv Radiol 2007;18(7):847–55.
14. Rhee TK, Lewandowski RJ, Liu DM, et al. 90Y radioembolization for metastatic neuroendocrine liver tumors: preliminary results from a multi-institutional experi-ence. Ann Surg 2008;247(6):1029–35.
15. Mayo SC, de Jong MC, Bloomston M, et al. Surgery versus intra-arterial therapy for neuroendocrine liver metastasis: a multicenter international analysis. Ann Surg Oncol 2011;18:3657–65.
16. Kelz RR, Fraker DL. Metastatic carcinoid: don't forget the surgical consultation. Surgery 2014;156:1367–8.